Sci

D1505217

21 X 5/05 √ 8/09 1/07

"Complete and helpful"

"*Coping with Limb Loss* is the most complete and helpful book that I have ever seen for the person who is trying to cope with an amputation. . . . The tone of this book is upbeat and friendly. . . . I strongly recommend *Coping with Limb Loss* to anyone who is experiencing amputation, either personally or in someone to whom they are close. It really opens a new area of understanding regarding the proactive application of coping skills to the situation of amputation."

G. Edward Jeffries, MD, FACS
Orthopedic Surgeon
Secretary, Amputee Coalition of America

"Important"

"This book is the only complete guide for the new amputee I have ever seen. It is a must gift from the family member or friend of someone who has suffered this trauma. And, it is an equally important resource for those trying to help."

The Honorable J. Robert Kerrey
United States Senator, Nebraska

Coping with Limb Loss

Ellen Winchell, PhD

Avery Publishing Group
Garden City Park, New York

Cover Design: William Gonzalez
In-House Editor: Marie Caratozzolo
Typesetter: Bonnie Freid
Printer: Paragon Press, Honesdale, PA

The medical and psychological information and suggestions presented in this book are not intended as a substitute for consulting your physician or mental-health professional. All matters concerning your physical health should be supervised by a medical professional.

Our language, unfortunately, has not provided us with a genderless pronoun. To avoid using the awkward "he/she" when referring to both genders, the pronouns "he," "him," and "his" have been used throughout this book. This was done in the interest of simplicity and clarity.

To protect the privacy of those individuals whose stories have been quoted throughout this book, fictitious names have been used.

Library of Congress Cataloging-in-Publication Data

Winchell, Ellen
    Coping with limb loss : a practical guide to living with
amputation for you and your family / Ellen Winchell.
      p. cm.
    Includes bibliographical references and index.
    ISBN 0-89529-646-2
    1. Amputation—Popular works. 2. Amputation—Psychological
aspects. 3. Amputees—Mental health. I. Title.
RD553.W56 1995
617.5'8—dc20   95-5445
                                                CIP

10 9 8 7 6 5 4 3 2 1

CONTENTS

Part III: Social Aspects

This book is lovingly dedicated
to all who demonstrate the remarkable resiliency of the Human Spirit
by transmuting their experience of physical and emotional trauma
to embrace life more deeply and joyously.

CREDITS

The information on "How to Choose a Prosthetist" on pages 37–39 has been adapted with permission of the Mutual Amputee Aid Foundation in Lomita, CA.

The insurance information on page 40 has been adapted with permission of Phyllis A. Bell Stong, Director of Support Services, Sabolich Prosthetic Center, Oklahoma City, OK.

The excerpt on page 41 is from *Prostheses and Rehabilitation After Arm Amputation* by L.F. Bender. Reprinted by courtesy of Charles C. Thomas, Publisher, Springfield, Illinois.

The excerpt on page 41 is from *Children with Limb Differences: A Guide for Families*. Reprinted by permission of the Area Child Amputee Center, Mary Free Bed Hospital and Rehabilitation Center, Grand Rapids, Michigan.

The excerpt on page 42 is from *The One-Hander's Book: A Basic Guide to Activities of Daily Living* by Veronica Washam. Reprinted by permission of the author.

The excerpt on page 48 is an adaptation of an audiotaped conversation with Tom Guth, C.P. It has been reprinted with permission.

The excerpt on page 79 is from *The Psychological Rehabilitation of the Amputee* by Lawrence Friedmann. Reprinted by courtesy of Charles C. Thomas, Publisher, Springfield, Illinois.

The excerpt on page 153 is taken from *Learning to Live Well with Diabetes*, International Diabetes Center, © 1991. Reprinted by permission of ChroniMed Inc.

The excerpt on page 166 is from *The Anxiety and Phobia Workbook* by E.J. Bourne. Reprinted by permission of New Harbinger Publications.

The excerpt on page 191 is from *Bodylove: Learning to Like Our Looks and Ourselves* by Rita Freedman, Ph.D. © 1988 by Rita J. Freedman. Reprinted by permission of HarperCollins Publishers, Inc.

The song lyrics found on page 202 are from
Ac-cent-tchu-ate The Positive
Lyrics by Johnny Mercer
Music by Harold Arlen
© 1944 (Renewed) HARWIN MUSIC CO.
All Rights Reserved. Reprinted by permission.

The excerpt on page 211 is from *Teach Only Love* by Gerald G. Jampolsky, M.D. and Claire Huff. Copyright © 1983 by Gerald G. Jampolsky, M.D. Used by permission of Bantam Books, a division of Bantam Doubleday Dell Publishing Group, Inc.

The excerpt on page 237 is from *Life After Loss: A Personal Guide Dealing with Death, Divorce, Job Change, and Relocation* by Bob Deits. Reprinted by permission of Fisher Books.

The excerpts on pages 258 and 268 are from *Building a New Dream: A Family Guide to Coping With Chronic Illness and Disability* by Dr. Janet Maurer and Dr. P.D. Strasberg. Reprinted by permission of the authors.

The excerpt on page 274 is from *The Body Silent* by Robert F. Murphy. Reprinted by permission of W. W. Norton & Company.

The discussion "Know Your Rights," found on pages 294–295, has been adapted from the National Easter Seal Society pamphlet PR-44 and reprinted with permission.

ACKNOWLEDGMENTS

Many individuals have contributed to turning the vision of this book into a reality, and to them I am greatly appreciative.

To the persons I interviewed who offered first-hand accounts of the experience of living with amputation. They allowed me into their inner worlds, discussing this most traumatic, life-altering event and its ramifications in every aspect of their lives. These people were incredibly generous in the sharing of themselves at deep core levels, and to them I am deeply grateful.

To Thomas Guth, C.P., of RGP Prosthetic Research Center in San Diego, California, who has been of invaluable assistance since the inception of this project. He provided prosthetic information and fielded innumerable questions. Tom is dedicated to advancing prosthetic design and function, which improves the quality of life for countless persons, including me. Other staff members of RGP who have lent their support and offered input include Jack Duckworth; Alan A. Ames; Troy Farnsworth, B.S., M.E.; Justin Norton C.P.; Charlene Rawls; Maria Ruff; and Mary Wendt.

To Harold Forney, M.D., an orthopedic surgeon with a special interest in amputation and prosthetics, who contributed much of the information on amputation surgery.

To G. Edward Jeffries, M.D., orthopedic surgeon and secretary of the Amputee Coalition of America, for his generous efforts and encouragement from the onset of this project. He revised the information on amputation surgery and suggested other significant revisions.

To Tom Watson, M.Ed., P.T., who is board-certified as a fellow by the American Academy of Pain Management, and founder of Watson Physical Therapy in San Diego, California. Much of the information on phantom limb phenomenon was derived from interviews with Tom.

To Mary Novotny, R.N., M.S., president of the Amputation Coalition of America (ACA), for her valued input and ongoing support of this project. I commend her for her countless hours of dedication to the ACA, which is bettering the lives of those with limb loss through its diverse services. I also wish to thank Noelle Broyelles, R.N., B.S.N., and Charles H. Cook, M.H.A of the ACA for their contributions. To the members of Amputees in Motion, a San Diego-based suppor group, who provided useful commentary and suggestions; to the member of the Mutual Amputee Aid Foundation, who graciously allowed me t adapt their excellent article, "How to Choose a Prosthetist;" and to Jack M East of the American Amputee Foundation (AAF), who allowed me t incorporate portions of the AAF glossary into this book.

As it was very important that the medical and prosthetic information i this book be accurate, I am sincerely grateful to John W. Michael, M.Ed. C.P.O.; and Jon Closson, M.D. for their careful review of medical portion of the text, and for their extremely useful feedback.

To all of the authors and their publishers who have generously grante me permission to quote or adapt portions of their works, as well as to th professionals who allowed me to interview them concerning areas of thei expertise. Among these people are Bob Gailey, M.S., Ed., P.T.; Willian Atchison, Ph.D.; Kathy Krohn, C.T.R.S.; Peter W. Thomas, Esq.; Michael D Yapko, Ph.D.; Blue Dunn, H.H.P.; Todd Huston, M.A.; Peter Kopko, D.C. Bob Wilson, executive director of the National Amputee Golf Association and the staff of the Area Child Amputee Center in Grand Rapids, Michigan

To Rudy Shur, managing editor of Avery Publishing Group, who ha been enthusiastic about this book since its beginning stage. His suggestion have been pivotal in reshaping the concept of this book. And his ready wi and keen sense of humor have eased the anxiety that accompanied my firs venture as an author.

To my editor, Marie Caratozzolo, for her personal warmth and profes sional expertise. She not only refined the text and smoothed its rough edges, she caught "boo-boos" and put up with revisions of the revisions The overall quality of the text is due largely to her.

For their love, support, and input, I am grateful to my dear friends and colleagues D. Jesse Peters, M.D., Ph.D., Dr. Sherri Goldstein, and Usha Cunningham.

To Oscar Ichazo of the Arica Institute, to Gurumayi, and to all of my other teachers for their guidance.

To my parents, Bea and Lou Glassman, for their unconditional love and ongoing support.

And finally, to my husband, Peter Gaines Winchell, without whose patience, support, and forbearance this book could not have been written. He gave me manuscript suggestions and helped with extensive editing. Most of all, Peter provided the unwavering emotional support that was necessary to complete this project.

FOREWORD

ong before Ellen Winchell and I became professionals interested in habilitation, we were friends. Ellen's near-fatal accident and loss of mb radically and unexpectedly changed not only her life, but the lives f those around her. The accident and the agonizing uncertainty of the ays that followed brought with them a dramatic demonstration of both fe's fragility and finitude. At the center was Ellen, deep in a coma and hysically battered beyond recognition. When she emerged, more than week later, her equanimity and obvious joy at life—even in the midst f her pain and suffering—were a complete surprise. The profound nse of peace that pervaded her interactions with us, I am convinced, sulted from her fully giving herself to each of us, even as she was near eath.

Thirteen years later, Ellen continues to give in profound ways. Her ving now reaches through this book, well beyond the circle of her close iends and clients. The focus of this book is coping with limb loss. It scusses the important medical, physical, psychological, and social issues at one will likely encounter in both the acute and recovery phases of nputation surgery.

Coping with Limb Loss is an excellent aid to the healing process. Its nguage is deceivingly simple and advice immanently practical. Born out her own struggles and successes, it is, as Ellen herself states, the kind of ok she wished had been available at the time of her accident.

With the sparkling enthusiasm that is the essence of Ellen, she brings to e the realities of medical treatment, rehabilitation, and social interactions including the words of others who have also experienced limb loss. Ellen ntly encourages those with amputation to take realistic control of their es through practical solutions based on sound principles. She shows that is possible to turn major trauma into an active affirmation of life that anscends physical limitation.

The spirit that animates *Coping with Limb Loss* is the same one that carried len through her own recovery process. The words of this book are not based on abstract theory. They are annealed in the fires of near tragedy and given selflessly. I highly recommend them to you.

David Jesse Peters, M.D.
Senior Fellow
Department of Rehabilitative Medicine
University of Washington
Seattle, Washington

INTRODUCTION

Thirteen years ago, my life was "in the pink." I enjoyed a career as a physician's assistant in a university-affiliated neighborhood clinic. I had just completed a master's degree in children's health and was investigating career advancement. My boyfriend and I were discussing marriage. I enjoyed my network of friends and family. Actively interested in the evolution of mind/body/spirit, I studied the martial art of T'ai Chi Chuan, and practiced meditation, calisthenics, and yoga. My boyfriend and I enjoyed long walks, camping trips, and "dancing our socks off."

One day, after leaving work at the clinic, my car developed mechanical problems on the freeway. The next thing I remembered:

> I am floating downstream in a current of energy, suspended in space, in total blackness. I feel a tremendous sense of well-being and am aware of being directed by loving nurturing forces from above. I come to a crossroads where I have a choice: Do I choose to go with the current's flow, or do I go in a different direction? Relying on the sense of well-being I feel and the healing energy from above, I choose to stay with that flow. I open my eyes and find myself in an intensive care unit, looking at my mother's face.

Upon emerging from this near-death experience, I learned I had just come out of an eight-day coma. I would soon discover that my life as I knew it was over. From that day forward, the results of that car accident would profoundly affect every aspect of my life.

I learned that I had been crushed between two cars , and that my body had been pinned face down on the freeway beneath a third car. Clinically dead-on-arrival, I had been resuscitated on the operating table. In addition to a fractured pelvis, ribs, skull, and right leg, and a collapsed lung, my left leg had been amputated above the knee. A close friend later told me that the only recognizable part of me was my hair.

I was not able to sit up for six weeks, nor could I walk adequately for nearly a year. Eventually the fractures and lacerations healed. And after multiple reconstructive surgeries, countless versions of artificial limbs, and years of physical and psychological therapy—here I am. During those initial years after the accident, my main focus was on the long road of physical and emotional rehabilitation.

Ultimately we must go through crises and traumas in our lives alone. No one could have had my surgeries for me. No one could have learned to walk again for me. No one could have looked into the mirror and experienced my reactions for me. No one could have felt society's response to me. And no one else could have integrated this experience and transmuted it into a healthy, vital orientation that embraced life.

I struggled internally with a myriad of emotional adjustment issues that my able-bodied friends and loved ones could not truly appreciate. Losing my limb caused me to feel very isolated, even though I had the invaluable support of loving family and friends rooting and praying for me. I drew deeply and profoundly on my connection with Spirit. Yet, there was no one who was able to say to me, "I'm like you. I know what you're going through. I know what it's like to have a limb cut off. I know what it's like to face those fears about the future."

Eventually, I was visited by a volunteer from a local support group for those with amputation. Although we shared many similarities, we were also different in many ways. Still, I began to learn there is life after amputation. I, in turn, then visited another woman who had an above-the-knee amputation. She had two small children to whom she had given birth after she lost her leg. This was very encouraging to me. She was also married—to a man with limb loss. Suddenly, I found myself confronted with fears about whether I would be accepted only by another who had lost a limb. After watching her awkward, lurching manner of walking, I cried with anguish. I did not yet have a prosthesis, and I imagined that that was how I, too, would walk.

Having these visits, and finding out what life was like for others in my situation, were critical to my recovery process. During these visits, many of the questions I had were answered, and many new questions were raised in areas I had not yet considered. I have since become a volunteer peer visitor and make home and hospital visits to women who have recently lost a leg. I continue to be amazed at the remarkable resiliency we human beings possess, and am impressed by each of our unique coping styles.

Years have passed since my own amputation. Emotionally, I am in a very different place today than I was in 1981. I still continue to "adjust" and to integrate my physical reality with daily living. However, I am now "a person living with an amputation" rather than "an amputee struggling to live."

The loss of my leg has profoundly affected almost every area of my life. Since that accident, I have discovered that the emotional challenges one faces after amputation are at least as great as the physical challenges. I have also found that there are very few written resources to help the person with limb loss deal with such adjustments. Following my limb loss, I craved practical information and sound advice about coping with the physical and emotional adjustments I was going through. I wanted to hear from others who had been there—others with amputation. How did they cope? How did they survive? Had they learned anything from the experience? Had they benefitted in any way? In short, I wanted a primer for those who had undergone loss of limb.

The scarcity of written resources in this area is appalling and amazing, considering that thousands of individuals undergo loss of limb each year. The idea for this book grew out of the recognition of this scarcity. I wanted to provide persons with amputation, their families, and interested others with basic information about the physical and emotional impact of limb loss, and coping strategies to aid in the adjustment process.

With these ideas in mind, I focused my doctoral dissertation in psychology on emotional adjustment to loss of limb (with the goal of writing this book). After extensive research, I conducted a series of interviews with people who had undergone amputation from many different walks of life. I talked at length with individuals ranging from children to senior citizens. Some of these people had lost a limb as the result of cancer, some as a result of trauma, and some as a result of vascular disease; others were born with limb abnormalities. These individual examples describe both struggles and triumphs in coping with this traumatic life-altering crisis. What is striking is how each individual makes meaning of his experience in his own unique way, and forges his own path in emotional recovery.

The meaning you make of your amputation is paramount to the quality of your life. This key concept is explored in detail in Chapter 15, "Making Meaning of Your Amputation." In my opinion, this is the most important chapter of this book.

I received my doctorate in psychology and now work in private practice. My life experience has been extremely helpful in counseling not only those who have lost limbs, but anyone who has experienced major trauma or loss in their lives. It is because of my life experience that I have chosen to write this book. I have learned much about myself and others, and about life's priorities. I wish to make a contribution to the lives of others. I wish to give something back to Life.

I have written the book I wish had been available to me after my amputation. My sincere hope is that *Coping with Limb Loss* will be of assistance to individuals with amputation, their families, and interested health-care professionals.

PART I

MEDICAL ASPECTS

1

INTRODUCTION
TO AMPUTATION

Who loses limbs? Why is amputation necessary? What are the issues that individuals must face? I had never given more than a passing thought to these questions until my own amputation. Suddenly and irrevocably I found myself a member of a group to which I never imagined I would belong. I discovered a segment of society with which I suddenly had much in common and yet knew nothing about. If you are like me, you will be curious to discover who these people are, why they lost their limbs, and what kinds of issues they have had to face. Most importantly, you will want to learn how these individuals cope with the life-altering experience of losing a limb.

This chapter addresses the basic "who," "why," and "what" questions regarding amputation. Other chapters in Part I address surgery, prosthetics, phantom limb phenomenon, and rehabilitation. Part II tackles, in great detail, the emotional responses resulting from limb loss, and describes how each individual discovers his or her own path of physical and emotional recovery. Chapters in Part III explore social aspects. Tools that can help in coping with recovery issues will be offered throughout this book to assist you in your own healing process.

CAUSES AND PREVALENCE OF AMPUTATION

No one knows exactly how many people have undergone amputation; the range of estimates is staggering—from 300,000 to more than 2.5 million in the United States. The National Center for Health Statistics estimates that 3,000 people per week undergo amputation surgery. Of all amputations, 90 percent are of the lower limbs. Of these, 50 percent are below the knee, 40 percent are above the knee, and 10 percent are hip disarticulations (removal at the hip joint). Due in part to the greater accident rate among men, there are many more males than females who undergo amputation. Although amputation is found in all age groups, most occur in individuals between the ages of fifty-one and eighty.

The four major causes of amputation, listed in order of prevalence, are: vascular disease and infection; trauma; tumors; and congenital deformities or abnormalities that require limb amputation for better function or appearance. Let's take a closer look at these major causes for amputation.

Vascular Disease and Infection

"I was being treated for diabetes, when I started to notice a numbness in my legs. One of my legs began to develop streaks and my toes began turning black. I knew it was something serious. My foot was always numb and cold, and I shuffled when I walked. I was referred to a vascular surgeon, who put me in the hospital the very next day. Tests confirmed that gangrene had set into one of my legs. It was a fast process—a period of six months. I had never realized how serious diabetes is. I was amazed when I went to the hospital and was notified that I needed amputation. As difficult as it was for me to accept, I knew that if I had to lose my leg, I was just going to have to learn to live without it."

—John

Conditions that impair circulation fall under the category of vascular disease. Half of this group is comprised of older individuals who have diabetes. A narrowing and hardening of the blood vessels can cause an inadequate supply of blood to the extremeties, resulting in dead or decayed tissue—an irreversible condition known as *gangrene*. Once a body part has developed gangrene, amputation of that part is necessary.

Gangrene can also develop in the presence of infections, such as those to which diabetics are especially susceptible. Overwhelming infections may accompany diabetes or follow some injuries. When these infections do not respond to vigorous treatment, amputation may be necessary.

Other situations can also necessitate amputation. Occasionally, a person will develop a severe non-treatable condition—ulcers or bone injuries that won't heal, disease complications, problems with blood flow, complications of neurological disorders, and conditions like frostbite—that may eventually lead to amputation.

Physical Trauma

"I was at work trimming palm trees. I was moving an aluminum ladder when I dropped it. I tried to stop the ladder from falling, but it hit the power lines and the power got me. When the initial electrical shock hit me, I passed out. I woke up on the ground with the paramedics reviving me. I jumped right up, and they had to sedate me. Because I was in shock, I felt no pain. I ended up losing my leg because of the severe electrical burn. My leg was just destroyed; it looked like a burnt stick. There was no chance of saving it."

—Grant

Physical trauma occurs mainly in individuals between the ages of twenty-one and fifty, and accounts for about 20 percent of all amputations. Generally, traumatic injuries are due to motor vehicle (car, motorcycle, bicycle) accidents. Other causes include severe burns (electrical, scalding, or fire related), explosions, and crushing injuries from tools or equipment. Trauma is the most common cause of childhood amputation (and most often the result of injuries from car accidents).

Some accidents may cause immediate limb amputation, while others may result in irreparable limb injuries for which amputation is the only option. As long as there is no other underlying health disorder, an amputated limb resulting from trauma usually heals quite rapidly.

Tumors

"I was thirteen years old. One day I noticed that my kneecap felt a little strange. A couple days later, it began to hurt. After the pain had persisted for a week, I saw my doctor, who sent me to an orthopedist. By then, my knee was really hurting; I couldn't walk without feeling pain. The orthopedist took some x-rays and discovered that I had a tumor. A biopsy showed that it was malignant. This entire chain of events had occurred in just three weeks! The cancer had come from nowhere and started growing really fast.

My doctor took me aside and told me that if his son had the same condition, he would want him to have the limb amputated because then the cancer would be gone. He talked with me about modern prosthetics and how improved they had become. With practice, I would still be able to get around. I took his advice. I decided that I would rather have one leg than be dead."

—Mark

Malignant (cancerous) and benign (noncancerous) tumors of the bones, blood vessels, nerves, and soft tissue account for about 5 percent of amputations. Cancer is the second most common cause of childhood amputation; it is the primary cause in those aged ten to nineteen. Malignancies of a long bone or soft tissue cause a need for amputation; lower limbs are more often affected than upper limbs. The most common type of cancerous tumor that may lead to amputation is *osteogenic sarcoma*. In the case of malignant tumors, amputations are usually performed higher on the limb than the location of the growth. This is done to prevent the spread of the cancer. In the case of benign tumors, sometimes the growth will destroy other body structures or become so large that there is a loss of function in the extremity. In either case, the extremity must be removed.

When cancer exists, the omnipresent issue, which looms far larger than the amputation itself, is the fear that the malignancy may not be arrested. In addition, the distressing process of going through the cancer treatments—radiation and chemotherapy—can be tremendously challenging.

Congenital Problems and Nonfunctional Extremities

"I was born with two very short, weak legs. Each leg had one toe instead of an entire foot. My legs were useless for walking. When I was almost three years old, I had both legs removed above the knees so that I could receive artificial limbs. I remember there was this boy who used to make fun of me all the time, and that is when I first realized I was different from other kids. My dad said that what really amazed him was that I never really took offense at the teasing. I just went to the boy and hugged him every time he said something really bad about me."

—Marie

Congenital limb abnormalities occur in about one in every two thousand births and are responsible for less than 3 percent of all amputations. The severity ranges from minor limb differences to the absence of all four limbs. The most common congenital limb deficiency is below-elbow. The most common lower-limb abnormality is partial or complete absence of the fibula (the smaller of the two bones in the lower leg).

Why me? Did my parents do something wrong? Could this have been prevented? Unfortunately there are no easy answers to these questions. In over 90 percent of affected children, the cause of limb deficiency is a *complete mystery*. Hereditary basis for limb abnormalities is found in only a small percentage of cases. Minor malformations of the fingers or toes may run genetically in a family. Certain syndromes are associated with absence of limb.

Most often the cause of limb abnormalities is related to failure of the formation of the developing limb bud. Why this occurs is often unknown. Abnormalities may be caused by "constricting bands" of tissue found around the limbs of the fetus. Thalidomide, once taken by pregnant women, is the only drug proven to cause abnormalities of developing limbs; it has long been taken off the market.

A thorough examination of a child with congenital limb differences is advisable to be sure there are no other limb, organ, or joint abnormalities, such as webbing of joints, extra fingers or toes, or a fusion of two or more fingers, toes, or joints. These conditions may be addressed through surgery. A child may have *nubbins* (rudimentary fingers or toes that do not grow to normal size). Nubbins may have nerve endings like fingertips; so, unless their presence becomes an emotional problem, they can be kept to provide tactile sensation.

Most children born with limb differences are otherwise completely healthy. Aside from orthopedic and prosthetic follow-up, they require the same routine pediatric care that any child needs. Genetic counseling for parents of these children can help to create peace of mind and aid them in future family planning. If no one else in the family line has been born with similar problems, most likely, family members will not be at risk for producing a child with limb differences.

For some birth defects in which the limb is congenitally absent, the person may be fitted prosthetically without needing surgery. A deformed limb may be nonfunctional; in these cases, the person (or his or her parents) may decide to have the limb removed, so that a prosthesis, which is more functional and cosmetically pleasing, might be used. Corrective surgery might also prove useful for the child who has congenital webs and contractures, the presence of extra fingers or toes (polydactylism), or awkwardly positioned feet or limbs that preclude the ability to walk. In some instances, the child is just as well off without surgical alteration, so careful judgment must always go into this type of decision.

Occasionally, a person will have an arm or leg that has ceased to function due to nerve damage or a disease process such as polio. In such cases, the person may decide to have the limb removed so he or she can use a functional prosthesis.

LEVELS OF AMPUTATION

Depending on the cause, amputations occur at different levels on the limb. The level or site of amputation refers to the location of the amputation on the affected limb. The amputation level partially determines the residual limb's functional ability, strength, and mobility.

The term *disarticulation* refers to an amputation that is at the level of a limb joint. Upper-limb amputations that occur between the wrist joint and the elbow joint are referred to as *below-elbow* amputations. Amputations located between the elbow and the shoulder are referred to as *above-elbow*.

Amputations between the ankle joint and the knee joint are known as *below-knee* amputations. Amputations between the knee and the hip joint are known as *above-knee*.

Lower-limb amputations include partial foot, ankle disarticulation (also called Syme's), below-knee, knee disarticulation, above-knee, hip disarticulation, and hemipelvectomy.

Upper-limb amputations include the following: partial hand, wrist disarticulation, below-elbow, elbow disarticulation, above-elbow, shoulder disarticulation, and fore-quarter.

Of course, any number of limbs may be affected. A person is said to have a *unilateral amputation* if one upper or lower extremity is lost, and a *bilateral amputation* if two upper or lower extremities are lost. The loss of one upper and one lower limb is referred to as a *double amputation*. Individuals with triple and quadrilateral losses have *multiple amputations*. Detailed information on the levels of amputation is presented in Chapter 3, "Prosthetics."

IN CONCLUSION

Losing a limb is a very personal matter. Your body is permanently altered and almost all aspects of your life are impacted. If you lose a limb, you may feel that no one else could possibly understand what it is you are experiencing.

This brief discussion of the causes of amputation have been presented in part to educate you, and in part for you to know that you are not alone. Millions of individuals have faced the challenges you now face and have gone on to lead rich, fulfilling lives.

2

Amputation Surgery

I awoke from a coma to discover a "fait accompli," a "done deal"—my thigh was swathed in bandages, and there was an empty space on the bed where my lower leg was supposed to be. As you can imagine, this was quite a shock, to say the least! If, like me, you have lost your limb due to trauma, you, too, may have had little or no choice about amputation surgery. However, many of you who require amputation will have some time to choose a surgeon and discuss the upcoming operation. Maybe you have already undergone one amputation and face another; if you were dissatisfied with your first surgeon, you might choose to interview others.

Before discussing the amputation surgery itself, this chapter begins with suggestions on to how to choose a surgeon. The very process of interviewing surgeons can be an important educational venture. By following the suggestions presented, you will be more at ease and better prepared for what lies ahead. If the cause of your limb loss was, at least in part, out of your control, then exercising some control with your own physical and emotional well-being can in itself be healing and empowering.

HOW TO CHOOSE A SURGEON

It is important to recognize that each surgeon has his or her own approach to amputation, and your specific medical requirement for amputation is unique. The following overview is intended to help you make a well-informed decision in choosing the best person to perform your operation.

In your search for a surgeon, the first question you will likely ask yourself is, "How do I begin?" The answer—by gathering referrals. Check with your personal physician. He or she may know of surgeons with good reputations for performing amputations. You can also check with a *prosthetist* (one who makes and fits artificial limbs) for referrals. Most major cities have an amputee support group, which may be a good source for recommending both surgeons and prosthetists. Rehabilitation centers employ specialists who might also be good referral sources. The Amputee Coalition of America can put you in touch with local support groups as well as surgeons with interest and expertise in amputation surgery. Call the Amputee Coalition at (800) 355–8772. The one place you should not look is the phone book. Most surgeons do not advertise.

Important Considerations

Once you have obtained your referrals, it is important for you to meet with the surgeons and learn more about them. Consider the following points during your interviews:

• **Does the surgeon have an interest in care for those with amputation?** In general, amputation should be performed by surgeons who are involved with your post-operative care. They should help you choose a good prosthetist, and be active in your rehabilitation. This type of surgeon is clearly preferable to one who just hands you a prescription for a prosthesis after the surgery.

Assess the surgeon's attitude toward amputation surgery. Does he or she think of it as a failure for not having been able to arrest an underlying condition? It is crucial that the amputation be viewed as constructive and positive, since it may afford you relief from pain, arrest a progressive condition, and perhaps allow you to better function with (or without) a prosthesis.

• **How experienced is the surgeon?** The experience of the surgeon who performs your surgery is critical. Find out how many amputations he or she has performed at the level that you require.

• **Do you feel a rapport with the surgeon?** Communication between you and the surgeon is important. Assess how well he or she is able to understand your needs and feelings. Communication should include discussion on the options for the level of your amputation, since this decision sometimes requires a judgment call—one in which you may have strong desires. Once again, the more you know about your medical options, the better chance you will have to obtain desired results.

• **Find out what to expect during surgery and recovery.** The surgeon should be very clear when explaining the upcoming surgical procedure and your post-surgical care—physical therapy and prosthetics. Know how often you will need to be seen for follow-up care. Will you be seen in the office or at a special amputation clinic, where there is a team approach to rehabilitation?

• **Know the surgeon's availability.** When can you call if questions arise? What should you do in the event of an emergency?

• **Can the surgeon refer you to groups and/or programs that will help you improve your life?** Can the surgeon put you in touch with such resources as gait-training clinics, support groups, counselors, sports groups, pain clinics, and nutritional guidance programs?

• **Discuss financial arrangements.** The cost affiliated with amputation surgery and follow-up care is quite high. When interviewing a surgeon, be sure to discuss the fee and know the schedule of payments for which you are responsible. Hospital and prosthetic bills will be high, as well.

Insurance coverage varies. It is important for you to review your policy and understand your coverage. If you have any questions, call your insurance representative. You might be interested to ask the surgeon's office staff to discuss its experience with your type of insurance.

Since there are so many factors to consider, it is a good idea to bring along a written list of questions when interviewing surgeons. Remember, there is no such thing as a silly question. You might also have a friend or family member accompany you on your interviews to listen, ask additional questions, and help you remember and sort out what you have learned.

Just as it is smart to use good consumer practices when choosing a new automobile or hairdresser, it is just as wise to apply these practices when choosing a surgeon. Once you have interviewed a few surgeons and have made your decision, have him or her put you in touch with a person of your gender who has had the same level of amputation that you require. (Your local amputee support group or the Amputee Coalition of America can also help put you in touch with such people.) It will help you immensely to talk with someone who has undergone a similar surgery.

UNDERSTANDING THE NEED FOR AMPUTATION

A well-prepared individual understands the need for amputation, and realizes that even though an artificial limb can never duplicate the wonders of a natural limb, it is still a better alternative than a nonfunctional or diseased limb. An amputation should be performed only if it improves your present condition. In some cases, the amputation is necessary as a life-saving measure, and although you may be losing a limb, the surgery is actually "constructive" rather than "destructive." The surgeon's goal is to construct the very best possible residual limb, so that after surgery, you will be able to function as well as possible.

The majority of those who require amputation do so as the result of vascular disease, and they are usually in a fairly serious situation by the time they are scheduled for surgery. Often they have been referred by an endocrinologist or vascular surgeon, and they may have a gangrenous limb that needs to come off immediately!

It is usually obvious when immediate amputation is required. Two indications may be present: intolerable pain and/or uncontrollable infection. While amputation is indeed a radical solution, it may be a necessary one.

In the case of infection, it is not always as easy to understand the necessity to amputate. For example, if you have a "rotten," severely infected foot accompanied by a high fever, even if you do not feel horrendous pain, amputation may be necessary to arrest the infection and save your life. If you put off the amputation, you may be in danger of eventually losing your limb at a higher level, due to the spread of the infection. Furthermore, it is usually necessary to remove the limb above the area of infection. For example, if you have a necrotic (dead) toe, it is possible that part of your foot or leg may need to be removed as well. You may wonder why the surgeon doesn't simply remove the toe. If the toe alone is removed and the infection recurs, it may be necessary to amputate even more of the foot than was originally planned.

Knowledge is a comfort and fosters rehabilitation. Lack of knowledge fosters fear. The more thoroughly you understand why you require an amputation, what will be done in surgery, and what the expected recovery and rehabilitation entails, the more active you will become in your recovery process. This participation fosters successful recovery. As an active participant in your own care, you will be better able to handle emotional reactions and cope with the far-reaching ramifications of the loss of a body part.

When a child's congenital condition requires amputation of a lower limb, the surgical procedure parallels that used for adults. Surgery is usually performed when the child is nine to ten months old. The wounds should be healed by the time the child is ready to walk. Children will try to walk, even with their limb abnormality. When they have learned to walk with a prosthesis, never having known anything different, they tend to experience fewer adjustment problems than those who lose limbs later in childhood.

Deciding the Level of Amputation

The goal of the surgeon should be the same as yours—to leave your residual limb at an optimal length in order to best function with or without a prosthesis. In most cases, the longest length is optimal; however, this is not always so. For example, an extremely long below-knee residual limb may be difficult to fit with a prosthesis if there is not enough room between the end of the limb and the foot.

Except during an emergency, the surgeon needs your written permission to amputate your limb at a particular level. He or she may also request your permission for amputation at a higher level on the limb, in case of a nasty surprise during surgery. This will eliminate the need to stop the surgery until your permission is obtained.

A lot of judgment goes into deciding amputation level. It is important for your peace of mind that your surgeon spend some time talking with you, explaining the medical reasons for your amputation, and confirming that everything possible has been done to preserve your limb. He should emphasize the positive—you are still a functional person; you are going to walk again, or use upper-limb capabilities; and eventually you can be physically active again.

Each person must be evaluated as a unique individual. Deciding the level of amputation is a very complex issue; it requires integrating your desires with the surgeon's expert recommendations. His or her judgment call is an example of what is known as "the art of medicine." The mechanics of surgery are frequently the easy part; the "art" is the hard part.

THE SURGERY

This section describes quite graphically how amputation surgery is performed. If you tend to be a bit squeamish when "blood and guts" are discussed, you may choose to skip over this section. If, on the other hand, you are curious to learn how an amputation is performed, then please read on.

A Transtibial Amputation

A *transtibial* (below-the-knee) amputation is the one most frequently performed; it includes any amputation that occurs between the knee and ankle. A transtibial amputation involves several features common to both upper- and lower-limb amputations, and is presented here as an example to illustrate the surgery in general.

In order to determine the level of amputation, many factors are considered. First, there is the clinical examination of the limb's color, temperature, and the condition of the skin. Hair growth on the limb, which is a sign of good circulation, is checked. Various tests are performed to check the blood flow to the skin, which is critical for healing. The final determinant of where to amputate is the appearance of the tissues—this is where the experience of the surgeon is very important. If these factors indicate that a transtibial amputation will work, the operation will be performed at that level.

The first incision is made through the skin. Next, the muscles are cut; smaller vessels are cauterized (sealed) to stop the bleeding, and larger vessels are clamped and tied with sutures.

Nerves require special treatment, because the cut end of a nerve will form a *neuroma*—a little ball of nerve fiber. Neuromas, which cannot be prevented, can get trapped in scar tissue or against bone, and can be painful if pressed by a prosthesis. During surgery, the nerves are cut off as short as possible allowing them to retract into the muscle, which pads them. Some surgeons inject the nerves with local anesthetic to decrease pain.

After the skin, muscle, blood vessels, and nerves are properly cut, the tibia is sawed through at the predetermined level. The fibula is cut next, approximately one centimeter shorter than the tibia. The tibia is carefully rounded off and beveled to eliminate any sharp edges.

After the bones are cut, the posterior muscle group, blood vessels, and nerves are carefully severed. Next, the surgeon "adjusts" the flaps of soft tissue to cover the bone, and usually inserts a drain. Carefully, the muscles and the muscle coverings (fascia) are sewn together over the end of the bone in a procedure known as *myoplasty*. The skin is then closed snugly over the end of the residual limb, completing the amputation. The position of the closed incision is very important for proper prosthetic fit and comfort, especially in below-knee amputations.

To optimize function for those who require *transfemoral* (above-the-knee) amputation, the muscles can be sewn to the bone through holes that are drilled in the bone. This procedure is called *tension myodesis*. Through this procedure, the muscles will be under some tension, which will help to maintain muscle strength and stabilize the femur (thigh bone) within the residual limb. Tension myodesis also enables better control of the residual limb for optimal prosthetic function. Your unique physical situation and needs must be individually addressed to provide you with the best outcome.

The Removed Limb

The section of the limb that has been removed is sent to the pathology department for microscopic tissue examination. In the case of a progressive disease such as cancer, the tissue is evaluated to be sure that the amputation has been performed well above the level of the malignancy. The tissue may also be studied to confirm the diagnosis that prompted the limb removal. If you provide special permission, your amputated limb may be studied further to augment knowledge of the disease process that necessitated the amputation. The pathology report is sent to your physician, and it will become part of your permanent medical record.

The limb is taken away and stored, according to strict guidelines for biohazardous materials established by the Occupational Safety and Health Administration (OSHA), until the time it is permanently disposed of, generally through cremation.

If your religious beliefs include the importance of being buried with all of your body parts, special arrangements can be made for the amputated limb to be buried in your cemetery plot. When you die, you will be buried along with your limb.

POST-SURGICAL EVENTS

The recovery period following surgery largely depends on the reason for the amputation. Individuals who have lost a limb due to an underlying problem with circulation tend to take longer to recover than those who have lost a limb due to trauma, cancer, or a congenital problem. The quality of circulation in the residual limb or the presence of infection also influences healing.

If you have had a "typical" below-knee amputation, your post-surgical progression of events will be roughly as follows:

1. In the operating room, a compression dressing, such as an ace bandage, an air splint, or a rigid cast will be wrapped around your residual limb. The type of dressing chosen will depend upon your surgeon's preference and your unique needs. Your surgeon may use an elastic compressive dressing or a rigid cast to help control swelling and promote healing. In some cases, a prosthetist will come into the operating room and apply a temporary prosthesis to the plaster or fiber cast. (This is not for weight-bearing purposes, but for a psychological boost.)

2. As soon as your pain subsides, enough of your general strength has returned, and your physician has determined you have healed enough to bear weight, you can get up and begin to ambulate with the use of a walker or crutches.

3. Once the IVs and drain tubes are removed, and you are in general good health, you can go home.

4. If healing is progressing well, the cast or dressing can come off and be replaced with a new cast or a dressing with good compression. The cast may be changed about every two weeks.

5. When your wound is well-healed, you should wear either a rigid cast dressing or, as an alternative approach, an elastic wrap. If you have the latter, you should be taught proper wrapping technique, so your residual limb can be rewrapped every several hours to insure optimal compression. You may use a rigid "stump protector" over the elastic wrap to prevent injury to your residual limb in case you fall.

6. After a few more weeks of healing, you can usually begin to have your first prosthesis built. The average time before an initial prosthetic fitting in a nonvascular case is six to eight weeks.

As mentioned earlier, some people can be fitted right in the operating room with a temporary cast that has a foot attached. It can be helpful psychologically to wake up and see a foot on the end of your leg. This doesn't always happen, though. It may be days after the surgery before you can have a prosthetic unit—a pylon (pole) with a foot on the end—placed on the rigid dressing of your residual limb. Once again, these choices are up to your surgeon and the availability of a prosthetist.

When your surgeon believes you and your residual limb are ready, you will be allowed to begin to bear weight. This timing varies considerably, based upon how well you are healing.

PAIN FOLLOWING AMPUTATION

It is absolutely normal to experience post-operative pain after amputation. After all, skin, muscles, nerves, and bone have been cut. Pain at the surgical site will decrease day by day. Your physician will generally prescribe strong pain medication. He or she may even give you anesthesia (in the form of an epidural block) to numb your residual limb following the surgery. After a few days, the strength of the medication can be tapered off, and you can take mild pain relievers until you are comfortable.

In addition to the obvious pain that is caused by the surgery itself, there are other pains commonly experienced after limb amputation. The typical onset of pain will vary with the underlying cause. These pains are often caused by one of the following reasons:

• **Neuromas.** When a nerve outside the spinal cord is cut or injured, the severed end of the nerve will form a neuroma—a ball of fibers that is surrounded by scar tissue. Some people tend to form larger neuromas than others, just as some people tend to form more scar tissue than others. If a neuroma is pinched or under pressure, it may cause pain. Pain from a neuroma most commonly occurs when you start wearing a prosthesis. During the operation, surgeons do their best to cut the nerves so the neuromas end up in areas where they are padded by body tissue and, therefore, not able to be pinched.

If you are experiencing pain from neuromas, there are multiple treatment options including socket adjustments, local injections, or surgical revision.

• **Pain from the Prosthesis.** An improperly fit prosthesis can cause pain. If the socket is too tight or too loose, the residual limb hits bottom, or a neuroma is pinched or compressed, you will feel pain. Adjusting the fit of the prosthesis can usually address the cause of these pains.

• **Skin Irritation or Infection.** If your skin has become irritated due to friction caused by the socket of your prosthesis, have your prosthetist adjust the socket. If the skin has become inflamed, if red streaking or fever develops, or if worrisome lesions appear, consult your physician to make sure your limb is not infected. If you have an underlying vascular disease, it is especially important to watch for these signs of infection.

• **Phantom Limb Phenomenon.** "Phantom limb sensation" and "phantom limb pain" refer to the strange, often painful, feelings you may experience in the part of your body that has been removed. These unusual physical sensations can include the feeling that your amputated limb is still present or in an unusual position. You may experience crushing, burning, stabbing, and/or shocking pains in your "phantom" limb.

Be assured that these sensations are very real and you are not going crazy. For more detailed information, see Chapter 4, "Phantom Limb Phenomenon."

PHYSICAL THERAPY AND FOLLOW-UP CARE

Optimally, physical therapy should occur before surgery in the non-emergency situation, and if good health permits. The goal is to teach proper transfer and gait technique. Otherwise, physical therapy usually begins the day after the amputation. Most people who have undergone lower-extremity amputation need upper-body strength, as well as general body strength to manuever crutches or a walker.

If you have had a lower-extremity amputation, you will likely begin your therapy with some range-of-motion and weight-lifting exercises while you are in your hospital bed. You must also learn to transfer yourself from the bed to a chair.

If you have been in bed for a few weeks, you may have developed *muscle contractures* (shortened muscles due to lack of use) of your opposite leg or hip joint. A physical therapist will help you get those muscles back into shape. If you are ready to walk on crutches, you may be given a temporary prosthesis and learn to use that, as well. For a more in-depth discussion on physical therapy, refer to Chapter 5, "Rehabilitation."

While you are in the hospital, your surgeon will probably come in to see you once or twice a day. Once discharged, you will go to his or her office for follow-up care. Next, you will visit a prosthetist for prosthetic fitting. If possible, it is recommended that you go to an amputation clinic or rehabilitation center for your continued care. At such clinics, you will find a variety of health-care specialists, such as physical therapists, prosthetists, social workers, and physicians (such as physiatrists). A team approach can serve to simplify the coordination of your care. If you live in a small community, you may not have access to such a specialized center. In this situation, your physician can assemble a team of professionals to meet your unique requirements.

Once you are progressing well, you will need less follow-up visits. However, because your residual limb will shrink, especially in the first year following surgery, socket adjustments may need to be made. Some doctors recommend that diabetic or vascular patients be evaluated more regularly. These visits are to ensure that the residual limb remains healthy, other limbs are all right, and the prosthesis fits properly.

IN CONCLUSION

Amputation is certainly traumatic, and something that no one would consciously choose to undergo. However, you can become better prepared for its eventuality if you take the proactive steps outlined here.

So take an active role. Start by making sure you understand the medical necessity for your amputation. Have a hand in choosing your own surgeon, and make sure you have full knowledge of the surgical procedure and recovery process. Be sure to ask questions about puzzling or troubling issues. Your active participation will help ease your mind about your limb loss and help you feel re-empowered about controlling your own health.

3

PROSTHETICS

"Before I lost my leg, I thought people who needed artificial limbs simply went to a big warehouse that was filled with prefabricated prostheses. I figured they were measured and then found a limb that fit; kind of like going into a shoe store. What a surprise! It was definitely a different experience from what I had imagined it would be."

—Kent

Mastery of an artificial limb can work wonders for you, both from a psychological standpoint, as well as a physical. Receiving a prosthesis (an artificial limb), and learning how to use it, can often restore much of your prior physical ability. After you have been using a wheelchair or crutches, or functioning single-handedly for a period of time, the use of an artificial limb can elevate you to new levels of freedom. A greater sense of independence and autonomy can be regained, which will help boost your self-esteem and provide an enhanced sense of well-being.

This chapter addresses whether or not a prosthesis is the optimal choice for you. It also presents the nuts and bolts of what is involved in the fitting and fabrication of an artificial limb. Prosthetic options for different levels of amputation are discussed, as well as areas of ongoing prosthetic and medically related research.

The physical and emotional aspects of learning to walk again or restoring upper-limb capabilities deserve special consideration. Chapter 5, "Rehabilitation," as well as the chapters in Part II are devoted to these aspects of recovery.

PROSTHETICS TODAY

Amputation has been a part of humanity's experience since the dawn of time, whether the result of disease, a traumatic accident, a war injury, or the punishment for some crime. As long as there have been individuals without limbs, there have also been artificial limb replacements.

The goal of an artificial limb is to provide its user with the most natural movement and function possible. Today, there is a great variation in prosthetic practice throughout the world. The two world wars plus the wars in Korea and Vietnam have focused attention on the plight of those with amputation. These events have raised the awareness of the need for emotional rehabilitation assistance from society, and have inspired the research and development of improved prosthetics.

In recent years, prosthetic improvements have allowed those with limb loss to enjoy a physical freedom that was never before possible. Dedicated professionals, committed to incorporating the latest medical and technological advances in prosthetic development, have bettered the quality of life for those with amputation.

Modern material and technology have allowed the evolution of arms and legs that are more natural in appearance and function, require less energy to use, and are much more comfortable than ever before. The most recent prosthetic advancements have taken place in three major areas—the development of lightweight, durable metals and plastics; the improvement of fitting methods, such as clear diagnostic sockets; and ongoing research and development of technological components, such as microprocessors and myoelectric parts. Today's prosthetics have enabled individuals to be more active physically, which provides a tremendous boost to physical confidence.

I am personally grateful for every little development. When I lost my leg in 1981, the first prosthesis I received was made of a hard laminated material, rendering it totally stiff and uncomfortable. The socket design made it difficult for my muscles to function in a normal way, so I lurched awkwardly from side to side when I walked. The prosthetic knee swung out unnaturally. The prosthetic foot had little spring to it, so walking took excess energy. I felt like I was encased in the leg of a mechanical toy soldier!

In sharp contrast, my current artificial limb is composed of a soft, flexible plastic that is so much more comfortable to wear. The "skin" on the cosmetic cover is more durable and lifelike. The socket design is more flexible, so it conforms, and the leg is better aligned, so my gait has greatly improved. The foot design enables me to expend less energy when I walk. My knee swings more smoothly and naturally. Each of these improvements has increased the quality of my physical life. Thus, at least from a prosthetic point of view, this is the best time in history to undergo an amputation.

FITTING AND FABRICATING A PROSTHESIS

The fitting and fabricating (building) of a prosthesis is both a science and an art. Each prosthetist has his or her own style of fitting artificial limbs, fabrication procedures, and opinions of what might best serve you. The opinions and practices presented here may be different from those of your own prosthetist. Know that they are meant to provide a general overview of what is involved in fitting and fabricating an artificial limb.

Be aware that proper socket fit and limb alignment are the most important considerations when fabricating a prosthesis. Directly responsible for comfort and usability, these two factors are more crucial than any other. Without proper socket fit and limb alignment it won't matter how sophisticated or state-of-the-art your prosthetic knee, ankle, foot, or anything else is.

It is wise to take into account the reality that no matter how wonderful your prosthesis is, it is not going to replicate exactly the wonders of a limb designed by Mother Nature. Nevertheless, a great deal of normal function and physical freedom can be regained.

Ideally, if you require amputation due to a health problem that is not life-threatening, try to talk with a prosthetist before your amputation surgery. If possible, tour the prosthetic facility. Get an overview of what to expect and gain a realistic view of what your prosthesis will be like. If you can, speak with others who have had similar levels of limb loss. This can be invaluable in learning what to expect.

Meeting Your Individual Needs

Before giving you a prescription for your prosthesis, your physician should have discussed your case with the prosthetist to hear his or her recommendation. By this time, you and the prosthetist should have had a thorough discussion in which you have reviewed your physical condition, the level of your amputation, and your desires for specific physical capabilities. The prosthetic options that are available to best meet your unique needs should have been discussed.

In your initial evaluation, the prosthetist (or other rehabilitation team member) should learn the reason for your amputation, and discover whether or not you still have health problems. In order to determine the kind of leg or arm that is best for you, it is important for your health-care professionals to be aware of certain aspects of your life including your lifestyle, hobbies, recreational activities, occupation, and special needs and desires. If you are already wearing an artificial leg or arm, your prosthetist may want to learn of any problems or shortcomings you may have found with it.

Stay abreast of the latest prosthetic developments. Become knowledgeable about what is available and the potential application issues for you. Amputation support groups can help keep you informed. The better educated you are as a consumer, the better position you will be in to go to your prosthetist and inquire about a new prosthetic option. Make sure he or she answers your questions fully. Your prosthetist should be able to tell you why a particular prosthetic option may work for some patients but not others. If a certain device is not appropriate for you, the prosthetist should explain why. However, if there is even a small chance that an option may improve your life, you should try it. Even one change, such as an energy-storing foot, can make a big difference in everyday comfort and function.

It is really your prosthetist's job to explain the available options. Before making any final decisions, your prosthetist should let you try out all of the component options that are applicable to your prosthesis. (In many cases, lack of interchangeability won't allow this.)

To further illustrate the concept of fabricating a prosthesis to meet unique individual needs, read the the following experience of a young, physically active man who underwent a below-elbow amputation.

"Soon after my forearm was removed, I went to a prosthetist. Although I was fairly ignorant in the area of artificial limbs, there were a few things that I knew were important to me. And I was very specific when discussing these needs with the prosthetist. First of all, I have always been a physically active guy and very hard on things, so my new limb had to be strong and durable. I also wanted to be able to continue fixing cars. I still wanted to drive to the desert. I still wanted to, well, do everything! And I knew I would, no matter what kind of limb they built for me. If the prosthesis was going to help me, I would use it; if not, I was prepared to leave it off.

At first, the prosthetist brought me a myoelectric hand that was attached to a forearm. Although it was state-of-the-art, it wasn't durable enough to fill my needs. We decided on an arm made totally of polyester urethane resin and carbon graphite (no fiberglass). I tried a steel hand, as well as an old-fashioned hook. I was able to voluntarily open the hook, but I needed rubber bands to close it. In my business I need to be able to control the amount of closing pressure I use to hold onto each thing I pick up. I might pick up a piece of glass, set that down and reach right over and pick up a ten-pound bunch of steel. Obviously, the same number of rubber bands isn't going to cut it. I needed to be able to control the closing force. Finally I decided on both the steel hand and the hook."

—Clint

As Clint's story illustrates, a prosthetist may be the expert at building and fitting artificial limbs, but you are the expert about yourself—your lifestyle, activities, and dreams for the future. A farmer, working mother, mechanic, business executive, sedate elderly person, and an athlete may all choose very different prosthetic components. Communication between you and your prosthetist is a key factor for success. Also, by actively participating in your own care, you will gain an increased sense of self-control, which is very important when your life has been radically impacted by loss of limb.

PROSTHETICS FOR CHILDREN

Children adapt well to using prosthetics. They are energetic, physically and emotionally flexible, eager to master new skills, and motivated to be as normal as possible. In the same way as adults, children utilize their prosthesis, not only to regain physical abilities, but also to restore their concept of themselves as a "whole" person. Children's emotional well-being, social confidence, and adjustment to school all appear to be strengthened when they use a prosthesis, although they can do very well without them. Since this book is directed primarily toward adults with limb loss, prosthetics for children are discussed only briefly.

When and if a child should use a prosthesis depends upon many factors, as does the specific choice of components. Parents, the child's prosthetist, and the child himself, may all have differing opinions about the benefits and drawbacks of prosthetic use. Many factors, beyond the scope of this book, must be considered before making choices about what is optimal for a child's unique circumstances.

One of the curious realities of deciding if and when to fit a child with an artificial limb is that the prosthetist often finds that he has to "fit" the parents as well as the child! A baby born with limb differences doesn't realize that he is different from any other child. It is the parents who are most painfully aware of their child's uniqueness. It is important that parents learn to differentiate their *child's* real needs from their *own* emotional ones.

Since a child grows and changes at a rapid pace physically, intellectually, and emotionally, his prosthetic needs will differ from those of an adult. There are special prosthetics and components designed for children. A prosthesis must be matched for a child in terms of his physical and developmental capacities. There will be starts and stops, and peaks and valleys, as parents explore what best suits their child's unique circumstances. Ultimately, it is the child who will set the pace and determine what works best for him.

CONSTRUCTING A CUSTOM PROSTHESIS

Prosthetics is an evolving field. Keep in mind that each prosthetist may utilize somewhat different procedures in the fitting and construction of custom limbs. The steps presented are to give you a general idea of the process involved.

Although there are different levels of amputation, there are many similarities in the fitting and fabrication methods used for upper- and lower-limb prostheses. In the discussion that follows, the procedure for creating a lower-limb prosthesis is presented.

General Progression of Events

The sooner you meet with a prosthetist after your surgery, the sooner you will be able to begin your rehabilitation with a prosthetic fitting and fabrication.

Although it is not usual, it is possible to have a prosthetist present in the operating room immediately following surgery. If you are a candidate for an immediate post-operative prosthesis (IPOP), a prosthetist can have a pylon with a prosthetic foot attached to your cast. Although you won't be healed enough to bear weight on it, psychologically, it is an advantage to wake up and see a foot at the end of your leg, even if it is not your own! It can be used to assist you to develop a normal walking pattern later on as you progress in your post-operative healing.

The first time most persons see a prosthetist for a fitting is two to three weeks following their surgery, or when the surgeon considers them healed. (This first device will be a temporary one that is used until the residual limb is completely healed and has stabilized in shape.) Those with vascular problems may take longer to heal—four to six weeks or more. Young children may be ready to be fitted for a prosthesis about a month after surgery, while the elderly may take six to eight weeks or so. One thing, however, is certain—the sooner you begin the construction of your prosthesis, the shorter your rehabilitation is likely to be. (This is especially true in the case of the elderly, who must minimize their loss of muscle tone.)

To help decrease post-surgical swelling of your residual limb, you will learn to wear a compressive sock called a "shrinker" or be shown how to carefully wrap your limb in an ace bandage. The use of a wrap or shrinker is very important. It is needed to help mold your residual limb into a conical configuration, which enhances prosthetic fit and comfort.

Your residual limb will undergo its own process of healing and changing shape, as it stabilizes over a period of six months or more. This change in limb shape is due to an interplay of factors. First of all, the muscles in the limb will atrophy (shrink) since they are not functioning the way they used to. You may gain or lose weight during the period following surgery. Loss of muscle tone is another common occurrence. However, once you start walking again, you will build back some of that muscle tone and probably return to your normal weight. For most people, this return to normal weight and muscle tone takes about six months; by then, the size of the residual limb should have stabilized.

With all of these limb changes, you may well be wondering how comfortable adjusting to a prosthesis will be. If you have had a recent amputation and it is the first time you will be walking with a prosthesis, there will be some pain. One reason is that you will probably be fit with a temporary-fitting prosthesis before your residual limb is completely healed. Until you are able to bear more weight, you may have to use crutches or another assistive device. Expect somewhat painful gait during the first month after surgery. As your limb heals, the more comfortable it will be to walk. If you experience pain that shows no sign of improvement after a week, there is probably a prosthetic problem. Return to your prosthetist for an adjustment.

Early gait training should be under the close supervision of a physical therapist and/or prosthetist, so that proper mechanics and good habit patterns can be learned. Learning to walk with a prosthesis requires developing new techniques. It's far better to develop good habits from the onset than try to correct bad habits later on.

Sometimes a temporary prosthesis will need to be refitted several times during the post-operative period, due to the the changing shape of the residual limb as it heals. After the six-month period following surgery, a final or definitive prosthetic device can usually be completed. By this time, you should see a marked improvement in comfort and in your walking.

The average person takes two to six months to learn how to walk well. If your amputation is below-knee, walking will be relatively easy, since you still have your knee joint. With above-knee loss, walking will require more effort, training, and perseverance, but it can be done successfully.

Generally, it takes a full year to become a "veteran." By the end of a year, you will likely be wearing a definitive prosthesis, which should require very little adjustment. While there are individual variations in the healing process and prosthetic needs, this one-year timetable is average. Each person rehabilitates at his or her own rate.

Prosthetic Socks, Silicone Inserts, and Socket Suspension Systems

Two ways to enhance the comfort of your prosthetic fit are through the use of prosthetic socks and silicone inserts. Residual limbs for those with below-knee amputation are often bony and not well padded with tissue; prosthetic socks provide the cushioning that these limbs require for added comfort. Most persons with above-knee limb loss do not need prosthetic socks since their residual limbs are generally well padded with tissue.

Originally, prosthetic socks were made of wool; and, for those allergic to wool, a cotton variety was available. Today, most prosthetic socks are made of a material blend—nylon on the outside and wool on the inside. The word "ply" refers to the thickness of the sock. Prosthetic socks generally come in one-, three-, five-, and six-ply varieties. If there is a loss or gain of volume in the residual limb, a person can adjust the ply of the sock. These socks are especially helpful after a recent amputation, when the residual limb is constantly changing in volume. Even some people with "seasoned" amputations sometimes discover that they lose residual limb volume during the course of the day. To maintain optimal prosthetic fit, these people are able to add or remove the right sock ply for maximum comfort.

Another way you can enhance socket comfort is through use of a silicone socket liner, which acts as a cushion or second skin. The intimate fit of the silicone helps eliminate the discomfort of the friction caused by the piston-like motion of the residual limb in the prosthetic socket. This silicone liner is rolled onto the residual limb in the same way that some women "roll on" their stockings. The design of the insert is a bit like the Chinese finger traps you may have played with as a child—once on the residual limb, the liner cannot be removed unless it is "rolled" off. This design insures secure placement. This liner may have a one to two-inch rachet pin on its far (distal) end; when a person steps into the prosthetic socket, the silicone liner "locks" into place. If the person wears prosthetic socks, a hole can be placed in the end of the sock to accommodate the liner's pin. This type of liner eliminates the need for straps.

The use of suction to hold the prosthesis in place eliminates the need for straps. There are two types of suction suspension systems. One is the silicone liner with the pin (discussed above), the other is a silicone liner with a valve located at the far end of the socket. The wearer applies a lubricant to the outside of the liner, steps into the socket, and releases the air by pressing on the valve release button. This creates the suction that holds the prosthesis in place.

STEPS FOR CREATING A LOWER-LIMB PROSTHESIS

After deciding on the type of prosthesis that best fits your needs, it is time to start your journey toward the fabrication of that limb. The following is a common, but by no means universal method of fitting and fabricating a prosthesis.

First, your residual limb will be casted in order to make a model. The model will then be modified to create space in certain areas to prevent bony or tender parts of your residual limb from bearing weight.

The fitting of a clear diagnostic socket that will hold your residual limb comes next. The fit of this socket is adjusted as you bear your weight into it. Next, alginate, the substance used to make dental impressions, is used to further refine the fit of the socket. Other aims of this fitting process are to balance the pressure on those areas of the residual limb that are designed to bear weight, and remove any pressure from the nerve pathways and arteries. This results in a better custom fit and increased comfort. Another model of the residual limb is then produced to incorporate these refinements. Next, a socket is made, and you can finally try out your new prosthesis!

An adjustable device will help align your leg so you can replicate a normal gait. During the weeks and months following surgery, your gait will undergo many changes.

The prosthetist will start you off with a temporary "preparatory leg," which will need continual adjustments until it fits you well and is in good alignment. You will probably wear this leg from one to six months or until the following changes have occurred: the muscles in your residual leg have developed or shrunk, your weight has stabilized, and your prosthetic alignment and gait are optimal.

During this period, you may try different knees or different feet to discover the one that is best for you. When you have worn your preparatory leg satisfactorily for over a month, it will be cloned or duplicated. A copy of the leg will be used to craft the definitive leg.

Although it will periodically undergo minor adjustments, your new prosthetic leg should last for some time. Of course, if you gain or lose a lot of weight, become pregnant, undergo surgery to correct a bone spur, for instance, or are extremely hard on your prosthesis through physical activity, it may be necessary to refit your socket and adjust your alignment more frequently.

PROSTHETIC OPTIONS FOR LOWER-BODY AMPUTATIONS

Some different levels of lower-limb amputation and their common prosthetic options are presented here. Below- and above-knee prostheses are discussed later in this chapter, as well as upper-limb prostheses.

Partial-Foot Amputation

If you have undergone a partial-foot amputation, you have many prosthetic options. One very popular prosthetic foot is composed of molded silicone and looks very much like a normal foot. It slips onto the residual foot like a slipper.

Syme's Amputation and Ankle Disarticulation

In a Syme's amputation, the entire foot is removed. The pointed ends of the tibia and fibula (bones of the lower leg) are flattened, and the heel pad is sewn back onto the flattened bones. The advantage of this type of amputation is that you can bear weight on the heel pad, and walk for brief periods of time without the aid of a prosthesis.

In an ankle disarticulation, the entire foot is removed. The tibia and fibula are left naturally pointed, and the heel pad is sewn back onto the pointed bones. This type of amputation is often performed on those for whom the trauma of additional surgery is undesirable, such as diabetics and those with some other medical condition. If you have undergone either a Syme's amputation or ankle disarticulation, you can be fit with a prosthetic foot.

Transpelvic Amputation and Hip Disarticulation

The term transpelvic amputation (formerly hemipelvectomy) refers to the removal of part of the pelvis, and, consequently, every connected structure of the lower extremity. There is no remaining ischium or "sit bone" (the lowest of the three bones that make up the pelvis), leg, or foot.

A hip disarticulation refers to amputation at the level of the femur (thigh bone). The pelvis remains intact.

A Few Words
About Weight Control

It is especially important for a person who wears a prosthesis to maintain a stable weight. Since the prosthesis is a custom-fitted device, a weight change of even five pounds may cause the socket to lose its intimate fit, which is necessary for maximum comfort and proper function.

People who are excessively overweight will likely have an additional problem—finding the extra energy needed for optimal use of their prosthesis. Their bodies are already carrying around the burden of excess weight.

So, watch your dietary intake! Good nutrition is essential for everyone's optimal health. Let your prosthesis be an added incentive for staying fit.

Transpelvic amputations and hip disarticulations are usually performed on those who have undergone severe trauma from an accident, or for those with cancer in related parts of the body. In extremely rare cases, an infant is born with congenital absence of these same body parts.

There have been a number of advances in prosthetic components in recent years. A variety of hip, knee, and foot options are now available for those with these amputation levels.

Prostheses for both transpelvic amputation and hip disarticulation are built with a very flexible socket. You "strap" yourself into the socket by wrapping it around your pelvis for a secure fit, and buckling the socket in either the front or back. Older versions of this type of socket were made of hard material and were very uncomfortable. The socket came up above the iliac crest (top of the hip bones), and the person's body would "piston" up and down in the socket as much as one inch with each step. That hurt! Additionally, the movement of the limb in the socket would, in effect, lengthen and shorten the leg with every step, and throw off the gait. Understandably, the vast majority of those who were fitted with this style of prosthesis eventually stopped wearing it.

Due to recent improvements in the design and material of this socket, it has become more widely used than ever before. The socket is now made of a soft, very flexible, opaque plastic that is "skin adhesive." This means that the socket material "sticks" to the body for a snug fit. With this type of socket, there is no need to wear a prosthetic sock. The socket grasps the person below their iliac crest in the fossa (indentation) of the pelvis, and wraps around to include the opposite hip. This is not only much more comfortable than the older socket version, but its snugger fit allows for a more natural gait.

These new sockets are also about 50 percent lighter in weight than the older sockets. This makes a huge difference in the amount of energy required to operate the limb.

Translumbar Amputation

A translumbar amputation (formerly hemicorpectomy) is usually performed on those who have undergone severe trauma from an accident, or for those with cancer in related parts of the body. The amputation is made through the lumbar vertebra (the lower back). This type of amputation is very rare. In such cases a person generally depends upon a wheelchair or a custom-made sitting seat for mobility. In extremely rare cases, an infant is born with congenital absence of these same body parts.

ENDOSKELETAL AND EXOSKELETAL COMPONENTS

You have the option of choosing "endoskeletal" or "exoskeletal" components for your prosthesis. An exoskeletal laminated socket is hard like fiberglass. (You might remember from biology class that an exoskeleton is a hard, outer structure like the shell of a crab.) We humans are not like crustaceans; we are endoskeletal, supported by our internal skeleton.

Key advantages to endoskeletal components are that they are light-weight, require few alignment adjustments, and have parts that are easily interchanged or replaced. A soft foam endoskeletal cover also has a more natural feel than a hard exoskeletal limb. The major advantage of exoskeletal components is their overall durability. These components last long and stand up to rough wear, such as that which occurs during certain recreational activities. Exoskeletal components are also able to endure strenuous physical movements such as kneeling.

The cosmetic appearance of artificial limbs has come a long way in a relatively short period of time. Examples include new types of "skin" made of durable waterproof material, which can be custom-matched to skin tone, and prosthetic feet that are so real-looking they even have toes and veins. Due to such improvements, it is more and more difficult to spot the wearer of an artificial limb.

SPECIALTY LEGS AND PROSTHETIC OPTIONS

There used to be more of a need for "specialty legs" than there is today. If, in the past, you wanted to go for a swim, you would have needed a special waterproof leg. If you wanted to go snow skiing, you would have needed a special foot setup to provide the correct ankle angle. Now, with the new prosthetic options available, most individuals do not need special limbs.

If you swim or jet-ski, you can obtain a customized prosthetic leg that is waterproof yet still useful for normal walking. If you actively participate in sports, the cosmetic cover of your artificial leg can be removed so it does not get torn during periods of physical activity. Most of the time, your prosthetic leg can be customized to help you perform just about any activity you desire. Therefore, if you have special needs, be sure to discuss them with your prosthetist, and together you might be able to work out a solution.

There are adjustable prosthetic feet that accommodate shoes of varying heel heights. This allows both women and men to wear boots or shoes of varied heel heights. The only problem with adjustable feet is that they are a bit tricky to adjust, and few individuals can do so with ease. Instead, some people choose to have interchangeable prosthetic feet, while others, for whom adjustable foot height is important, have two legs made—one high-heeled, one low-heeled. Some convert their spare limb to the desired heel height.

Different options are requested by individuals depending on their unique cultural or personal needs. For example, in some Eastern cultures it is important that those with above-knee amputations are able to bend the joints of their prosthetic knees so they can sit cross-legged on the floor.

For those with bilateral above-knee amputation, there exist prostheses that are known as *stubbies*. Stubbies are essentially sockets that fit the residual limb with prosthetic feet or a "rocker platform." This design eliminates the need for knees and other more-complex intermediate components. These walking devices are much easier and safer to use than full-length bilateral above-knee prostheses. Some individuals who have bilateral above-knee amputations choose to wear stubbies when they begin learning how to walk again; when physically able, they progress to full-length artificial limbs. Occasionally, a person will choose to be fitted with stubbies to accomplish certain tasks more easily, such as repairing a car or boat, or working in the garden. Some individuals, however, consider the loss of height personally or socially unacceptable and will strongly reject this type of limb.

If you are physically active and participate in certain sports, it may be advantageous to have an ankle rotator placed in your prosthesis. If you are a golfer, for example, this rotator may help improve your golf swing.

These are just some examples of the many, varied prosthetic options available today. You can see why it is so important for your prosthetist to know all of the activities that are important to you.

If a certain artificial limb or prosthetic option is not available at your prosthetist's facility, but you feel that it might improve the quality of your life, what should you do? *Ask for it anyway!* Together, you and your prosthetist can discuss your request and decide whether it is realistic and appropriate for you (in terms of both comfort and cost). *Remember, very basic components might be better for your individual needs than "so-called" state-of-the-art options.*

BECOMING AN EDUCATED CONSUMER

Due to the growing number of prosthetic options, it is important for you to gather as much information as possible before you make any major decisions regarding your prosthesis. The more you think of yourself as a health-care consumer and research that which is best for your unique circumstances, the better off you will be.

In addition to the information you get from your prosthetist, you can learn about the latest prosthetic options through a variety of other sources. Speak with others with amputation in your local and national support groups, and as well as those you meet at your prosthetist's office. Many support and consumer groups publish newsletters that include updates on prosthetic developments, as well as referral sources for additional information. (For more information on support groups, see Chapter 17, "Developing your Support System.")

The National Office for Orthotics and Prosthetics is an umbrella organization that houses the following three organizations:

• **The American Academy of Orthotists and Prosthetists (AAOP).** Composed of professionals in the fields of orthotics and prosthetics, the function of the AAOP is to provide advanced, continuing education and improved quality of prosthetic and orthotic care.

• **The American Orthotic and Prosthetic Association (AOPA).** Composed of professionals in the fields of orthotics and prosthetics, the AOPA is a trade association that represents the vast majority of prosthetic and orthotic businesses.

• **The American Board for Certification (ABC).** The ABC is an independent body that issues credentials for orthotists and prosthetists. Criteria for certification includes rigorous written, oral, and practical tests, and continuing education requirements. For a prosthetic facility to be certified by the ABC, it must have at least one certified prosthetist on staff; it must also meet certain accommodation requirements, such as wheelchair access and private fitting areas.

The AAOP, AOPA, and ABC will send you written introductory material upon request. To contact any one of these three organizations, send your correspondence to:

1650 King Street — Suite 500
Alexandria, VA 22314
(703) 836–7118

• **National Association for Advancement of Orthotics and Prosthetics (NAAOP).** This nonprofit trade association is composed of prosthetists, orthotists, and consumers. Individuals with amputation are among the members of NAAOP's board of directors. Dedicated to improvement of life for those with amputation and other disabilities through technological advancement, NAAOP is also active in lobbying and legislation, education, and advocacy.

1275 Pennsylvania Avenue NW — 3rd Floor
Washington, DC 20004–2404
(202) 624–0064

A reminder—by all means, it is important to become well-educated about your prosthetic options; but, *it is also important to remember that the most advanced technology available might not be necessarily the best solution to your unique prosthetic needs.* For example, a simple mechanical prosthesis may fit your needs better than a state-of-the-art myoelectric limb.

CHOOSING NOT TO USE A PROSTHESIS

A prosthesis is not always the best solution following amputation. Some individuals have found ways to compensate for their lost limb and may not feel the need for a prosthesis. This is most common in those with upper-limb loss. If you still have one fully functioning arm and hand, with practice, you can learn to perform almost all necessary daily tasks.

Choosing not to use a prosthesis can stem from a number of other reasons as well. Some of the most common reasons are presented below.

• **Medical Contraindications.** If you have medical contraindications, such as vascular failure in the residual limb or severe neurologic disease, obviously, the use of a prosthesis does not make sense. A prosthetic limb is also inadvisable if you don't have the energy necessary to operate it.

• **Severity of Amputation Level.** Generally, it is hard to compensate for lower-limb loss without a prosthesis. (It is difficult to hop a long distance on one leg.) In general, the higher the loss and the closer the amputation is to your trunk, the less perfectly function can be restored. There are certain levels of lower-limb amputation that are so severe, an extreme amount of energy is required to walk with the prosthesis. If you have such a loss, you may find it more efficient to move with the aid of crutches or a wheelchair.

This same logic applies to those with severe upper-limb amputation—above-elbow or shoulder disarticulation. The amount of focus and energy necessary to operate the gadgetry for two or three prosthetic joints can be overwhelming. In this situation, the choice to become one-handed is common.

No matter what your level of amputation, only *you* can decide if it is worthwhile to use a prosthesis. Be aware that some people with high levels of amputation, manage to thrive using artificial limbs.

• **Intolerance to Pain and Discomfort.** There is a very rare minority of individuals who have an extraordinarily low tolerance for discomfort or pain. If, after receiving the most optimally fit limb possible, you feel discomfort that is unbearable, you may opt not to use a prosthesis.

• **Inability to Accept a Prosthesis.** There are a number of people who, for various reasons, just cannot accept wearing a prosthesis. Whether the reasons are physical, mental, or emotional, if you are one of these individuals, your choice deserves to be respected.

• **Poor Fit or Poor Choice of Components.** Some individuals reject their prosthesis due to improper fit or poor choice of components. If you fall into this category, I encourage you to try again. Together with a prosthetist, discover what changes (if any) can be made to improve the quality of your artificial limb. A well-fit, comfortable limb can make a world of difference.

• **Unrealistic Expectations.** Some people have been poorly educated about the realities of a prosthesis—appearance, function, capabilities, and limitations. These people may develop unrealistic expectations that cannot be met when they actually receive their prosthesis. Frustration and disappointment can cause rejection of the limb.

Be sure to request and receive a thorough education about the realities of prosthetic wear and component options. To maximize your prosthetic outcome, be sure to receive good training in learning how to use your new limb.

• **Selective Use of the Prosthesis.** Some people choose to wear their prosthesis selectively. For example, they may wear their limb at work or when in public, but choose to take it off when at home and use another form of mobility such as crutches or a wheelchair.

If your circumstances make it necessary for you to use crutches or a wheelchair, or if you simply choose to do so, you can still have a rewarding, successful life.

HOW TO CHOOSE A PROSTHETIST

The Mutual Amputee Aid Foundation suggests that the best way to start your prosthetist selection process is through referrals. Your surgeon, personal physician (or physiatrist), or members from your support group can usually recommend good prosthetists. If there is someone of your gender and age group who has your level of amputation, be sure to talk with that person.

There are other important things for you to consider as well, such as the prosthetic facility. Is it conveniently located? (Remember, you will be returning regularly for prosthetic adjustments.) Along with location, what are the office hours? Do they fit into your schedule? Are evening and/or weekend appointments available? What are you supposed to do in case of an emergency?

The quality of communication with your prosthetist is a crucial factor. Is he or she able to understand your needs and feelings? Communication should also include discussing possible component options that might be good for you. Remember, your prosthesis will be custom made and should suit your specific lifestyle needs. Once again, the more you know about your care, the better your chances are of getting good results.

The prosthetist should explain each step in the fitting and fabrication of the prosthesis. This should include an approximation of how much time will be spent in adjusting the new limb.

The experience and education of the prosthetist is also critical, especially if you are a candidate for newer techniques, such as improved sockets and myoelectric limbs. Many progressive facilities exist. Be wary of "old-time" prosthetists who are not interested in up-to-date technological advancements. With an older-type prosthetic limb, you will still be able to have restored limb function, but the limb may not be as comfortable or functional as it could be with a modern prosthesis.

It is wise to discover how much experience the prosthetist has had making limbs for others with your level of amputation and needs similar to your own. For example, it is different meeting the special needs of a child than those of an adult. If you have an upper-limb loss and the prosthetist has mainly fit those with lower-limb loss, he or she may not have the experience necessary to ensure optimal fit and function of your limb.

Investigate the certification of both the prosthetist and the facility. In most states, prosthetists are not licensed like doctors and nurses, but they should be certified by the American Board of Certification (ABC). See page 35 for more information on the ABC.

Make sure of all financial arrangements before letting anyone start working with you. Know the schedule of payments for which you will be responsible. If cost is an issue, be sure you understand the services and component options that are included in each proposed price.

Can your prosthetist introduce you to additional services that might improve your life? For example, can he refer you to mutual support groups, emotional-recovery counselors, sports groups for those with disabilities, and/or pain clinics?

Since there are so many factors to consider, you might want to bring a written list of questions (or checklist) on your interviews. Remember, there is no such thing as a silly question. You have entered what is, for you, unchartered territory. The right prosthetist can be an excellent guide who can address many of your questions and concerns, so feel free to tap into his knowledge and expertise.

The very process of interviewing prosthetists is an important educational venture. What you learn from your interview should help prepare you for the road ahead. Exercising control over your own physical and emotional well-being, by actively participating in your own health care, can in itself be healing.

FIRST OFFICE VISIT WITH THE PROSTHETIST

When you arrive for your first office visit with the prosthetist, it is natural to be a little nervous. Prepare yourself. There are a number of things you can do to help increase your comfort.

Consider bringing someone along with you for emotional support. A family member or close friend can be invaluable in helping you ask relevant questions and remembering the information that was presented. Afterward, he or she can serve as a sounding board to help you sort out the experience of your first office visit. It is also a good idea to leave small children at home, if possible. It is best to be able to focus your attention without any distractions.

Arrive wearing a compressive cover, such as an elastic wrap or shrinker sock, on your residual limb. If you have a lower-limb loss, wear your usual shoe and bring its mate for your prosthesis. Also, wear or bring a pair of shorts to make the fitting easier. If you have an upper-limb amputation, wear a tube top.

Be sure to bring your prescription and x-rays, if requested. Also, bring along your health insurance information. It is a good idea to contact the office staff prior to your appointment and ask if they have any other suggestions to facilitate your first visit.

COST OF PROSTHESES

The cost of prostheses, whether for upper or lower limbs, varies with type and components. Cost may also vary widely depending upon local overhead.

Consider the following: Are you going to have an energy-storing foot or a Flex Foot, which costs about three times as much? Are you going to use a roll-on silicone liner for suspension, or are you going to use a strap? A relatively simple, basic prosthesis for a low level of amputation in an inactive person may cost only a few thousand dollars. The higher the amputation level, and the more active the person, the more expensive the prosthesis.

Basically, the cost of an above-knee prosthesis is roughly twice as much as a below-knee prosthesis. A prosthetic device for a hip disarticulation is generally 20 percent more expensive than one for an above-knee.

Generally, an above-elbow prosthesis costs twice as much as a below-elbow prosthesis. A prosthetic device for a shoulder disarticulation is roughly 20 percent more than one for an above-elbow.

Myoelectrics can triple the cost of a standard upper-limb prosthesis.

Keep in mind that many optional components are difficult to operate and often unnecessary. Carefully consider your priorities and select only those functions that are important to you. In most cases, if your residual limb changes in size or shape, you will have to replace only the socket. If you are young and active you will probably get anywhere from three to five years use out of the limb's components. The less active you are, the longer the components will last. Many with amputation want a spare prosthetic limb for various reasons. Women often like to have both a low-heeled and high-heeled leg to accommodate different shoes. Many with amputation do not like to be seen at work or other public places without their limb, and they desire a spare to use when their other one is being repaired.

Insurance

Insurance coverage for prosthetics varies widely, and the insurance industry is constantly changing. A great variety of plans exist, ranging from private insurance to managed-care options to government-assisted programs. If you have no insurance and little money, check with your state social services department to discover if there are programs available to assist you with prosthetic costs.

Each insurance plan offers differing benefits at differing costs to the consumer. Due to this variance in coverage, it is highly recommended that you enlist the expertise of your prosthetist's office staff to assist you in dealing with your insurance company. They have experience working with a variety of insurance plans and can help ensure that you get maximum benefits.

It is critical for you to understand the prosthetic benefits offered under your specific insurance plan. Answers to the following types of questions are important: Are prostheses covered under my policy? (The definitive prosthesis or just a temporary device?) Is preapproval or predetermination required in my policy? If so, what specific information must be furnished? Am I free to choose any provider? If only the initial prosthesis is covered, does this mean the first one I receive or the first prosthesis that is billed to this insurance company? Are replacements, repairs, and supplies covered under my policy? Is there an annual limit ("cap") or a lifetime limit for prosthetic services? What is the benefit schedule? Is there a deductible? What is my coinsurance liability? Is there a process of insurance appeals? Be sure to request a copy of those parts of the policy specific to your concerns.

When contacting an insurance company by phone, *it is very important* to keep a record of the call. *Always* write down the name of the person to whom you have spoken, their department, direct phone number, and date and time of the call. Be sure to have any insurance-related terms you do not understand defined. Keep notes of the topics discussed.

THE UPPER-LIMB AMPUTEE

In years gone by, a person's usefulness was amputated along with his hand. A man who lost his hand, lost his hope. Indeed, amputation was often used as retribution and punishment, particularly for thieves, and the crude devices that replaced lost limbs became a symbol for evil men, like the legendary Captain Hook. Most amputees became beggars, outcasts reflecting the psychological and social trauma that to this day accompanies loss of limb and means of livelihood.

In recent years, however, we have seen tremendous progress in the field of prosthetics. New materials and technology have made it possible to fit almost every patient with a functioning prosthesis, regardless of the level of amputation. . . . Presumably a person who has lost an arm can now look forward to a more normal life than was ever before possible.

L.F. Bender, M.D., M.S.
Prostheses and Rehabilitation After Arm Amputation

The experience for both those with upper- and lower-limb amputation is tremendously traumatic, in that a crucial part of basic anatomy is lost forever; however, immediately following the amputation, upper-extremity loss is often more emotionally devastating. This is due, in part, to the loss of sensation and function, and because of how visually apparent the loss is. (People tend to look first at your hands and arms, not at your feet and legs. Lower-limb loss can be camouflaged by shoes and clothing.) Another reason that adds to the devastation of upper-limb loss is the symbolism associated with hands. The following excerpt, taken from *Children with Hand Differences: A Guide for Families*, illustrates this point:

Rings worn on fingers symbolize love, friendship and commitment. We associate our hands with assistance and competence when we say, "I need a hand with this," or "Can I give you a hand?" Hands express affection and friendship. Hand gestures are used to express feelings and are part of our communication with others. Hands, along with faces, are the most readily visible parts of our body, so any form of difference is easily noticeable.

Adapting to Being One-Handed

Your hands do so many different things—they are so versatile. Yet, even if you are missing an upper-limb, you can still function very well. Many people use their prosthetic arm as nothing more than a "paperweight" to do such things as hold paper in place so they can write, or hold an orange steady so they can peel it easily. When you think about it, you will discover that you do most things one-handed anyway; your other hand really just helps out!

Most persons with upper-limb loss will eventually adapt as well as those with lower-limb amputation, but their initial shock is generally greater.

You will discover your own unique ways to adapt. Of course, the level of your amputation will impact your residual limb's remaining function. It will be easier for you to make adjustments if the amputated arm or hand is not your dominant one.

You will find ways to compensate for your limb loss by using your remaining arm and other body parts. Artificial limbs perform many normal functions. I have watched little children with myoelectric limbs grasp tiny items, play ball, and roughhouse with other children, without losing a beat.

Having an apparent physical difference, such as an upper-limb loss, can be socially awkward for others, who may not be sure how to interact with you. If you notice that others are ill at ease around you, you can diffuse their tension by saying something like, "This is how I do such and such." The more relaxed you are, the more relaxed others will be, and the focus will shift from your missing limb to normal interaction. For example, if your right hand is missing, you can initiate a handshake with your left hand.

In *The One-Hander's Book: A Basic Guide to Activities of Daily Living* (New York: The John Day Company, 1973), Veronica Washam, who herself has one hand, states:

> As your confidence increases, you will be tackling activities usually regarded as being only for two-handers, such as piano playing. Depending upon where your interests lie, you can learn, or relearn, the techniques for swimming, carpentry, sewing, driving a car, and other things, and generally function as efficiently as your friends, neighbors, family, and co-workers. It may take you a little longer to perform such activities, particularly in the beginning, but with practice, you will not be far behind. Your patience, effort, and determination will be rewarded by efficiency, renewed faith, and restored independence.
>
> Most of all keep your sense of humor alive! . . . We who are one-handers must always remember that our attitude about ourselves largely determines the world's attitude towards us.

Occupational therapists are trained to teach you how to accomplish everyday tasks. They are creative problem solvers and can be an excellent resource. The occupational therapist can make you aware of special tools and assistive devices that are designed to make your life a bit easier.

If you choose to use a prosthetic arm, it is important to get one as soon as possible. If you go too long without an arm, you may become "one-handed," due to the new habits you develop. Most with upper-limb loss who choose to wear a prosthesis, often want to start with a limb that is cosmetically pleasing; however, once they become accustomed to wearing a limb, they end up with something more functional.

If you have undergone amputation of both upper-limbs, it will be necessary to learn to accomplish many physical tasks of everyday living— things that are often taken for granted. Some self-care activities such as eating, dressing, and keeping yourself clean will require assistance from others. This loss of independence and subsequent physical dependence on others, may be especially difficult to handle emotionally. If you have bilateral upper-arm loss and are going to be using prostheses, the sooner you are fitted, the easier your adjustment process will become.

Partial-Hand Prostheses

Most partial-hand amputations are due to accidents. Generally, you can function extremely well with a partial hand, and there is often little or no need for prosthetic assistance. This is fortunate, since there currently exists no myoelectric or mechanical partial hands that really work well. With partial-hand loss, the only time you might want a prosthesis is either for cosmetic purposes, or in order to use your hand as a useful tool.

Most of the time, a partial-hand prosthesis functions like a tool, accomplishing a number of tasks for which it was specifically designed. An "opposition post" may be worn to restore the invaluable function of the opposable thumb and fingers, which allows the wearer to grip items more easily. For example, if you desire to pick up and use a shovel at work, a prosthesis can be designed to allow you to do just that.

Presently, there is no prosthesis that is capable of providing the ability to feel sensation. If, like most with partial-hand amputation, you still have fingers remaining, you will still have the ability to feel. Partial-hand prostheses are designed to allow you to continue feeling sensation with your remaining fingers.

If the cosmetic appearance of your hand is especially important, you can wear a natural-looking prosthetic glove (with no functional ability). The trade-off for the glove's improved appearance is that it can interfere with the hand's function by blocking the sensation of the remaining fingers. For some, such as those who interact with the public in white-collar jobs, this trade-off may be acceptable. So your choice of a partial-hand prosthesis is a matter of individual preference.

Mechanical Upper-Limb Prostheses

"My prosthetist told me, 'We built a limb for this guy who lost his arm below the elbow during World War II. He can pick up an ash out of an ashtray, move it around, then set it back down without crushing the thing! When you can do that, you're a pro.' It sounded pretty impossible to me. But guess what. I was able to do it in three days!"

—Clint

The type of limb an individual is willing to accept is sometimes influenced by culture. In Europe, and especially in Latin America, it may be socially unacceptable if a prosthesis does not look like a natural hand. In fact, most myoelectrics have been developed in Europe, because individuals generally will not accept a prosthetic hook. The United States is one of the few countries where people are willing to accept a limb with good function, even if it is at the expense of appearance.

More recently, however, fewer and fewer Americans are accepting hooks. They feel that if they can have computers in their cars, why do they have to have hooks on their hands? However, there are certain individuals—car mechanics and others with jobs involving manual dexterity—who do utilize hooks.

There is nothing wrong with that old-style hook. It operates by using a harness that is connected to the other shoulder and upper trunk, and cables that are directed by shoulder movement. The most common and simplest hook-gripping device uses a rubber band that keeps the two fingers closed together; so, when you are relaxed, the hook is normally closed in a gripping mode. A little lever opens the "finger" on the hook. This lever is connected to a cord that is attached to a small strap that runs around your opposite shoulder. Hook operation is simple and natural—when you reach forward with your prosthetic arm, the cord is pulled and the hook opens. When you bring your arm back toward your body, the tension on the cord relaxes and the rubber band pulls the hook closed.

Myoelectric Upper-Limb Prostheses

What in tarnation is this new-fangled myoelectric stuff anyway? Explained simply, myoelectric technology uses electronic sensors to pick up the feedback of muscle-fiber contractions as muscles move naturally. The sensors activate the motors that automatically control the action of the prosthetic limb.

In other words, muscles contract when they receive messages, in the form of electrical impulses, from the brain. Surface electrodes, which are embedded in the prosthesis, can pick up a signal as small as the "firing" of one muscle fiber. This information is transferred to the myoelectric hand or elbow, so that it will respond by moving in a natural way. The "inside" muscles of the myoelectric arm generally bend the elbow or close the hand. The "outside" muscles of this arm generally extend the elbow or open the hand.

Myoelectric prostheses are here to stay; they have been around long enough to have proven themselves dependable and useful. Most myoelectric research has been conducted on arms. This is partly because, unlike a leg, an arm does not have to bear weight, so the electric motor in the limb does not have to be as strong.

It is common to put on a below-elbow myoelectric limb and use it right away with very little training, because the muscles required for its use are the same ones you use to open and close your hand anyway. With a myoelectric prosthesis, you do not have to know where your hand is to know what it is doing, so individuals can use it very well in a variety of positions. Both mechanical and myoelectric above-elbow prostheses can be held in place on the residual limb with a suction socket. Below-elbow prostheses are often "self-suspending"—they are held in place on the residual limb by contouring the socket to align with your remaining bones.

It is not always necessary to wear prosthetic socks with either above-elbow or below-elbow prostheses; both may utilize flexible sockets that are housed in carbon graphite frames. With this type of construction, if there is a size change in the residual limb, only the socket needs to be changed, not the entire prosthetic limb.

Durability of Prostheses

Upper-extremity prostheses last longer than lower-extremity types, which must carry more weight and bear the stresses of walking. Today's myoelectric limbs rarely break down—on the average, they are in the shop for repairs only a few days a year. One drawback of the myoelectric limb is that it weighs a bit more than the mechanical type. However, researchers are currently addressing this problem. Other drawbacks of myoelectric limbs are that they react slowly and make some noise.

Because of the physical changes that your residual limb will undergo after amputation, most individuals choose to wear a conventional limb for about a year before they are fitted for a myoelectric one. The socket for a myoelectric prosthesis has a very intimate fit, and if your residual limb atrophies (shrinks) or develops more muscle, the limb will not operate properly.

The decision to wear a mechanical upper-limb prosthesis versus a myoelectric one is really up to you and your individual circumstances. One is not necessarily "better" than the other.

Options, Options, Options!

There are various combinations of options for an above-elbow prosthesis. The choices presented here are only a few of the many that are available. So be sure to have an in-depth discussion with your prosthetist to become educated about the choices you have, based upon your specific physical needs and individual circumstances.

Warning! These options can sound confusing. I suggest you read them slowly and consider them carefully.

Your above-elbow prosthesis can have a myoelectrically controlled hand with one of two options: a mechanical elbow, or an elbow that is myoelectrically controlled. When using a myoelectric hand with a myoelectric elbow, both hand and elbow are controlled by the same electrodes. Once the myoelectric elbow is locked in position, the electrical control switches from the elbow to the hand, which allows the hand to open and close.

Your above-elbow prosthesis can also have a mechanical hand or hook with a mechanically controlled or a myoelectrically controlled elbow. These options are in addition to a mechanically controlled elbow with a mechanically controlled hook. All of these combinations have advantages and disadvantages, so it is advised that you discuss all available options with your prosthetist to choose the options that are best for you.

HIGH LEVELS OF UPPER-BODY AMPUTATION

High levels of upper-limb amputation include *shoulder disarticulation* and *forequarter amputation*. Let us take a look at these amputation levels and their prosthetic options.

Shoulder disarticulation refers to an amputation in which the entire arm is removed, but the shoulder is left intact. This type of amputation is generally performed on those who have undergone severe trauma from an accident, or for those with cancer in related parts of the body.

If you have had a shoulder disarticulation and desire to use a prosthesis with myoelectric components, be aware that, due to missing shoulder muscles, you will have to master unnatural movements to operate the electrode sites in the arm in order to lift the elbow and open and close the hand. It is quite tricky, and requires coordination and much practice on your part. For this reason, only about half of those with shoulder disarticulation choose this type of prosthesis.

A forequarter amputation refers to loss of the entire arm, shoulder, and shoulder girdle. Like a shoulder disarticulation, this type of amputation is performed generally in conjunction with a tumor removal or as the result of a severe trauma from an accident. Only a relatively small percentage of amputations fall into this category. At this level of amputation, there is often no residual limb remaining; prosthetic use is uncommon, but not impossible. A "shoulder cap" is often recommended for those with forequarter amputation. It serves as a "filler" so upper-body clothing hangs more evenly, improving general appearance.

Depending upon individual degrees of comfort, some individuals with these high levels of amputation choose to mask their limb loss with a cosmetic prosthesis. Others choose to wear no limb at all.

LOSS OF BOTH UPPER LIMBS

If you have lost both upper limbs, you can still do well. Of course, the artificial limbs cannot give you your original freedom; however, you can still feed yourself, groom yourself, and take care of your personal hygiene. You can still do everyday things around the house. Different items can be adapted so you can hold them better. With determination, you can do a lot. Even though it will take more work than with a unilateral limb loss, you *can* function well with a bilateral loss. It is highly recommended that you read the works of Reverend Harold Wilke, a man who was born without arms and who has adapted beautifully. (See page 329 in the "Further Information" section.)

Acceptance of your physical reality and a good personal attitude are critical in affecting your emotional recovery. The many factors involved in emotional rehabilitation, as well as specific coping skills, will be presented in subsequent chapters, along with examples of well-adjusted, successful people who have lost more than one limb.

AREAS OF ONGOING RESEARCH AND DEVELOPMENT

While prosthetic development is progressing in slow, steady incremental steps in some areas, it is making significant advancements in others. These developments may someday prove to be great news for those with amputation. Some of these include:

• **"CAD/CAM" Technology.** In the upcoming years, Computer Aided Design (CAD) and Computer Aided Manufacturing (CAM) will likely play an active role in the prosthetic industry. For example, some prosthetists already use this system of computer imaging to modify prosthetic sockets. Through this technology, the image of your natural limb can be copied, then reversed, so that a laser can cut a cosmetic cover for your prosthesis.

• **The Microprocessor "Smart" Knee.** Research is now being conducted to further develop an "intelligent" knee that offers greater walking stability to the user. Unlike a conventional artificial knee, this smart knee makes possible a more natural range of walking speed without conscious effort on the part of the user. This is accomplished through the use of a microprocessor. Microprocessors are small circuitry designed to process impulses (input) and turn them into information (output). The input is received from sensors in the knee, which register the movement of the artificial shin. This input is converted into information that will help the wearer control walking speed. The first models of this type of knee are already commercially available.

• **Restoration of Sensory Feedback.** Still being researched and developed, pressure transducers have been incorporated in the sole of the artificial foot, which send tingling sensations to the residual limb. Through this it is possible to receive a limited amount of sensory feedback. This information tells you when and how much weight you are bearing on the foot, and whether you are putting pressure on the heel or toe. This may produce a heightened sense of security when walking. In the future, sensors that transmit heat and cold might be incorporated into this system.

• **The Myoelectric Knee.** In layman's terms, a myoelectric knee is something a "bionic man" would wear. The electric components of this knee interface with impulses from the body to produce more natural control and movement of the prosthetic limb. To be more specific, when the muscles contract in your thigh, they send a message through an electrode in the form of an electrical impulse. This impulse activates the motors that automatically move the myoelectric knee. When you fire your muscles, a "myoelectric lock" fixes the knee and heel in a position that prevents you from falling as you walk. Eventually, the whole prosthetic limb may be controlled myoelectrically. You won't even have to think about your gait while walking!

While prosthetics may never be able to match the marvels of human biology, advancements are coming at a rate never before seen. The "science fiction" of today may become the reality of tomorrow.

THE IMPORTANCE OF A POSITIVE ATTITUDE

As in many other areas of living, your attitude and the meaning you attribute to your experiences are as pivotal to your well-being as the actual physical processes you are undergoing. Chapter 15, "Making Meaning of Your Amputation," is devoted to this concept.

To conclude this chapter, read the words of certified prosthetist Tom Guth on the importance of attitude as it affects your success with prosthetics:

> Attitude is one of the most important aspects in the fitting and successful use of a prosthesis. If a person doesn't really want an artificial limb and isn't willing to put the necessary effort into rehabilitation, the best limbs in the world won't change that.
>
> A person has a healthy attitude when he regrets what he has lost, and realizes that what we can do will never completely replace it. If he works hard, and we work hard together, he will be able to achieve an acceptable level of function. (This may take six months to a year.) He may not be able to do everything he did before, but he may be able to do most things. He has to accept this as a reasonable goal. He must also accept that this process is not going to be easy. He must realize that although he will keep improving, there will be plateaus he'll hit, when he thinks he's not going anywhere, or it will seem like he's slipping backwards.
>
> So we prepare our patients by making them aware of these factors and by giving them as much information as we can about what to expect. And we always encourage positive attitude.

This does not imply that a person with an excellent attitude can overcome a poorly fit or poorly aligned prosthesis. It does emphasize that a positive attitude not only promotes your well-being, it also helps optimize your prosthetic success.

4

PHANTOM LIMB PHENOMENON

"When my legs were first amputated, it felt like they were still there. In fact, I can remember being in the hospital right after the operation. I was sitting on the side of the bed when the doctor came into the room. I stood up to shake his hand and fell on the floor! I thought I still had both legs!"

—Frances

"Out of the clear blue sky, I felt instant pain! It was as if somebody had taken a strand of barbed wire, wrapped it in a figure eight around my ankle, and tightened it! There wasn't anything I could do. It wasn't like a cramp or a charley horse where I could have gotten up to walk it out—I just had to wait. I still occasionally get phantom pains, but not as bad as I used to."

—Kent

No, you are not going bonkers. You are not imagining things. It is quite possible to continue to feel the presence of your limb after it has been removed. *Phantom limb sensation* refers to the physical impression that an amputated limb is still there. Phantom sensation is normal after surgery and encompasses any feeling or sensation that might have been felt in the missing limb before surgery. The range of sensations varies from simply feeling that the leg is still present, to a tingling or unpleasant itching. The phantom sensation is so genuine, individuals often imagine the missing limb still possesses normal functions such as movement or weight-bearing capacity. For most, phantom limb sensation gradually diminishes in intensity within the first two years following surgery, and usually recurs under stress.

Unlike phantom limb sensation, *phantom limb pain* actually hurts! The intensity, type, and duration of pain varies; some individuals may feel sharp, tingly "pins and needles" or electric shocks. Others may experience burning, piercing, shooting, cramping, crushing, or agonizing pain. The good news is that it is very rare for a person to have disabling, agonizing phantom pain that persists over time.

The vast majority of individuals with amputation experience some type of phantom sensation, phantom pain, or both. A person who has pain in his residual limb will often have phantom pain. Phantom limb phenomenon commonly occurs in those whose nerves have been cut or torn from the spinal cord, such as in the case of paraplegics and quadriplegics.

It is important to understand that surgical pain at the amputation site is natural and to be expected. This is different from phantom limb pain.

CAUSES OF PHANTOM LIMB PHENOMENON

So, what causes these bizarre sensations and pains? There are various theories as to what physiological mechanisms actually cause phantom limb phenomenon. Those presented here are certainly not definitive. Hopefully, our knowledge will continue to increase as new research sheds light on this mysterious occurrence.

First, let's discuss a few concepts about our basic physiology that might better help you understand the causes of phantom limb phenomenon. Simplistically speaking, pain is "all in your head" no matter what the actual cause of that pain is. In other words, sensations of pain are ultimately *interpreted* by the brain, even when these sensations are originally perceived in another part of the body. There are certain areas in the brain that register and interpret information that relates to individual body parts. For example, a specific part of the brain "feels" sensations that arise just in the foot.

Nerves are very specific in what they do. Pain nerve fibers can sense pain only; they cannot, for example, sense heat or coldness. Similarly, a vibration nerve cannot register pain, and a temperature nerve cannot feel deep touch. This specificity of nerve function is analogous to the fact that you do not expect your eyes to hear. At the end of the sensory-information pathway, nerves lead to an area in the brain's cerebral cortex in which feeling is accurately sensed. Studies have shown that if specific areas of the central cortex of the brain are stimulated, then the person will perceive certain sensations.

Any sensation that was felt when the limb was still intact, is still within the nerves that carried those feelings. These same nerves are still present in the residual limb, as is the part of the brain that registered the messages from those nerves. So it is not hard to imagine that a person with amputation might still experience a wide range of sensations from the residual limb.

Theoretically, there are two causes of phantom limb pain. One cause is due to ingrained memories. If a limb has been amputated, the subconscious part of the mind remembers that the limb was once there, and it can recreate certain types of uncomfortable sensations. This is referred to as *central pain dysfunction*.

The other cause of this pain is the result of certain free-floating nerve endings in the residual limb. Two of these nerve endings, in particular, pick up sensations and transfer that information back to the brain. If these nerve endings become chronically stimulated, the information may be transferred in a manner very similar to a broken record that repeatedly clicks back and forth. Technically, this is a type of *peripheral pain dysfunction*, sometimes referred to as a *noxious sensation*.

In other words, nerves in the residual limb receive pressure information through special receptors; this pressure can sometimes be interpreted as pain. The nerves, which originally went all the way to the distal (far) end of the body, are being stimulated closer to the body, but still "remember" the messages as if they originated in the missing part of the limb. The central pathway that carries the information from the remaining limb to the brain can become "short circuited" and carry the same information repetitively. Even though there is no actual stimulus, the sensation keeps repeating itself.

Variations in Phantom Limb Sensation

Phantom limb sensation can manifest itself in a variety of ways. In order to illustrate this diversity, several persons who have undergone amputation describe their experiences with phantom sensation.

"I felt phantom sensation immediately after my amputation. It was very bizarre! Although both of my legs were gone, I had the feeling that my knees were in a flexed position, as if they went straight down through the bed to the floor. The sensations weren't painful, just very obviously present. My amputated arm and hand felt like they were in a slightly flexed position."

—Leslie

"Sometimes it feels like my hand is still there and my fingers get stuck together in odd positions. It is as if the muscles and everything are still there, so if I think about it hard enough, I can move the phantom muscles and other parts. It's uncomfortable in that I can feel it all the time; but I've learned to not pay attention to it."

—Clint

"I feel like my missing leg is still there a lot of the time. If I think about it, I can actually feel it. Right now I'm sitting down and I feel that both my feet are flat on the floor."

—Mark

"During the first moments of consciousness after my surgery, it felt like my amputated leg was up in a sling. It wasn't painful—just an exhausting muscular ache. I kept asking people to put pillows underneath the missing leg. That's how strong and real the feeling was. Although the phantom sensation diminished with time, I still feel it occasionally. It's as if my amputated leg is asleep, and there is an energy there. There are certain muscles I feel I can move in the missing limb when I contract my stump."

—Marcy

Variations in Phantom Limb Pain

The following examples are provided to reassure you that phantom limb pain *does* hurt and is indeed real. If you experience this phenomenon, be assured that you are not alone. Also note that the pain experienced is different for each individual and may differ in type, intensity, and duration from episode to episode.

"Immediately following amputation, my phantom pains were so bad I just sat and rocked back and forth. The pain was stabbing, horrible, and constant! It felt like my foot was still there and was being twisted off. I was given drugs to stop the pain, which further upset me because I was afraid of getting hooked on them. Then one night I begged God to stop the pain before I lost my mind! Miraculously, the pain stopped just like that."

—Jill

"During the first six months after my operation, I often had phantom pain when I was trying to sleep at night. Out of nowhere, I would feel an electric shock. It was weird. I had to take sleeping pills for awhile just to get some sleep."

—Bob

"After my leg was amputated, I sometimes experienced sharp pains in my missing foot, leg, and in back of my knee. When I first got these phantom pains, it drove me crazy. I was miserable. When the pains became very sharp, I took pain pills. Sometimes I wrapped a towel around my residual limb, then I tapped on the stump to help desensitize the nerves. It seemed to help for awhile."

—Grant

"After sixteen years of being an amputee, I began to experience phantom pain in my missing leg. The pain began shortly after I started riding a life cycle, which put more pressure on my stump than it was used to. For several days I was in severe pain. On one day in particular, I was getting little shocks every fifteen seconds. After several hours I was going batty; it was horrible; I was freaking out! I couldn't understand why, after all these years of being an amputee, this was happening now. Hot baths and a heating pad on my stump seemed to relax the muscles a bit and ease the pain."

—Marcy

TREATMENT OF PHANTOM LIMB PAIN

There exist psychological, pharmacological, physiological, technological, and nutritional ways to treat phantom pain. Wow! Does this give you the impression that there are many avenues to relief? Although many treatment methods exist, their success varies tremendously from person to person. The following treatment methods are just a sampling of what is available. Your own physician, physical therapist, or pain specialist may have additional suggestions.

If you have episodes of phantom pain, experiment with different methods, then stick to those that work best for you. Treatment methods can be used separately or together. Combining methods is often more successful than using just one. *Always check with a health-care professional before initiating a treatment or combination of treatments for phantom pain.*

It may be that phantom pain is something you must learn to live with, along with the other discomforts and inconveniences that inherently accompany limb loss. Fortunately, with the passage of time, most phantom pain either resolves itself or occurs less frequently.

The following treatment methods for phantom pain are presented by category for easy comprehension. Obviously, many of the methods fall into more than one category.

Stress Reduction

Understanding that phantom pain is normal can, in itself, help decrease discomfort. Knowing that there are steps you can take to diminish the pain can further reduce any anxiety you may feel.

Anxiety can manifest itself in physical and emotional ways—apprehension, fear of losing your mind, rapid heartbeat, sweating, and muscle tension. These responses can intensify the experience of pain. You can prevent or counteract anxiety by living a healthful lifestyle, which should include the following: sound nutrition, exercise, good self-esteem, and the use of coping skills. All can contribute to your overall well-being.

Biofeedback is one tool that teaches you to relax, decrease stress, and alter physiological responses through the use of electrical monitoring devices. Progressive muscle relaxation, guided visual imagery, meditation, and medical hypnosis can be used alone or in combination with biofeedback. Remember, the brain *can* be trained to overcome pain, whether or not that pain is due to a physical cause.

Medical Treatment

Mild pain relievers such as aspirin, acetaminophen, and ibuprofen are often sufficient to help alleviate phantom pain that is not severe. If your pain level is beyond tolerance, consult your physician for stronger medication. Be aware, however, that stronger medications, such as narcotics, often have undesirable side effects (loss of effectiveness, addiction), so it is preferable to explore other methods first.

Some physicians choose to prescribe short-term use of antidepressants to treat phantom pain. No one knows exactly why these medications work. What is known is that some types of antidepressants raise the level of a substance in your body known as *serotonin*. Others raise the level of *norepinephrine*. Heightened levels of serotonin and norepinephrine promote enhanced feelings of well-being, while decreasing symptoms of anxiety and depression. As antidepressants are long-lasting, they are generally taken once a day. However, because they may have significant side effects, it is important to discuss their benefits versus their possible negative effects with your physician.

Research has shown that acupuncture and the use of an acuscope have also been used successfully in the treatment of phantom pain. Endorphins, the body's natural pain killers, are released through the insertion of acupuncture needles or electrical currents at certain points on the body.

Altering Physical Activity

The degree of your physical activity may have an effect on your phantom pain. Distracting yourself from focusing on the pain by becoming involved in some type of activity is a beneficial tactic. Conversely, decreasing your involvement in an activity that has been found to increase the incidence of pain should provide relief. Experiment to discover whether an increase or decrease in physical activity works for you.

Working with the Residual Limb

In some individuals, pressure sites develop on the end of the residual limb when the prosthesis is not properly fit. These areas can get inflamed and nerves can become irritated, causing referred pain. The prosthetist can treat this pain by adjusting the socket of your artificial limb to relieve pressure sites.

For some, increased pressure on the residual limb, such as that which comes from wearing a shrinker sock, may bring some measure of relief. Sometimes, just wearing a prosthesis stimulates the residual limb and diminishes phantom pain.

Desensitization of the residual limb has been known to help reduce phantom pain. As the limb heals, be sure to massage it. Wearing prosthetic socks and keeping the limb wrapped with a compressive dressing may help decrease some of the sensation.

Moderate heat, which increases circulation, can decrease phantom pain discomfort. This can be achieved by taking a warm bath, or by applying a special "moist" heating pad (available in drugstores) to the residual limb.

A pasty mixture of alum and rubbing alcohol applied to the residual limb is a traditional treatment that many people have found helpful for reducing phantom pain. This mixture helps desensitize the free-floating nerve endings, while it toughens the residual limb itself.

Nutritional Awareness

Some people who experience chronic pain may find that they crave certain foods such as avocados, chocolate, and leafy green vegetables. Certain amino acids found in these foods help produce the body's endorphins, which are natural pain killers. Sometimes when the body is depleted of these amino acids there will be continuous pain. You may choose to be evaluated by a physician who has a special interest in nutrition, a dietician, or a nutritionist to determine if amino acid supplementation might be appropriate for you. Other ways to improve your diet and increase your feeling of well-being should also be determined.

Technological Treatment

Your physical or occupational therapist may suggest that you explore some of the following methods for treating phantom limb pain. Some of these treatments require a prescription from your physician.

• **Ultrasound.** This means of transmitting inaudible sound waves at a very high frequency is effective in breaking up inflammation of the nerve endings in the residual limb. The sound waves enter the body and create friction, which massages cells and fibers beneath the skin. The friction also causes some mild heat, which promotes relaxation. The blood rushes to the area, bringing nutrients and carrying away cellular waste. This increased blood activity helps heal the cells.

• **Pulse Magnetic Resonator.** This device gives off magnetic impulses that align certain molecules in the body, decreasing the release of chemicals that produce pain. The impulses emitted from this device actually penetrate the entire limb on which it is placed. Treatment is neither painful nor irritating; it is similar to the magnetic resonance imaging (MRI) often performed at hospitals for diagnosis.

• **Transcutaneous Electrical Nerve Stimulator (TENS) Unit.** The TENS unit provides relief by simply interrupting pain messages to the brain through counterstimulation. The TENS unit is often placed at the end of the residual limb by the therapist. It can also be placed on the patient's lower back to treat a leg amputation, or on the neck for the treatment of an arm amputation.

• **Interferential Current Unit.** This electrical stimulation unit penetrates three to four times deeper than the TENS unit. It desensitizes the nerve endings, decreasing the irritation that is produced through them. Compact units are available for home use.

• **Microstimulator.** Similar to a TENS unit, the microstimulator uses a different amount of electrical current. Electricity is measured in amperes (amps). A TENS unit works with milliamps, while a microstimulator works with microamps. Since a milliamp is a thousandth of an amp, and a microamp is a thousandth of a milliamp, you can see that a microstimulator uses a current that is about a thousand times more delicate than the current emitted by a TENS unit.

Microcurrent stimulation works on certain types of cells and promotes energy transfer to help the healing process. It works on a subsensory level— some people don't feel it at all, while others feel only a small tickle. This treatment has shown great promise with patients who have severe pain. In some cases, it has been known to cause prolonged improvement, rather than temporary relief. There are several varieties of microstimulators on the market. Most are smaller than a pack of cigarettes and can be easily used at home.

• **Cold Laser Therapy.** This treatment method, also called *low laser therapy*, is another effective nonsurgical treatment for phantom pain. This therapy works through the production of photo-biological stimulation, which releases a variety of enzymes that can decrease inflammation and stimulate healing. The laser can also be applied to acupuncture points. Cold laser therapy is currently used in Europe and a few selected centers in the United States.

• **Surgery.** In extreme cases of pain, surgery may be performed to block the nerve endings. Your extremity will still move and function normally, but you will not feel any sensation in the residual limb. Understand that this surgery is risky! Pain is often the body's way of making sure you do not hurt yourself. By taking away the feedback that feeling provides, you may damage your limb without knowing it.

An experimental surgical procedure known as DREZ has been performed with some degree of effectiveness. In this procedure, the "dorsal root entry zone" of the nerves is severed. This zone is where sensory input comes into the spinal cord. Severing nerves at this level dampens some of the information that normally would be sent to the cerebral cortex, and so decreases pain. As the DREZ procedure is still in the experimental stage, the length of its effectiveness is unknown.

With this variety of technological treatments to choose from and with new ones being developed, hopefully, one method will help you find relief from phantom limb pain.

Pain Treatment Centers

If you experience continuous phantom pain, and the treatment measures you have tried do not provide relief, seek assistance from a pain treatment center. It is especially important that you seek relief when the intensity or duration of your pain interferes with your ability to carry out work, enjoy life, or interact freely with family and friends.

Pain treatment centers or clinics are staffed with multi-disciplinary professionals who are experts in dealing with chronic and acute pain. Growing numbers of these centers are popping up across the country; many are associated with teaching hospitals. When looking for a pain treatment center, be sure it is staffed with at least four of the following types of practitioners: anesthesiologists, psychologists, psychiatrists, physicians, chiropractors, acupuncturists, nutritionists, physical or occupational therapists, massage therapists, and biofeedback technicians.

IN CONCLUSION

If you are one of the many persons who experiences phantom limb phenomenon, take heart. Remember that phantom sensation, while feeling admittedly weird, does not hurt. And if you experience phantom limb pain, know that there are many measures you can take to find relief. As you have read, some individuals have come up with their own novel approaches for relief; perhaps you will, too.

When exploring treatment modalities, keep this advice in mind—if the methods you have used to relieve your pain have not worked, then try something else. In any event, phantom pain is likely to diminish by itself over the course of time. With improved technology and a better understanding of the body-mind connection, phantom pain may even be fully treatable or preventable in the near future.

5

Rehabilitation

The word rehabilitate means "to restore." After surgery, your rehabilitation goal should be to restore yourself in body, emotions, mind, and spirit. Your amputation should be simply one aspect of your life, not the central one. The realities that accompany your loss of limb cannot be made to disappear; but, through rehabilitation, their negative effects can be decreased.

This chapter presents several facets of the rehabilitation process including recovery goals, the concept of a rehabilitation team, and the importance of being an educated health-care consumer. Selected topics such as residual limb care, prosthetic training, and emotional adjustment to your first prosthesis are also included.

THE TEAM APPROACH TO REHABILITATION

Ideally, there should be a team approach to your rehabilitation, in which each member of the team contributes his or her expertise. The team should be custom-tailored to meet your specific needs, based on your physical, emotional, psychosocial, and vocational requirements. Working with well-coordinated experts can increase the quality of your care and significantly shorten the overall length of your rehabilitation. In some locations, this type of approach is available in specialized amputation clinics or rehabilitation centers. If you live in a small town or rural area, there may not be a large enough patient population to support such a facility. In this case, your physician can cooperate with some other professionals who will assist with your rehabilitation. In this way, you can still receive quality care.

Team Captain—YOU!

Always remember that you are the most important member of the team. You are the expert of your own needs, and your active participation will be a major factor in your physical and emotional recovery.

Since it is likely that there will be several health-care professionals involved in your rehabilitation, you might want to ask one of them to help you coordinate your team. This will help you avoid needless duplication of services; it will also help provide a broad overview of your needs, so you can best attend to areas that might otherwise fall through the cracks.

When choosing team members, think of your specific needs. For example, if you have diabetes, it might be wise to include a nutritionist on your team to help you with a proper diet. If you do not fully understand your medical treatment protocol, your physician or a nurse might be a good choice. Perhaps you are athletically inclined and do not know how to re-enter the world of sports—a recreational therapist might help you get into condition and come up with ways you can adapt to sports and other recreational activities.

Remember, by being active in your rehabilitation, you will be exercising control over your life. This can be a great comfort, especially if your experiences with limb loss have trampled your sense of autonomy. You have lived through bodily changes and medical procedures that have been, at least partially, beyond your control. Being clear about your goals, and making sure that they are yours and not someone else's, can be very empowering.

Physician

The physician is often the popular choice for coordinating the members of a rehabilitation team. It is important that your physician has an interest in working with those with amputation. He should understand the complications that can follow amputation, and have knowledge of residual limb care. He should be able to guide you when choosing a prosthetist, as well as a physical and/or occupational therapist.

It is your physician who will write your prescription for a prosthesis, as well as for physical or occupational therapy. Although it is not absolutely necessary, it can be helpful if he is connected with a special clinic for those who have undergone amputation. The physician is often a good choice for helping you select the other members of your team.

A physiatrist is a physician who specializes in physical medicine and rehabilitation, and is an ideal choice for your team. A physiatrist might follow you from the time of your surgery through the time you have a satisfactory prosthetic limb.

Physical Therapist

The role of a physical therapist in your rehabilitation is very important. A good therapist can build your confidence, especially if he has worked with others who have mastered the new skills that you must learn. He can answer many practical questions about accomplishing physical tasks in everyday life.

When is it a good idea to begin physical therapy? The sooner the better!

Even before your amputation surgery, you can meet with a physical therapist and learn how to use assistive devices such as walkers, crutches, and/or wheelchairs. Ideally, whether you have lost an arm or a leg, it is good to work on strengthening both your upper and lower limbs. If you are undergoing lower-limb amputation, you will need strong arms to bear the weight of your crutches or walker, or to push your wheelchair.

If you require a wheelchair, either temporarily or permanently, the physical therapist will teach you how to navigate ramps and uneven surfaces, and how to maneuver through doorways. If you need to use a "transfer board" to get from the bed to a wheelchair, or from the wheelchair to another seat, once again, it is the physical therapist who will show you how. The physical therapist is also the one who will teach you how to "wrap" your residual limb with a compressive bandage, or house it in a special compressive sock as it heals.

You should be undergoing physical therapy while your prosthesis is being made. This will help prevent muscle contractures (shortening of the muscles) in your residual limb, which can limit both the strength and range of motion necessary for optimal control of the prosthesis. If you want to increase your overall strength and muscle tone, the physical therapist will design a conditioning program specifically for you.

How often you receive physical therapy will depend, of course, on your overall physical condition, type of amputation, and kind of prosthesis. If your physician does not recommend that you meet with a physical therapist, let him know that you want to do so!

If you are in a rehabilitation facility, you might work with a physical therapist two or three times a day. If you are in a regular hospital, you might receive therapy once a day. As an out-patient, you might go into a clinic for physical therapy anywhere from three to five days a week.

Some persons with lower-limb loss (especially below-knee) may be told that a prosthetist is the best one to teach them to walk again. This is not always optimal. You will recover sooner and avoid picking up bad habits if you get good feedback from a physical therapist. A physical therapist who is skilled in the area of prosthetics will be able to note any problem you may be having in your therapy and determine if it is due to your prosthesis. The therapist's feedback will be given to your prosthetist, who will then make the necessary adjustments.

To make your life easier and safer, the physical therapist might make suggestions for architectural changes in your home. For example, depending on your needs, he might suggest building ramps, adding a seat in the shower, replacing the shower head with a hand-held variety, reworking cabinet pulls for ease of operation, and removing rugs that might cause you to skid.

The expertise of a good physical therapist cannot be denied. He should be an invaluable member of your rehabilitation team.

Occupational Therapist

The roles of the occupational therapist and the physical therapist often overlap. An occupational therapist who is experienced in working with amputation often specializes in helping those with upper-limb loss. He helps you to develop upper-body strength and overall conditioning programs. If you have lost an upper limb, an occupational therapist will help you learn to operate your prosthesis. He is an excellent resource to help you adapt to the activities of daily living.

The training time for learning to use an upper-limb prosthesis will likely be longer than it is for a lower-limb device. This is especially true if the upper-limb training includes learning how to adapt a hook or myoelectric limb, or how to use the prosthesis in your vocation.

Since the emotional trauma of losing a hand or arm can be greater than losing a lower-limb, the occupational therapist often provides much-needed emotional support. He may also help make an assessment of your vocational goals.

Recreational Therapist

A recreational therapist can assist you in developing a healthy leisure lifestyle. He can introduce you to activities such as wheelchair sports, skiing, and swimming or other water sports—activities that you may not have considered. He will explore activities in which you may have special interest and determine if you might be able to participate in these activities.

A recreational therapist can serve as a bridge from the practice and integration of new skills you have learned in physical or occupational therapy to their real-life use. For instance, he might take you to a park where you can practice maneuvering your wheelchair, walking on uneven surfaces, or accessing a public bathroom.

Whether a recreational therapist helps you get involved in a community recreation program or shows you how to enjoy an activity at home, his goal is the same—to help you become active and fulfilled in your leisure time.

Chiropractor

A chiropractor has a specialty in maintaining the integrity of the neuromusculoskeletal system. Ambulation with a prosthesis is dependent upon biomechanics. A chiropractor can help your body stay in proper alignment in view of the stresses imposed by prosthetic use. He can be effective in treating back and neck pain, and other symptoms associated with misalignment.

Nurse

A nurse can visit you while you are in the hospital and accompany you on your ongoing clinic visits. He can help you by providing direct nursing care for any underlying medical disorder, such as diabetes or peripheral vascular disease. He may also educate you to better care for yourself. A nurse can also do the following:

• Teach you to alternate your body's position to help prevent muscle contractures.

• Show you how to hygienically care for your residual limb to keep it in optimal health and prevent skin problems.

• Serve as a bridge between you, your physician, and other members of your rehabilitation team.

• Provide ongoing emotional support during your physical healing, and psychological and social adjustment.

• Answer questions and allay fears that you or your family may have.

Although some people do not feel nurses are necessary members of their rehabilitation team, others consider them to be invaluable. You and your physician or other team members will have the job of deciding what is best for you and your individual needs.

Prosthetist

You will likely form a long-term relationship with your prosthetist, since he is the one who will fabricate, repair, and replace your artificial limb over the course of your lifetime.

The prosthetist will ascertain when your residual limb has atrophied (shrunk) enough and has assumed a stable enough shape to be fit for your first prosthesis. He will fit and fabricate your prosthesis by following your physician's prescription.

As prosthetists are often more aware of current prosthetic technology than physicians are, your prosthetist may want to advise your physician about your prescription. You might try to arrange a meeting between you, your prosthetist, and your physician. Together you can decide on the best prosthetic device for you.

For a more in-depth look at the role of the prosthetist, refer to Chapter 3, "Prosthetics."

Nutritionist or Dietician

If you have special dietary requirements related to an ongoing medical condition, such as diabetes, a nutritionist can help you come up with a sound dietary plan. Of course, anyone can benefit from good eating habits. A nutritionist can help you modify your current eating habits to improve your overall health, prevent future problems, and increase your energy level.

Massage Therapist

Trauma leaves its marks in the body tissue. The "memory" of pain is also stored in the tissue as muscle tension and connective tissue shortening. Seek out a massage therapist trained in "deep tissue release" and skeletal realignment. He can address the imbalances in your musculo-skeletal system and help prevent future problems. Even more general types of massage that increase circulation and relieve muscular tension are advantageous. Aside from the physical benefits, it is valuable to discover that you can expose your body to nurturing touch and feel safe. This aids in self-acceptance of your body. The American Massage Therapists Association (AMTA) can refer you to licensed practitioners in your area. Write to the AMTA at 820 Davis, Evanston, IL, 60201, or phone (708) 864–0123.

Social Worker

A social worker has expertise in referring you to the appropriate social service agencies and other community resources to help you meet your specific needs. He can help coordinate the financial assistance you may be entitled to in order to help you cover the very high cost of hospitalization, medical and prosthetic care, and vocational training. Depending on your individual circumstance, financial assistance may come from a variety of sources—third-party payors and/or state and federal agencies.

The social worker can set you up with a "homemaker" while you are recovering and learning to adjust to your new lifestyle. A homemaker will provide additional assistance in helping you carry out the everyday tasks of living.

Psychologist

Recovering emotionally from amputation can be as challenging as recovering physically. A psychologist or other type of psychotherapist can assist in teaching you coping skills and in facilitating your emotional adjustment to loss of limb. For more information on the many ways in which a counselor can assist you in emotional recovery refer to Chapter 16, "Seeking Professional Counseling."

Vocational Rehabilitation Counselor

Your limb loss may have affected your ability to continue the job or career you had prior to amputation. Chances are, you may need to learn how to perform the same tasks in different or new ways. If, however, your job requires physical feats that are now beyond your physical abilities, you will need to change fields completely. Vocational rehabilitation counselors can assist in job placement and retraining (if necessary). For more information concerning the effects of amputation on vocation, please refer to Chapter 21, "Vocation."

Spiritual Counselor

A spiritual counselor can be of great solace. He can assist you in finding the meaning in your amputation experience, defining your sense of purpose, and bolstering your beliefs. He can help you discover a community of like-minded individuals who provide support and help you reinforce your faith. For more discussion on the role of spirituality in your healing process, see Chapter 15, "Making Meaning of Your Amputation."

RESIDUAL LIMB CARE

Learning to care for your residual limb should be an integral component of your ongoing health care. The following discussion focuses on three areas: desensitization of the residual limb, the importance of good hygiene, and solutions to some common skin problems that are caused from wearing a prosthesis.

Desensitization

When a recently amputated limb is healing and adjusting to confinement in a prosthetic socket, it must adapt to new stresses. In the case of a lower-limb amputation, the residual limb must become accustomed to bearing weight in ways that nature never intended. As your residual limb heals and undergoes readjustment, it will be quite sensitive to the touch.

Desensitization of the residual limb can be accomplished in a variety of ways. You can repeatedly tap or press on the limb, rub it with a terrycloth towel, or move it around in a container filled with rice or beans. The idea is to gradually get the limb accustomed to touch and pressure. Remember, in order for you to wear your prosthesis daily to master its use, it must fit comfortably.

Hygiene

Hygiene for your residual limb should be similar to cleaning and caring for any other part of your anatomy. Since the prosthesis requires a snug fit that does not allow air to circulate, bacteria build-up is inevitable. If ignored, the bacteria can lead to unpleasant odor, clogged pores, infections, or even cysts. It is, therefore, wise to clean your limb daily with an antibacterial soap or mild antiseptic cleanser. And it is important to remove the soap or cleanser gently yet thoroughly, so the residue does not irritate your skin. Due to the lack of air circulation between the residual limb and the prosthetic socket, perspiration can also be a problem. Most people learn to live with it. However, if you are bothered by excessive perspiration wetness, you can apply an antiperspirant containing aluminum chlorhydrate to your limb. A special cream, specifically for this problem, is also available and can be ordered through your prosthetist.

The prosthetic socket also deserves special attention. Be sure to keep it clean by carefully washing it with soap and water then drying it thoroughly (myoelectric limbs can stop functioning properly if they get very wet). If your socket has a soft prosthetic cover, care must be taken not to cut or tear it (especially during physical activity). Common sense should rule.

Common Skin Problems

Due to the pressure and rubbing of the prosthetic socket, skin irritation of the residual limb is a common occurrence. Even small irritations can build to a point at which you can no longer tolerate wearing your prosthesis. Areas of irritation can also cause other serious problems, such as infections. So it is important to remove the cause of the skin irritation as soon as possible. You may need to temporarily stop wearing your prosthesis while you are healing. Your prosthetist may be able to adjust your socket to relieve the cause of the problem. Also, the use of a powder or lubricating lotion may help decrease the friction caused by the socket and, therefore, ease skin irritation. (Of course, this does not apply if you are wearing a prosthetic sock.)

If continuous rubbing causes an area to blister, know that there are special dressings available to cover the area and allow healing to occur. It is better to leave a blister alone rather than open it, since the skin serves as a protective cover, and removing it may open the way to infection.

If the skin is so irritated that it becomes raw, gently cleanse the area, then apply an antibacterial ointment. If the area becomes inflamed (red, warm, swollen, painful), shows signs of possible infection (pus or other discharge, rash, or red streaks), or if you develop a fever, consult your physician at once.

As for anyone, it is best to be cautious when discovering anything unusual about your skin. So if you develop any suspicious lesions (unusual-looking areas of skin tissue), consult your regular physician or a dermatologist at once.

If you are not wearing your prosthesis for an extended period of time, some form of compression, such as an elastic shrinker sock, should be worn on your residual limb to prevent edema (swelling of the tissue), and to ensure proper residual limb shape. If your limb is swollen, raising it onto a pillow and resting it in that position should help decrease the swelling. If you use any type of prosthetic or shrinker sock, it should be washed and changed frequently.

MASTERING NEW SKILLS

"Suppose while your friends are playing basketball, you sit on the sidelines and try to convince yourself that you don't want to play. Don't become comfortable with that! Just get out there and do it—even if you look stupid. After a while, you'll get the hang of it.

Suppose you're missing a couple fingers so you stop eating oranges because you can't peel them. Every time you see an orange you'll feel bad. But if you learn how to peel that orange, you will feel a great sense of accomplishment. Learning to do little things like that makes a lot of difference."

—Mark

When you have lost a limb, there are a number of new skills you will need to develop to make your life a bit easier. Mastering these skills will boost your sense of competency and well-being, which will enhance your self-esteem. You may have to learn to walk again, or grasp and lift objects with your new prosthesis. Self-care tasks that you had taken for granted, such as washing your hair or getting dressed, might need to be approached in novel ways.

Learning new skills is humbling in that part of the learning process includes trial and error. As a child, you gradually learned to do such things as tie your shoes and add a column of numbers without thinking twice of how you accomplished these feats. Remember when you first learned how to ride a bike? You tried the new skill and failed, made adjustments and tried again. With each failed attempt, you continued to adjust and practice until you succeeded. It is important to maintain this basic, innocent attitude when trying to master any new skill.

You will need to call upon your patience and develop what is called in Zen meditation a "beginner's mind." It means that you must be as open and curious as a child. Allow mistakes to serve as feedback. Be playful, explore, and experiment as you learn new skills.

New skills require practice. Maintaining an attitude of self-tolerance and having a sense of humor can help ease the process:

"Laughter is one of the best medicines in the world. Learn to laugh at yourself. I turned around too quickly one day as I came in the door and fell into the trash can. It was some sight! You know, I won't move that can because every time I see it, I remember not to swing around and lose my balance. It taught me a lesson. Once you adjust and learn to laugh at yourself, you'll have it made!

Stop feeling sorry for yourself. Push yourself. Go ahead and try! You'll be surprised at how good you feel with every little step you make—like walking through the house by yourself, or going down steps for the first time. With each new thing I do, I think, 'This is great! That wheelchair is sitting over there because I can't find anyone who could use it.' I'm independent and feel great about my future. I've learned to love life again."

—*Jill*

Remember, there is no such thing as failure—only feedback. Can you remember when you learned how to read? You began by sounding out one letter at a time, then you moved on to combinations of letters until you were finally able to read a word. Remember how elated you felt? Well, it is not much different when learning new skills as an adult. So give yourself permission to approach the task of learning new skills with childlike wonder. You might even have a good time.

PROSTHETIC TRAINING

The reality is that even when you recover well from the amputation surgery, are fit with a state-of-the-art prosthesis, and learn to walk or use your upper prosthetic limb as well as possible, the prosthesis *cannot* match the function, sensation, or cosmetic appearance of a natural limb. The whole experience of being fit with a prosthesis and learning to master its operation is unnatural and awkward. Therefore, it is critical to understand how your artificial limb functions and how to use it properly.

Upper-Limb Training

Occupational therapists tend to specialize in treating upper limbs. So if you have upper-limb loss, you may choose to work with one. (Of course, there are many physical therapists who also work well with upper-limb amputation.) As always, it is important to ask the individual therapist what kind of experience he or she has had working with others who have your level of limb loss.

With upper-limb amputation, it is especially important for you to strengthen not only your residual limb, but also the remaining limb, which will be relied on more than ever. The therapist can develop an ongoing program that includes muscle toning, strengthening, and flexibility exercises specifically for you.

Many individuals function beautifully one-handed. If you do so, or your level of upper-limb loss is very severe, you may choose not to use a prosthesis. If, however, you are going to use one, it is critical that you learn to master it as soon as possible to avoid becoming functionally "one-handed." There is a great temptation to develop one-handed patterns of function when a prosthesis is not available, making it more difficult to integrate the use of the prosthesis into normal activities.

When you first get your prosthesis, you must become oriented with it and learn how it operates. Practice putting it on and taking it off. Gradually, you will master the prosthetic control for such functions as positioning the limb and opening and closing the terminal devices.

You will have to practice the skills that underlie everyday activities, such as picking up and releasing objects of varying sizes, textures, and weights, then apply these skills to everyday tasks—grooming, eating, dressing, writing, etc. During this time, you will have the opportunity to build good habits that will last a lifetime; so take your time and learn to perform repeated activities as smoothly and naturally as possible while using minimum stress and energy. Like those with lower-limb amputation, the length of time those with upper-limb loss require physical therapy will vary, depending on overall physical condition, level of amputation, and type of prosthesis.

Before you are fitted for a more complex prosthesis, it is a good idea to be fit with a conventional prosthesis following your surgery. This is worn as your residual limb undergoes the expected changes in tissue volume and shape. With a conventional prosthesis, you can wear prosthetic socks to take up the changes in tissue volume, so you will always have a limb to wear. If you have also chosen to use a myoelectric limb, you can be fit once your limb volume and shape have stabilized. You will then have your conventional limb to use as a spare, or to wear in special situations such as those in which the limb might become wet.

Lower-Limb Gait Training

Gait training is necessary to learn to walk as normally as possible with a prosthetic limb, while expending the least amount of energy. Logically, the higher the level of amputation, the more complicated it becomes to use a prosthesis, since more components are needed to restore function to each joint that has been prosthetically replaced.

Gait training is broken down into the components of walking, and begins by simply practicing how to balance while wearing your prosthesis. (For your safety, during the initial stages of gait training, you will probably be positioned between two parallel bars.) Next, you will learn to shift your weight from side to side. Once you have mastered these steps, you will practice shifting your weight forward, then backward with one foot placed in front of the other. Gradually you will progress through each stage of walking, mastering each step before moving on to the next.

Your goals should include such things as learning how to walk on various terrains including ramps, hills, and stairs; being able to stand up from prone and sitting positions; getting in and out of cars; and modifying your driving techniques.

EMOTIONAL REACTIONS TO A FIRST PROSTHESIS

"At first I didn't want an artificial leg because I was afraid it would hurt. I refused to even try. One day, my doctor told me that he had his leg 'done' thirty-five years ago and has been waltzing ever since. I didn't know what he was talking about until he pulled up his pant leg! Seeing his prosthetic leg made all the difference to me. I decided then that I would give prosthetics a try. Now, my leg is the first thing I put on in the morning and the last thing I take off at night."

—Jill

Although many with amputation are physically able to wear a temporary prosthesis shortly after the surgery, a small number may not be emotionally ready and will need a longer period of mourning for their lost body part. It may take from several weeks to several months before some people are willing to even try a prosthesis.

After the initial trauma of the actual amputation and any underlying condition that necessitated it, the fitting of the first prosthesis, for many, is the second most emotionally charged experience. Any illusions about an artificial limb being just like a real one are countered by the harsh reality of the limitations of the prosthesis. Feelings of helplessness and frustration are common.

Other common initial reactions to a new limb include disappointment, depression, and impatience. Many have voiced surprise at the discomfort or pain involved in the fit of the prosthesis, as well as frustration with walking as compared to using crutches. The fear of falling and lack of confidence are other common reactions. If individuals cannot incorporate their limb loss into their body image, they will have trouble adjusting to the use of a prosthesis.

Even with a prosthesis, some people—due to decreased function and increased energy requirements for using the new limb—find themselves physically less active than they were before amputation. On the other hand, there are many who are able to rise above the obvious drawbacks of an artificial limb. Although limited, the restoration of physical ability and increased mobility provide freedom and independence.

Attitude Toward the Prosthesis

"Before I was injured, I was into football and wrestling—a real jock. My first prosthesis was so terrible that I threw it away and walked on crutches instead. Two years later, I started ski racing. All the other skiers with lower-limb loss wore artificial legs and wondered why I didn't. Until then, I had no role model to show me what could be done with a prosthesis, and I realized that I had given up on wearing one too quickly. I decided to give it another try.

My new prosthesis was more comfortable, more functional, and more flexible than the first one. I became more agile, and found myself walking better than I did with crutches. Now I live day-to-day like someone who has no physical disability.

Unfortunately, I have an artificial leg, but that has nothing to do with excelling.
Now nothing holds me back. I just look at many things as physical challenges."

—Grant

"Getting my leg was enjoyable. It was a challenge. It meant I was going to be able
to walk again on my own! I knew that I might walk with a limp, that I might be
limited, but at least I was going to walk and regain some of my independence. Oh,
it was so great! It was like a new birth for me, a new lease on life."

—Jill

Some suggest that the most helpful attitude you can have towards your prosthesis is to consider it a "part" of you. Thinking of it this way, rather than as a separate device like a walker or crutches, might better serve to restore your body image. Others consider a prosthesis simply a helpful tool. How you choose to think of your prosthesis is up to you. You might explore how it feels to consider your prosthesis in different ways. If your present way of viewing your prosthesis enhances your body image and self concept, then stick with it; if not, why not try altering your perception?

Accepting Reality

During your rehabilitation, you will have to deal with two basic realities that accompany most prosthetic devices: discomfort and fatigue.

Even at its best, a prosthesis is not always comfortable to wear. Muscles and tissue are called upon to bear weight in ways not intended by nature. The sensations that are experienced while wearing an artificial limb can range from very comfortable to terribly annoying to outright painful. Generally, as your residual limb becomes accustomed to bearing weight and gets used to friction, it will become less sensitive. In some cases, calluses will develop on the limb, making the prosthesis more tolerable.

Along with discomfort, you will have to deal with fatigue. Because using an artificial limb requires more energy than a natural limb, you must channel some of the energy that would ordinarily be spent on other endeavors into using your prosthesis. Additionally, you will need to pay conscious attention to controlling your artificial limb, which, in itself, is tiring; this is especially true at first, until you develop good habits and skills.

Thus, you will likely find yourself tiring more rapidly than you did before your limb loss. It is a kind of "double-whammy"—during rehabilitation, you need the energy to wholeheartedly participate in your recovery process, yet you may find yourself more worn out by simple tasks than you used to be.

But here's the good news. You will feel less worn out as you develop good skills and habits. Discomfort and fatigue, although common during the rehabilitation process, will lessen as you master the use of your new limb and improve the level of your overall fitness.

Patience, Self-Tolerance, and Practice

"I remember standing there with my husband after I had put on my legs for the first time; I was seeing him at the wrong level! The legs were too long!
Learning to walk again was exhausting and very discouraging. It seemed like a physical impossibility to stand, let alone balance, let alone ever be able to walk. Getting legs and learning to walk was an obnoxious process. It was certainly not like walking had ever been. But I had no alternative. It was either learn to walk or sit in a wheelchair for the rest of my life."

—Leslie

Because the prosthesis is a mechanical device, its performance is vulnerable to flaws in design and fit. Its use also depends on how well you have learned to control it, which may be affected by your physical condition. When learning to use your limb, accept the fact that you will experience some initial difficulties. If you have lower-limb loss, expect that you might occasionally fall and walk with an awkward gait; if you have upper-limb loss, you may have difficulty picking up or releasing items. If you are a perfectionist, or expect to "get it right" the first time, here is a wonderful opportunity to learn to relax and allow the learning process to take its own time. A good sense of humor helps!

Before I lost my leg, I studied the martial art of T'ai Chi Ch'uan. Its graceful, ballet-like movements belie its applicability as a tool for self-defense. My teacher was quick, subtle and artful. During each and every class, he would repeat the great secret of mastery: *"More practice, more relax . . . more practice, more relax . . ."* Many times, as I stumbled or lurched while learning to walk again, I would recall his sage advice. I urge you also to take it to heart.

YOUR REHABILITATION OUTCOME

There are many ways in which you can "take the bull by the horns" and improve the results of your rehabilitation. For you to be "restored" to a well-rounded, balanced lifestyle, your efforts must address all planes of your being—physical, emotional, mental, and spiritual.

Your rehabilitation is an area in which you can exercise great influence, and thus restore a sense of control over your own well-being. Some of the most valuable ways to do this include the following:

• **Receive the best possible medical care.** This includes a thorough education of any underlying medical condition, understanding and accepting the necessity of your amputation, and becoming involved in a coordinated rehabilitation program.

• **Develop a solid emotional support system.** In addition to your network of family and friends, you may find strength through involvement in a support group composed of others with amputation.

• **Return to active participation in your community.** This could include meaningful work, as well as social and leisure activities. (If necessary, get assistance in overcoming any tendencies you might have to withdraw socially.)

• **Maintain a positive attitude and self-acceptance.** Work to counter any limiting patterns of thoughts, beliefs, or behavior. Delve within yourself to define your sense of purpose. Consciously choose to make positive meaning of your amputation experience.

• **Learn coping strategies.** Increase your ability to deal with your emotions and the inevitable challenges that arise.

Your positive attitude, motivation, and active participation are the key factors in maximizing your rehabilitation and returning to a full, satisfying life. The more responsibility you take in your recovery program, the better the results.

Some Words of Caution

As an active participant in your rehabilitation, you will have a great deal of impact on your recovery. However, allow me to give you a few words of caution. We sometimes have the mistaken notion that if we "give it all we've got," everything will turn out exactly according to our wishes; if it doesn't, we may tend to blame ourselves. The perfect outcome does not always occur, even when you have given it your best effort. And it is unfair to subject yourself to feelings of guilt as a result.

Cut yourself some slack! Go easy on yourself! Accept the fact that there will be times when you are going to fall short of your expectations; on the other hand, know that there will be those times when your achievements will far exceed what you had dreamed possible. Therefore, the best course of action is to let go of preconceived ideas and be satisfied in knowing that you are doing the best you can for yourself.

Evaluating Your Rehabilitation

As mentioned earlier in this chapter, your rehabilitation goals should be to restore yourself in body, mind, emotion, and spirit. You should strive to live your life in such a way that your amputation is just one aspect of your life, not the central one. The ultimate success of your rehabilitation depends upon your unique physical, emotional, and mental make-up. Individuals with severe physical limitations can adjust as well or even better than those whose limitations are less severe. The realities that accompany your loss of limb cannot be made to disappear; but, through rehabilitation, their negative effects can decrease, and you can enjoy your life again.

You will know that your rehabilitation is progressing when your emotional balance, health, and physical ability have begun to be restored. This is evidenced through such factors as successful use of your prosthesis, wheelchair, or other assistive device; participation in an ongoing program of self-care; and the return to a satisfactory role within your family and community.

Another sign of successful rehabilitation is that you are more accepting of your physical differences. Your amputation is integrated into your life so that it impinges very little upon the enjoyment you get from your family and friends, or the satisfaction you derive from your job. In general, your life is more normal than it was right after your amputation. You have discovered a way to make peace with and derive positive meaning from your experience, which allows you to enjoy a full, rewarding life.

GET INVOLVED

The general public has become increasingly aware of the importance of being an educated consumer. The benefits of making educated decisions when purchasing goods or spending money on services is obvious. It is equally important to be educated when dealing with health-care products and services.

As a person with limb loss, do not take a subservient role and surrender your health-care options to others. It is up to you to learn about governmental benefits that may be due to you; you are the one who must become aware of current prosthetic advancements and other assistive devices to meet your unique needs.

An intelligent health-care consumer gets involved in advocacy, peer-support, and self-help groups. Become active in the removal of social prejudice and discrimination (including such things as architectural barriers).

It is vitally important for you to take an interest in issues that involve amputation. Your interest will help ensure that you receive the best health-care products and services, as well as optimal health-care related legislation to enhance the quality of your life and the lives of others. Grass root support can make a big difference in the outcome of a bill or the availability of a product.

Everyone has his or her own level of interest and the time to devote to such issues. Know that although it does not take long to write a few letters or place a phone call, such simple actions can make a difference in your life or the lives of others with amputation or another disability.

If you decide to get involved, follow the recommendations of Peter Thomas, Esquire, who lobbies in Washington, D.C. for disability-related issues. He suggests the first thing you should do is become educated. This is done through the following:

• **Know the issues.** Learn about issues pertaining to health-care reform; they could affect your future! Where can you get information? The National Rehabilitation Information Center in Silver Spring, Maryland, has a wealth of information concerning rehabilitation and financial issues, as do state vocational rehabilitation offices. Local and national amputee support groups are other sources of information.

• **Get copies of health-care bills.** Contact senators and congresspersons for copies of health-care bills in which you are interested. If you have any questions after reading the bills, contact the office of your national or local representative for answers.

• **Write letters.** Write letters to obtain more information or to state your concerns to individuals or organizations that can make a difference. A few such organizations are the Amputee Coalition of America, the American Amputee Foundation, the National Association for Advancement of Orthotics and Prosthetics, and the National Center for Medical Rehabilitation Research. To stay informed, get on the mailing lists of these groups. (For addresses and phone numbers, see "Groups and Organizations," beginning on page 323.)

Once you have become educated, become an educator. You might choose to begin sharing your knowledge and/or concerns at a local level. Attend support-group meetings, go to hospitals, or join and network with an existing organization. Request meetings with local and state officials to discuss important issues. If you live near Washington, D.C., try to meet with national representatives to advocate for your cause. Let your elected officials know what is important to you. Your voice does make a difference. Elected officials know that for every letter and phone call received, there are thousands of others who feel the same way. Legislators do listen.

Taking an active role in this area of your life will help empower you with self-determination and dignity. By becoming active in addressing issues that impact those with amputation, you will gain a voice in influencing the quality of your future.

THE ROAD TO RECOVERY

At some time in your life, you have probably heard of "the road to recovery." This concept has some interesting applications to understanding the process of rehabilitation.

On your road to recovery, the more accurate your map and other significant information, the shorter your journey will be. Your choice of traveling companions can make a tremendous difference in the quality of your trip. Good companions can provide much-needed understanding and compassion, as well as shared laughter.

Make sure that your vehicle is well-prepared for the trip. A thorough safety check is always a good idea; better to find out about a worn break or a cracked fuel line at home, rather than in the middle of nowhere. And remember, by talking sweetly to your car, you may be able to coax out additional performance that you would never get by pounding on the hood and cursing!

Each day and each mile can reveal hidden wonders when you are open to them. Be sure you do not become so fixated on your final destination that you miss opportunities to appreciate the passing landscape. With a light heart and determination, keep your destination clearly in mind. But above all, whenever possible, enjoy the journey itself.

PART II

PSYCHOLOGICAL ASPECTS

6

PSYCHOLOGICAL IMPACT
OF AMPUTATION

Treating the psychological problems faced by the amputee often has more significance to his life than the quality of the surgery or the nature of his prosthetic device. . . . The disability entailed by amputation either of an upper or lower limb is far more the result of individual and social attitudes than it is with loss of function. . . . It is the loss of ability to relate psychologically, socially, sexually, and vocationally that inhibits amputees most.

Lawrence Friedmann, M.D.
The Psychological Rehabilitation of the Amputee

Even when you have recovered from surgery and are adapting well to the physical changes resulting from your amputation, you will discover that paying attention to the physical aspects of your recovery is simply not enough. *You are more than merely a physical body.* As a human being, you are multidimensional—mental, emotional, and spiritual elements exist in addition to the physical. Because you deserve to enjoy the best possible quality of life, you must address all aspects. Your self-concept and body image; relationships with others; recreational and vocational activities; roles within your family, community, and society as a whole are all affected.

This chapter provides an overview of the psychological impact of amputation, and includes a special section on children with limb differences. Your attitude and the meaning you attribute to your amputation will greatly impact the quality of your life. These concepts are explored in Chapter 15, "Making Meaning of Your Amputation." In other chapters in this section, emotional responses to loss of limb are explored in greater depth, and specific strategies and tools for coping with your emotions, self-concept, mental outlook, and belief systems are presented.

EMOTIONAL RESPONSES

The emotional responses to amputation are as complex and unique as each of us is individually. Present at any given time can be an array of feelings such as shock, disbelief, anger, frustration, sadness, guilt, self-pity, revulsion, shame, hopelessness, helplessness, bitterness, grief, despair, depression, anxiety, fear, panic, and a sense of being overwhelmed. If your amputation was performed as a life-saving measure (to arrest the spread of a disease, or as the result of a trauma), you might feel relief and a certain measure of peacefulness. No matter what the cause, a part of your body is gone, and with it, your self-concept and way of life has become permanently altered. Concerns about your physical ability, social acceptability, sexuality, and vocation are to be expected.

Almost all individuals experience shock when faced with the reality of losing a limb; many experience total disbelief. The shock can be most severe when the person sees his or her residual limb for the first time, especially if it is coupled with the presence of phantom limb sensation or phantom pain. Other common responses can range from revulsion, horror, and self-pity to relief and happiness. Some persons regard their loss of limb as punishment for their behavior, which results in guilt and shame.

The effects of amputation are highly individual and can include periods of depression or hyperactivity, anxiety and nervousness, crying spells, and substance abuse. Other reported responses include the inability to cope with everyday problems, feelings of resentment and/or lack of trust in others, general apathy towards life, and increased physical illness.

Some experience temporary "personality changes" in response to their new stresses. For example, they may be more critical or demanding, more anxious, emotionally volatile, or more withdrawn. Be assured that most individuals do return to their former "good natures."

The extent to which you experience these painful responses is based upon your unique makeup. Your reactions may range from feeling little or no impact on your well-being and enjoyment of life, to an overwhelming sense of personal loss. If you and your loved ones can recognize this intense range of emotional responses as a natural part of the healing process, it is often a big relief.

Challenges

Along with having to cope with your emotional responses, you have a tremendous number of new realities to assimilate following amputation surgery. Personal, physical, economic, and societal challenges must be faced.

We often take the "normalcy" of our bodies for granted—I know I did. I took my two legs for granted, just as I expected the sun to rise each morning. If your limb is amputated, you will need to adjust in areas that you never would have considered. For example, I can remember being stunned when I learned that as someone with an above-knee amputation, I would have to climb stairs in a different way. I had to begin by taking a normal step with my intact leg, then follow by swinging my prosthetic limb in a sideways arc to avoid hitting the step. This was a very big deal for me; no matter how normal I looked when I walked, my abnormality was painfully evident whenever I climbed stairs. I was crushed!

In a similar way, it might be emotionally difficult for someone with upper-limb loss to shake hands with his left hand, or wear a wedding ring on the opposite hand. It may be equally difficult to have to learn to write and manipulate objects with a hand that is not the naturally dominant one.

Loss of a limb deprives you of physical sensation and normal upper- or lower-limb function. Even with a prosthesis, you will experience greater energy expenditure and limitations in movement. No matter how excellent the fit or how state-of-the-art the components, the current prosthetic limbs are still a far cry from the beauty and function of the limbs you were granted as your birthright.

At the same time, you are left with a permanently mutilated limb. In addition to a possible underlying medical condition, you might also be experiencing surgical pain, phantom pain, neuromas, or muscle spasms.

Pace of living, recreation, and perhaps vocation, may be altered. Your relationships with your family, friends, and colleagues may be impacted. Your financial resources might be strained. Discrimination by employers, as well as friends and strangers, must be addressed. For some, fears of an altered lifestyle, as well as fears for future health, must be met, or emotional debilitation may develop.

FACTORS THAT AFFECT PSYCHOLOGICAL ADJUSTMENT

A number of factors will influence how well you adjust to loss of limb. In general, your responses will depend upon your prior life experience, your overall psychological make-up (including how well you cope with challenges), and the unique circumstances of your amputation.

The circumstances under which your surgery was performed provide an emotional filter through which you perceive your amputation. Reactions, which vary according to the cause of the amputation, can range from profound grief to a sense of relief. These physical and psychological differences are presented and illustrated with the words of individuals who have lost limbs due to varying circumstances. You may find yourself identifying with some of these individuals, and feel comforted to know that there are others who have shared experiences similar to your own. By the way, the people interviewed in the following discussions have coped well with their limb loss and are currently enjoying their lives.

Trauma

Generally, in the case of trauma, there is little or no time for emotional preparation. You may emerge from surgery forced to cope with the fact that your well-functioning limb is suddenly gone forever.

In my own case, one moment I was a healthy, vital twenty-eight-year-old woman, enjoying a full, active life when a car accident changed my life forever. I emerged from a coma to discover that, along with numerous other injuries, my left leg had been amputated above the knee. I must admit that it took me years to recover emotionally.

Here follows the experience of two others who lost limbs due to sudden trauma:

"I was twenty-nine years old, just months from finishing my training as a physician. My husband and I were traveling in Europe when our car stalled on a railroad track. Without any warning, a train came. While scrambling to get out of the car, I fell onto the tracks. My husband tried to pick me up. He had me in his arms when the train hit; the impact blew us apart. The car fell on top of me and I was shoved down the tracks.

I was cognizant of being able to breathe with this crushing weight on top of me. I can remember being put into the ambulance, and seeing someone pick up my shoe with my foot in it. Somehow I realized that one of my legs was not attached. I saw the ambulance attendant pick up a sleeve of my shirt with my arm still inside. I really thought I was dying, so I just decided to accept it. I knew that this was the end, and it wouldn't do any good to scream. It turned out that one leg and one arm were totally severed. My other leg was irreparably crushed; it wasn't worth trying to save."

—Leslie

"I had just turned thirty years old. I was riding my motorcycle, when a car drove into me, crushing my right arm and right leg. As a result, I went through a series of bone and skin grafts—fourteen operations in seven months. I was going downhill pretty fast. I had to decide if I wanted to go through more operations over the next few years, with an outcome that, at best, would mean possibly saving my leg for appearances only. So I said, 'No contest! Just take it and let me get on with my life.'

I will always have certain negative thoughts about the amputation. Mentally, things might have been different for me if I had lost my leg immediately. If I hadn't tried to save it, though, I would have always wondered."

—Kent

Vascular Disease

You may have experienced a prolonged period of illness, pain, and disability before losing a limb to vascular disease. Even before amputation, you might have perceived yourself as disabled. During your illness, you may have realized that amputation would be necessary, perhaps as a life-saving measure. Such circumstances would have prepared you somewhat for amputation, and might have helped you adapt more quickly to your loss than it would to a trauma victim.

Yet, no matter how well prepared you are, and no matter how much relief the amputation brings, losing a limb is still no piece of cake. Even people who have begged their orthopedists to remove their limb due to severe pain or disability still experience profound shock and a sense of loss following the surgery. They will go through the full grieving process. The person with peripheral vascular disease may have impaired circulation of other limbs, as well as cardiac and cerebral impairment; there may be justified fear of losing the opposite limb, developing heart disease, or having a stroke.

Note how the following individuals resigned themselves to the necessity of their limb loss:

"I was sixty-one years old and was experiencing a gradual worsening of my vascular disease. I had to have open heart surgery; the surgeons used a vein from my leg. After the surgery, numbness set into my leg. I had no feeling in my foot, and I couldn't wiggle my toes. Within just a few days, my leg was amputated below the knee. I knew I had to learn to take it all in stride. I adopted the attitude that if my leg had to go, it had to go. And I would do all that I needed to do to adjust to my amputation."

—Jill

"Fifteen years ago, I had fallen down on my knee and an infection developed. I told the doctor, 'I can walk only so far, and then the pain becomes so bad that I can't stand it!' X-rays showed that most of the arteries in my leg were clogged. I had no idea! After the doctors operated, my leg turned white, which meant that it wasn't getting enough blood. After five days, I had to have my right leg amputated.

Five years later, a toe on my left foot began to turn black; eventually the doctor amputated part of that foot. Two years ago, my foot started hurting again. The doctor said he had to amputate again, just below the knee. I said, 'Anything to get away from this pain!'"

—Frances

Tumors and Cancer

If you have been diagnosed with cancer in a limb, and an amputation is necessary to arrest the spread of the malignancy and save your life, your surgeon will probably want to operate as soon as possible. Although cancer and benign tumors are the cause of only 5 percent of all amputations, cancer is the primary reason for amputation in young people between the ages of ten to nineteen.

Your status as a person with cancer is unique; even when amputation is performed, you may not know if the disease has been halted in its entirety.

You may still be undergoing radiation, chemotherapy, drug therapy, or other treatments that may have horrendous side effects. In fact, many persons find the side effects of chemotherapy harder to deal with than the amputation itself. Fear of further spread of the disease or death may understandably provoke anxiety and depression, making adjustment more difficult.

Here is how Bob and Judith describe their experiences upon discovering that they had cancer and that amputation was necessary. At the time of their interviews, both were living with the uncertainty of whether or not their cancer had been arrested.

"I was jogging along the beach and my leg began to hurt. The pain didn't go away. The next day, I went water-skiing and my leg just gave out; it turned out to be fractured. An x-ray showed a dark area, and a biopsy was done. I learned that I had cancer, and that I probably would have to have my leg amputated above the knee. A second opinion confirmed that my leg could not be saved.

I was shocked—I couldn't believe it. I worried how people would look at me without a leg, and wondered what I was going to do with my life. I had been very active. I was really upset, and then I put it out of my mind. The day of the surgery, I was very calm; it was as if I wasn't going to have the amputation at all. The realization came afterward—my leg was really gone!

I was told I'd be fitted with a good prosthesis and I knew I would be able to do things again. I wasn't too worried. Chemotherapy has been the worst part. I still have four treatments left. Other people are in control of my life. It's so hard being sick, losing my hair. I feel really drained. I'm scared of dying.

There is no guarantee, even after I finish the chemotherapy, that all the cancer will be gone. I try not to think about not knowing the outcome. I also know that I could go into the street and get hit by a car. I just try to enjoy my life now and live day by day. What has kept me going is just wanting to live. I think of the good days I do have, because I want more of them."

—Bob

(Note: It has been four years since Bob's chemotherapy ended, and he is doing quite well.)

"I was twenty-one years old and working as a waitress. I noticed a constant pain in my foot. I went to a general practitioner who told me that I had a bone spur, which he treated with cortisone. After three months my foot still hurt. I went to a surgeon who took x-rays of my foot. After reading the x-rays, he said, 'Honey, you don't even have a heel bone.' A malignant tumor had destroyed the entire heel!

My surgery was a week later; an amputation was performed just below the knee. Luckily, I didn't need any chemotherapy, and I was able to go on from there. So far, things have gone fine."

—Judith

Congenital Absence of Limb

Although prenatal tests may reveal the presence of limb abnormality in some cases; generally, limb deficiency is not discovered until birth, when it is a colossal shock and a devastating blow to parents. Of course, the newborn takes his limb differences in stride; it is parents (and often the hospital staff) who have the hardest time adjusting initially.

In most cases, congenital absence of limb is not hereditary; the cause is a mystery, although some instances are known to have a genetic basis. In some individuals, the cause of the limb abnormality is due to abnormal fetal development in which the "limb bud" does not grow properly. For more information refer to Chapter 1, "Introduction to Amputation."

OTHER ADJUSTMENT FACTORS

The following is an overview of other factors that may affect your emotional adjustment to limb loss. The ramifications of these factors are discussed at length in other chapters in this book. For example, were you forewarned of your surgery? Was there time for you to prepare for it? Do you believe that you were even partly responsible for the extent of your disease or injury? What was your age at the time of your limb loss and how much time has passed since your surgery? What is your general state of health? Are you experiencing a lot of pain (phantom and/or other)? What is your relationship with your treating physician? Are you utilizing a team approach to your recovery? Are you using (or do you plan to use) a prosthesis or other assistive device?

There are yet other factors that will influence your emotional responses to your amputation. Some of these include the strength of your emotional support system; the state of your financial resources; the meaning you attribute to your limb loss; your general attitude; your expectations, beliefs, and values; your ability to cope with physical, emotional, mental, and spiritual challenges; your self-image and self-esteem; your need for social approval; your ability to accept the reality of the limb loss; your flexibility in revising your expectations and goals; and your desire to reintegrate into society.

All of these factors influence your capability to adapt to the changes wrought by amputation. How well you have handled challenges in the past is often a tip-off to how well you will cope with your limb loss. Thus, coping ability is determined, in part, by the many factors mentioned, by your former life experience, and by the nature of the experiences you meet after amputation. If you have good self-esteem, past life successes, and many sources of fulfillment, you will probably find it proportionately easier to accept this new loss, and to adjust to your new reality.

STAGES IN THE ADJUSTMENT PROCESS

In adjusting emotionally to loss of limb, you may advance from shock and numbness, to denial, to a range of turbulent emotions, to depression, to eventual acceptance of your loss; however, not all individuals follow this progression. The order may vary; stages may be omitted. In fact, some people may never reach acceptance. However, most individuals discover their own unique path in accepting the disability and integrating it into the totality of their lives. You will, too.

In *Atlas of Limb Prosthetics* (St. Louis, MO: Mosby Yearbook, 1992), John C. Racy, M.D. presents a review of the adaptation process to limb loss, for which he uses a "four-stage" model. This model emphasizes certain issues that tend to arise at various points in the recovery process.

The four stages in the adaptation process following amputation are:

1. Preoperative Stage

Before your amputation surgery, you began the grieving process, which is an integral part of your healing. Even if you have been looking forward to the surgery as relief from pain and suffering, it is natural to feel anxiety. You may worry about the impact of your amputation in terms of pain, function, general health, and finances.

You may have concerns about the impact on your daily life in terms of physical abilities and your ability to maintain prior roles in your family. Your financial fears may be heightened by the medical costs involved with your health care. You may have concerns about changes in your self-concept and body image, as well as how your limb loss will affect your intimate and other relationships. Since you have entered a "new world," you may have questions about the surgery itself, about how your limb will be disposed of following the operation, about prosthetics and other assistive devices, and about other things you never would have considered had you not faced limb loss.

During the preoperative stage, there is time to prepare yourself for surgery. (Obviously, this does not apply to cases of sudden trauma, or when a severe disease, such as cancer, requires immediate surgery.) During this period, clear information can help erase fear of the unknown, as well as ease the way for your recovery. It is important for you to realize that your amputation surgery is reconstructive rather than destructive; its goal is to restore you to maximum health with the highest level of physical ability.

Careful explanation of the surgical procedure, as well as the plans for your physical recovery, including physical therapy and prosthetic care, can help decrease anxiety.

To promote your acceptance and inner peace, it is important that your surgeon takes time to answer all of your questions, as well as those of your family members. Remember, no concern of yours is too small to mention. (Please refer to Chapter 2, "Amputation Surgery," for more information concerning this stage.)

If you have limited physical ability due to a deformed or diseased limb, a prosthetist can help you understand how an artificial limb can provide you with more ability than you currently possess. Tour a prosthetic facility; speak with your future prosthetist; meet with others, especially those who are the same sex, similar in age, and who have the same level of amputation as you. These actions can aid you in your physical and emotional recovery.

2. Immediate Post-Operative Stage

The immediate post-operative stage is the short period just after your surgery. For me, this stage began when I emerged from a coma to discover that, among my multiple injuries, one leg had been amputated; the sheet was flat where my leg should have been. If your amputation was the result of severe trauma, you will have your own version of this experience. However, even if you are "prepared" for your surgery or look forward to ending the pain or suffering due to an underlying condition, waking up to the reality of amputation is still a rude shock.

During this stage, you will undoubtedly be concerned with pain, function, and complications. As part of your grieving process, you may be disoriented or in shock; you may feel numb, or find yourself in denial. This time is generally more difficult for those who have lost limbs due to sudden trauma than it is for those who were prepared for their surgery. For a more detailed discussion of this stage, refer to Chapter 8, "Mourning Your Loss."

3. In-Hospital Rehabilitation Stage

During the in-hospital rehabilitation stage, the initial focus of your concerns might be on physical pain, phantom limb phenomenon, disfigurement, and other health issues. As a defense mechanism to cope with the challenges you now face, you may experience denial, which might manifest itself in a variety of ways, such as bravado, competitiveness, elevated mood, wishful thinking (the limb might grow back), withdrawal, regression, and even humor. As your grieving process continues, sadness and other emotions may emerge as you mourn for your loss of limb, loss of lifestyle, and dreams of how your life might have been. Refer to Chapter 8, "Mourning Your Loss," for additional information on this stage.

Your recovery can be aided during this stage by the early fitting of a prosthesis. The love, support, and acceptance of your family and friends can be invaluably reassuring. I remember how loved ones, such as my parents and boyfriend, had the ability to "soothe my soul," so that I felt somehow, eventually everything was going to be all right. Meeting others with a similar level of limb loss who have coped well can provide a great boost. Seeing is believing.

4. At-Home Rehabilitation Stage

When you return home from the hospital, a different level of reality will set in. You will not be under the intense focus of your rehabilitation team; your day will no longer be as rigorously scheduled as it was in the hospital. I can remember saying to myself when I first returned home, "So, this is the way my new life will be!"

At first, you may feel elated to be home. This may soon be followed by an emotional "letdown." Some depression during this period is to be expected. You may also feel a variety of mixed emotions including frustration, anger, anxiety, and fear, as well as relief and gratitude for being alive.

During this stage, it's important to stay motivated, so keep up your physical rehabilitation process (physical therapy, prosthetic fittings, and other health-related care). This will increase your overall health and physical ability.

This stage creates a new wave in the process of grieving your loss. During this period, some persons act overly dependent and rely on others excessively, while others, in an attempt to assert their independence, refuse even the most reasonable offers of assistance.

Your goal during this stage is to begin reintegrating yourself into the activities that make for a "normal life." You may find yourself extremely vulnerable to the responses of others while you reformulate your self-concept, so it is critical that others treat you as "whole"—the same person you were before your limb loss—and that you resume your normal role in the family.

As you progress in your physical and emotional recovery process, you will reach greater and greater levels of acceptance of your physical realities. (It is important to note that acceptance of your reality does not mean you have to like or approve of it.) You learn to integrate alterations in your lifestyle. You recognize that life is not all smooth sailing, that stress may temporarily cause you to regress. You re-engage yourself with family, friends, and your community. You resume pursuing the fulfillment of your life goals. You know that your worth is unaffected by the number or shape of the limbs you have, so you are secure within yourself. Refer to Chapter 5, "Rehabilitation," for more detail about the recovery process, and to Chapter 13, "Self-Esteem," for more information about the concept of acceptance.

DEFENSE MECHANISMS AND COPING STRATEGIES

As a young child you developed "psychological defenses" to help you deal with life's stresses and to assist you to survive in your family and environment. When you undergo amputation as an adult, your psychological defense systems are well established and will naturally come into play. Initially, you may not be aware of your defenses, since they often work at a subconscious level. Through reflection, however, you may be able to analyze how your defenses have attempted to protect you.

Here are just a few examples of defenses. In order to cope, you may *displace* the anger you feel about your loss onto others, causing you to be angry with them. If you are upset at the sight of your residual limb, you might *project* your own response onto others and assume that they feel the same way. Through the use of *denial*, you may act as if your amputation has had absolutely no effect on you at all. For further protection, you might find yourself withdrawing from social encounters, or refusing to look at your residual limb.

Thus, your reactions to your amputation may include a wide variety of intense feelings, as well as the activation of defense mechanisms that were developed long before you lost your limb. Defense measures can be useful to you, especially at first, for they serve to shield you from unbearable emotions or overwhelming reality. However, if maintained too long, they can interfere with your acceptance and healing. When this is the case, psychological counseling can aid you in the acceptance of your loss, and help you develop new strategies and skills for coping.

Your ability to cope with the ups and downs of life before your amputation often parallel your ability to cope with the changes wrought by limb loss. Losing a limb does not change who you are as an individual. Your character and personality are already established. There are unique patterns in the ways you respond to the stresses of everyday living and to crises. If you have coped well with challenges in your life before your limb loss, you are likely to cope well now and still enjoy your life. If you have viewed past crises as opportunities for growth, you will continue to do so now. If you are the kind of person who generally has an optimistic outlook, a positive sense of "self," and a confidence in your coping abilities, it is likely that you will have an easier time adjusting to your loss than if you are pessimistic, insecure, or a believer that your worth depends on physical appearance or abilities.

LIMB DIFFERENCES IN CHILDHOOD

If you grew up with limb differences, over the years you have developed your own ways to cope with and integrate these differences into the totality of your life. Whether your condition was congenital or due to amputation, like your adult counterpart, you had to learn to cope with physical, psychological, and social challenges. You were additionally challenged to master the normal developmental tasks of childhood. You had to find ways to establish your place in your family, with friends, and among classmates. At the same time, you had to address medically related concerns—surgery, hospital stays, numerous visits to health-care professionals, and time spent in physical therapies—along with all of the physical discomforts and indignities involved. You had to learn to master your physical circumstances. You had to deal with the curiosity and ignorance of others in a world that is wary of those who are "different" from the norm.

Initially, parents of children who are born with some type of abnormality must deal with shock and despair, along with a host of other painful emotions such as anger, grief, loneliness, self-blame, shame, confusion, and sadness. They must learn to assimilate this new reality and adjust their dreams and hopes. They have much in common with adults who have recently undergone amputation and have had to deal with that loss. Parents of a child with limb differences, as well as other family members, must undergo their own adjustment process.

Each family's approach to child rearing is unique. A healthy self-concept is the basis for any child's ability to cope with challenges. When parents lay a foundation of unconditional love and acceptance for their children, it allows the children to feel good about themselves. A child who grows up in this atmosphere knows that he or she is capable, loveable, and worthy, and will likely become a secure, confident adult who can handle whatever comes his or her way.

How Children Adapt to Congenital Differences

Many children who are born with limb differences state that they have had a relatively easy time adjusting since they have no memory of living any other way:

"I think it is easier to be born without a limb than it is to lose one later in life. I was born with deformed legs. Never having known anything else, I was able to adapt to my situation quickly. I think if you lose a limb when you're older, it's probably harder, because you have to start all over again."

—Marie

"I got an artificial leg when I was a year old and learned to walk with it from the beginning. When I got a little older, I knew my leg was different from the other kids' legs, so I always wore long pants to keep it hidden. But I got used to my differences early in my life. It must be such a shock to lose a leg later in life. I had time to adjust. I feel I can do anything. Nothing can stop me!"

—Kent

Many people who were born with limb differences echo these sentiments. However, they still go through periods in which they grieve their differences and wish it might have been different. They still may undergo a range of emotions similar to those who undergo amputation later in life. They may rail out against God and the fates. They may lash out and blame themselves or their parents.

Children's Emotional Responses to Amputation

Amputation will have differing impacts on children, depending upon their state of psycho-emotional development. A toddler faces different challenges from a child in grade school or from those of a teenager. Many adults who underwent amputation as children, reflect that they feel fortunate for having had intact limbs as long as they did, compared with those born without limbs.

Like adults, children experience a broad range of emotional reactions to their limb loss including shock, fear, anger, denial, sadness, grief, depression, shame, guilt, and self-pity. They may express their feelings directly or through their behavior (or misbehavior). Parental acceptance of their child's feelings will affirm the validity of their emotional responses, and will help the child to better accept himself or herself. This will accelerate the grieving process.

There are many other ways in which the psychological effects of amputation on children and adolescents compare to those of adults. Fears about missing body parts, changes in physical appearance, and the effects of the limb loss on the activities of their daily lives, begin before surgery and continue afterwards. Like an adult, children must go through a process of reformulating a positive body image and self-concept. They must find their own way of making meaning of their limb loss and integrating it into the totality of their lives.

How well children cope depends upon several factors: their unique character and personality, prior life experience, the severity of their physical condition, and the strength of their support system. If children have a solid foundation of good self-esteem, they will have a far easier time adjusting to the stresses that accompany amputation. Children may feel guilt for causing their family more work, or they may feel like they are now a burden. It is important to relieve them of this unnecessary anxiety through reassurance. Empathy, love, and acceptance all assist the healing progress and minimize emotional scars.

Emotional recovery is complicated when loss of limb is due to a disease process, such as cancer. In this particular circumstance, amputation is only one aspect of the treatment; the child may also have to undergo chemotherapy with all of its dreadful side effects. Compounding this is the uncertainty of whether or not the cancer has been arrested. This is a heart-wrenching experience for the whole family.

Children go through a grieving process that is similar in many ways to that of adults. Out of necessity, they must begin to adapt rapidly. It is natural for them to worry if friends and classmates will accept them. If they had a circle of friends before their surgery, they will likely be accepted afterward. Girls, in particular, worry about how natural their prostheses look, and whether or not they can still wear current fashions and dress like their friends. Both boys and girls wonder how their loss of limb will affect their social lives and physical abilities. In general, the sooner a child returns to his or her normal daily routine the better.

Family Support

Family support is of inestimable value. Growing up we draw solace and strength from the love, comfort, and acceptance provided by parents and siblings. The truth is that no one knows a child's capacity, not even the child, until he "pushes the envelope" and finds out for himself. If parents have provided a solid foundation of love and acceptance, fostered self-esteem and self-acceptance, and encouraged a willingness to take risks, they have given their children deep, healthy roots from which they can grow.

Home life, school, and friendships are the bedrock of a child's world. Children are emotionally nourished by their interactions with friends. Competencies grow and world view is broadened through their experiences at school. When children are at home, they are within a loving, supportive sphere of influence. When out with friends or at school, inevitably, they will encounter teasing. The degree to which they feel comfortable about themselves will enable them to disentangle their sense of self-worth from the petty meanness of a small minority of children. Children usually weather the social challenges they face and often grow up with enough extra confidence to surmount almost any obstacle in their path.

The psychological effects for a child and his or her family deserve special consideration beyond the scope of this book. Check with your local library and bookstores for more information on raising a child with special needs; the "Further Information" section beginning on page 327, suggests some excellent resources. If you are the parent of a child with limb differences, I encourage you and your family to join a support group that will put you in touch with others who face similar challenges. Such groups provide the opportunity to exchange practical information with others, to decrease your sense of isolation, and to allow you and your child to interact with children with limb differences who are thriving. Your child's health-care providers may be able to put you in contact with others in similar circumstances. Joining special sports groups is another way to meet people like yourselves.

A Child Like Any Other

A child is normal aside from his or her limb differences. When treated as such, the message given is: *Life goes on. You are still the same person you were before the amputation. Who you are "on the inside" counts more than the number or shape of your limbs. You are still a capable individual. You are still an integral part of this family, and we hold great hopes and dreams for you.*

Thus, children with limb differences must learn to cope with physical, psychological, and social challenges, as well as master the normal developmental tasks of childhood. Children are remarkably resilient and resourceful. Most adjust well to living with their differences. They are far more similar than dissimilar to other children. The totality of who a child is encompasses so much more than his or her physical body. As children learn to adapt, their differences will recede in importance and become just another aspect of what makes them unique.

IN CONCLUSION

"I remember wondering, 'Why did this happen to me? What did I do to deserve this?' I thought, 'This sucks. I don't need this.' But I could think about it all I wanted to, and I'd still have one leg—so I just had to deal with it."

—Mark
(lost his leg to cancer at age thirteen)

When you lose a limb, everyday ordinary reality grinds to a screeching halt. Suddenly you must face your own mortality. You are presented with the awesome challenge of meeting your limitations head on. You must reevaluate your goals. You must learn to integrate this profound loss into your life; you must move on. This process can be incredibly rich in meaning; it can provide an impetus for a deepening of both character and appreciation of life.

Some individuals do very well, whereas others need extra help in assimilating the loss, and finding meaning in their lives. Some get so caught up in their own despair that they get stuck in their recovery process. Therefore, along with the loss of full physical freedom, there lies the danger that being "an amputee" may become a way of life, rather than just one aspect of it. There is a profound difference between a person who identifies himself primarily as "an amputee," and someone who identifies himself as "a person with amputation." It is my sincere hope that this book will assist you in becoming the latter, so that you can move forward and continue to enjoy your life.

Amputation is a harsh reality that presents new opportunities for inner growth and richness in living. Yet, a life lived with limb loss is not necessarily qualitatively "better" or "worse" than any other. It is how you live the life you have, and the meaning you impart to the happenings in your life that determines its quality.

7

Coping with Your Emotions

Amputation is bound to launch you on one of the wildest rides of your life—a roller coaster of emotions. On this ride you may sink to the lowest depths of despair and climb to the highest peaks of love and joy. These emotions can be upsetting, especially if they are intense and you are not accustomed to dealing with your feelings. Compounding this difficulty is the need to attend to your medical care, as well as changes in your self-concept, relationships, lifestyle, and perhaps, vocation.

This chapter helps you understand the nature of emotions in general, and offers practical suggestions and exercises to help you identify and enlist your emotions as allies in your recovery process. The principles presented can apply to any situation in which you discover your emotions "are getting the better of you." Subsequent chapters in Part II explore the most common emotions elicited when one undergoes amputation.

WHO'S IN CHARGE—YOU OR YOUR EMOTIONS?

Are emotions out there floating about in the atmosphere until you wander into one? Do you catch emotions like you catch the flu or some other contagious disease? Can someone else "make" you feel anger, envy, sadness? Of course not! Emotions arise within you; you are their originator. You have the power to recognize what it is you are feeling. And if the feeling is undesirable, you ultimately have the power to do something about it.

Many otherwise intelligent, capable people believe they have little or no control over their emotions. They act as if they are at the mercy of these intense feelings and are totally subservient to them; they follow their emotions every dictate. Some people wallow in their pain or glorify it in order to get attention. Others use their emotions as excuses for not getting on with their lives. Perhaps you know soap opera kings or queens who are so absorbed with their own dramas that their lives have become narrowed by their self-indulgence.

At the other end of the spectrum are those who deem emotions worthless, and do their best to override them with intellect. These people display implacable calm; nothing seems to ruffle their feathers. Unfortunately, they risk missing out on both the joys and the sorrows that render depth, texture, and dimension to life.

The truth is that as human beings, we are responsive to both inner and outer stimuli. If something triggers an emotional charge, it is our nature to respond emotionally, physically, intellectually, and spiritually (in the area of values and beliefs). For example, when we are criticized, we tend to respond by becoming angry and defensive, or perhaps by feeling bad about ourselves. If we are complimented, we tend to respond by feeling good.

The ways in which some people try to avoid painful emotions can be a bit desperate. Some may try to distract themselves from their feelings through intense activity or sleep; others may numb themselves with alcohol or drugs. Becoming detached from emotions does indeed serve to temporarily separate oneself from an uncomfortable experience. However, when we repress, deny, or disassociate ourselves from our emotions, we shut down a valuable part of ourselves that adds richness to life. Rest assured, until you make peace with the issue that triggered the emotion, that initial emotional response will surface again and again.

So, it is wise to learn to enlist your emotions as your allies in the process of gaining self-knowledge and maturity. Recovery from physical and emotional loss requires courage and a willingness to take action on your own behalf. It is your responsibility; no one can do it for you. No matter how much someone loves and supports you, you are the only one who is actually living your experiences and feeling your emotional responses. You are the only one who can "heal" you. Learn from your emotions and grow through them.

Keep Emotions in Proper Perspective

Somewhere between following your emotions' every dictate and repressing or denying your responses lies a middle ground. Accurately assessing and acknowledging your emotional responses can add depth and richness to your life. Keep in mind, however, that although your emotional responses provide useful information, they do not include *all* of the data necessary to make well-balanced, objective decisions.

Consider the emotions that are provoked while you watch a well-crafted film or television program; consider the pull on your heartstrings while you witness a fundraising event that compels you to donate money. Your feelings are being manipulated. Remember, your feelings are *subjective;* they originate inside you. By all means, listen to the messages that your feelings tell you; however, be sure to look at the whole picture; consider factors that lie outside your subjective responses. This will provide you with a better-balanced overall view of objective reality.

RESPONDING TO EMOTIONALLY TRIGGERING EVENTS

As a human being, your nature is to respond to both inner and outer stimuli. When an emotional charge is triggered, you respond on four levels—physical, emotional, intellectual, and spiritual (your belief system). Each of these factors may have an impact on the others. Let's briefly examine these levels.

1. **Physical.** Sections of your brain and nervous system regulate your physiological responses to feelings. For example, when you feel fear, the "flight or fight" response is triggered. Your heartbeat quickens, mental activity and metabolism speed up, and there is an increase in your blood's glucose level. These physical responses prepare you to take action.

   If you are under physical stress, such as that which is brought on by illness, amputation surgery, or the process of physical rehabilitation, your emotional threshold may be lowered, causing you to respond more intensely to stimuli.

2. **Emotional.** You may experience one emotion, or a variety of emotions that are blended together. Sometimes an event will trigger an emotional response that is below your level of awareness. Feelings may seem to arise "out of nowhere," yet in fact, they are rooted somewhere in your current or past experience. As with physical stress, emotional stress can intensify feelings.

3. **Intellectual.** What you "tell yourself" about internal or external circumstances greatly influences what you feel. Your thoughts are colored by your beliefs, level of physical well-being, and life history. More information about self-talk is found in Chapter 13, "Self-Esteem."

4. **Spiritual.** Your system of values and beliefs also influences your emotional responses to stimuli. For example, if you believe that all of life is a struggle, your recovery will likely reflect that belief and also seem like a struggle. If you believe your life has less value because you have lost a limb, your actions, interactions, and sense of inner peace will reflect this belief.

You can tune into each of these four dimensions to help you understand and diffuse the underlying triggers of your painful or puzzling emotional responses. Do this by first noticing the point at which your emotional reaction has arisen. Ask yourself, "What's going on in my body? What are my feelings? What are my thoughts and underlying beliefs about what has occurred?" Armed with this information, you can then correct or challenge erroneous or nonproductive thoughts or beliefs that have been hindering your well-being.

Withholding or Denying Feelings

As a child, you may have been taught that certain feelings such as anger, jealousy, and disgust are not acceptable. You have probably learned to control these "socially inappropriate" feelings. For example, you may choose not to yell at your boss (even when you are very angry) because you value your job.

You may fear that if you express your feelings, you might lose control and run amuck; you might say or do something you will regret. These fears are generally unfounded. Feelings that have been pent up for a long time are bound to be intense; and yet, as you express these feelings, you will notice their intensity diminish and you will experience vast relief. Compare this process to steam that has built up in a whistling tea kettle. By carefully letting the steam out, the whistling gradually abates.

Some people unconsciously convert their fears into physical symptoms on which they can focus their anxiety, rather than experience their feelings in a more direct fashion. This is referred to as *somatization*. Denying or withholding feelings may contribute to psychological or physical problems such as bodily tension, anxiety, disease, a depressed state, high blood pressure, and ulcers.

Physical Clues

Being in touch with your feelings enables you to experience authentic responses to life. However, this is not necessarily an easy task. Many people have lost touch with the ability to accurately identify what it is they are feeling. You may find yourself unable to clearly express your feelings at the appropriate time, which may leave you emotionally impoverished, feeling flat, empty, or numb.

You might have several emotions present that conflict with each other. It is important to "sort out" these feelings. Before you can express your feelings to yourself or to others, you must first identify them. Often, your body will give you clues. It is common for your body to tense in areas that correlate meta-phorically with your emotional blockages. Notice areas of tension. Is your jaw clenched with withheld anger? Are the muscles in your neck and shoulders tight because you have been carrying "the weight of the world"? Do you have a pain in the neck? Are you having a "gut reaction"?

If you are not exactly sure what you are feeling emotionally, tune into your body. Do you feel heat, coldness, tightening, or clenching? In what area of your body are you experiencing such physical reactions? Does the feeling shift or change? Often, awareness of your true feelings will emerge if you pay attention to these kinds of physical responses.

Circumstances Do Not Cause Reactions

There is a commonly held misbelief that the circumstances we encounter cause our reactions. "She made me angry." "The weather made me cranky." "My boss infuriated me!" These are such common phrases that we may believe them without even realizing what we are actually saying.

It is really very simple to prove that external circumstances do not cause your emotional responses; rather, it is your interpretation of those circumstances. Imagine a situation in which several individuals receive similar rude, insensitive comments concerning the fact that they have amputation. One person may be furious, one may feel hurt, another may shrug off the ignorant comments, while a fourth may respond with humor. Since different people have different responses to the same circumstance, it is illogical to believe that their reactions are caused by the circumstance. Reactions are caused by *their interpretation* of the circumstance.

Several people can witness the same event, but each will interpret the meaning of that event differently. This is partly because we tend to *project* meaning onto events, based upon our unique filters of perception. These filters are composed of the way we perceive information through our senses, our beliefs, and our life experiences.

Recognizing the fact that you create your own interpretation of reality is the first step in gaining mastery over your emotional well-being, no matter what life throws your way. You can become the master of the way you respond to circumstances in your life, rather than allowing circumstances to master you.

EXPRESSING YOUR FEELINGS

After you have identified your feelings, you can choose what to do with that awareness. Often, just identifying the feeling is healing in itself. You may find that vague feelings of uneasiness and anxiety dissipate simply by identifying your emotions.

Acknowledging and then releasing your emotions allows you to progress with your emotional recovery. Different people are comfortable with different ways of expressing their emotions. You may find one or more of the following techniques helpful in your own life.

Share Your Feelings with Others

Sometimes just being able to express your true feelings, fears, and vulnerabilities with someone who supports you can be tremendously healing. Expressing your feelings to others is a way to share information or to get troubling emotions "off your chest," so you can let them go and move on. Friends or relatives who are willing to be good listeners can be tremendously helpful in assisting you sort through your feelings and work out your conflicts. And they do not have to offer solutions; it can be healing in itself for you to feel "understood" by someone with an empathetic ear who cares about you. The best presentation I have found that addresses how to communicate simply and effectively, and how to develop active-listening skills is *P.E.T. Parent Effectiveness Training* by Dr. Thomas Gordon (New York: Plume Books, 1975).

Release Physical Tension

If you don't take care of your physical body, it is more difficult to be able to enjoy positive emotions. Remember that all emotions are directed through your body. If you feel out of sorts emotionally, you need to look at the "basics" of your body. How are you breathing? When some people are under stress, they breathe irregularly, which saps their vitality. If you are one of these people, become aware of your breathing and take deep, relaxing breaths when you feel stress. It is also important to recharge yourself by getting an adequate amount of sleep. Physical exercise revs up the oxygen flow through your system; the resultant emotional state of vitality can help you meet life's challenges. Refer to Chapter 12, "Stress" for more information on how to enhance your physical health and well-being.

Releasing the accumulation of physical tension that results from intense feelings is beneficial. This allows your body to dissipate its adrenaline response, so you feel more relaxed and calm. Choose any physical outlet that appeals to you. Running, hitting a tennis ball, and vigorous exercise are a few effective outlets that are particularly useful during those times when it is counter-productive to act out really strong feelings such as anger and rage.

Have a Conversation with Yourself

Another useful approach for sorting out your emotions involves having a dialogue with the aspects of yourself that are in conflict or confused. You can separate your conflicting internal voices by using any one of a number of methods. For example, you can sit in a chair and verbally express one of your emotions. With each new emotion, switch to another chair. Create a verbal interaction between yourself and the emotions. If you are not comfortable talking out loud, try writing a dialogue between yourself and your emotions—like a play.

Externalizing your emotions allows you to untangle conflicting messages you might be giving yourself. By "talking" with your emotions, either through verbalization or the written word, you can discover what the "positive intention" of that emotion is. Does it serve you in some way? For example, guilt may serve to motivate you to change negative behavior. Anger may motivate you to take action. Since emotions such as anger and guilt are unsettling, ask yourself how you can come up with more constructive ways to give messages to yourself that serve the same positive end. Then you can work out alternative solutions to satisfy the intention.

Once you have learned the lesson(s) of your response, you might imagine yourself in similar situations to the one that triggered your response. You can imaginally "play" with different responses. This type of exercise makes it easier to break habitual patterns of response, so that you have more internal freedom in your future responses.

At first you might feel a bit silly having a conversation with yourself, but these feelings will rapidly give way as the benefits of the exercise become apparent.

Have an Imaginary Conversation with Others

Have an imaginary dialogue with someone who has upset you, and say all the things that might cause further blowup if actually said to that person. In this dialogue, you can do or say anything you want, since you won't actually hurt anyone as a result of your words or actions. Acting as the other person, you can respond as you believe they might respond. In this way, you may also come to understand the other person's point of view, which will allow you to release some of your intense feelings.

Keep a Journal

Writing in a journal is another way to sort through muddled feelings. There is something about the process of writing that allows you to gain new insights and understanding about yourself, to experience emotional release, and to create a bit of distance from your concerns.

You can enhance this process by imaginally asking the part of you that represents your "internal wisdom" to assist you. Some refer to this as their inner voice, intuition, inner teacher, or internal guide. Ask this part of you to help answer troubling questions or provide new approaches to your concerns. This technique invites your intuition to kick in so you gain better access to your own internal wisdom.

ACCEPTING YOUR FEELINGS

Many of us have been taught to deny our true feelings, or to hide them so as not to make others uncomfortable. Many psychotherapists share the following gem of wisdom to their distraught clients—*the only way out is through*. This statement implies that, when appropriate, you should allow yourself to fully experience your feelings in the present moment. For instance, if you are feeling angry, be angry; if you are feeling sadness, allow yourself to experience that sadness; if you are feeling frustrated, let yourself feel that frustration. Don't talk yourself out of *feeling* your feelings.

It has been said, "What we resist, persists." It is a fascinating phenomenon—when we give ourselves permission to fully experience our feelings and honest responses, the emotions "play themselves out" much more quickly than if we resist or suppress them.

Objectively speaking, there are really no negative or bad emotions. Like beauty, negativity is in the eye of the beholder. There are no feelings that are inherently correct or incorrect. At times, in the appropriate context, there is a place for every emotion. For example, when your personal boundaries or values have been breached, it is appropriate to feel angry; when you are exposed to bigotry and stupidity, it is appropriate to feel indignation; when you have experienced a loss, it is appropriate to feel sad.

When you acknowledge and accept what you truly feel, you can then make an accurate assessment of your emotional responses, and use that information to give direction to your behavior. It is important for you to trust the wisdom of your being. This perspective allows you to appreciate your ability to respond emotionally, and will help promote self-acceptance and personal growth.

Honestly Assess Reality

Many of us have never learned how to accurately assess reality. We tend to make it worse or better than it really is; we may leave out or deny pertinent information. In other words, we tend to lay distorted beliefs on top of what is actually happening. It is very difficult to get where you want to go if you don't know where you are to begin with. For example, you may know you want to travel to Denver, but if you don't know the city you are in now, you won't know which direction to take to reach your destination.

So, too, you must honestly learn to assess that which has been lost, altered, or what remains the same due to your amputation. Every once in a while, it is a good idea to stand back from your situation, as though you are an objective witness, and observe your life. What is it that you see? What is the actual reality, the full multidimensional perspective? Once you have accurately assessed your current reality, you can take more meaningful steps toward achieving your recovery goals.

It takes courage to examine yourself with honesty. You may, however, be surprised to discover all that you have going for you. Life becomes much richer when you accept the darkness along with the light. By doing so, you accept and acknowledge your own humanity.

Enlist Your Emotions as Allies

Every emotionally charged response carries within it a nugget of treasure. Emotions let you know areas in which you may be "stuck"; they provide invaluable feedback that lets you know where to take the next step in clarifying areas in your life that need to be pacified or healed. Thus, your emotions can serve as internal checks that allow you to tune into destructive thought patterns and limiting beliefs that must be adjusted to keep you on track and in emotional good health.

Feelings can also be used to energize you so that you may carry out desirable actions. They are great motivators. When you feel "on top of the world," such as when you are in love or feeling joy, you believe that you can accomplish practically anything (and have the energy and will to do so).

Thinking of your emotions as allies will free you from believing that you are at their mercy. You can use them as tools to serve you. Your life will become fuller and you will experience enhanced well-being and happiness.

When you find yourself feeling an intense emotional reaction to a circumstance, know that you are actually experiencing a moment of power. Expressing that emotion might be destructive to others or hurtful to you; instead, use the information that you glean from your response to point you in the direction you need for clarity and peace of mind. Perhaps you need to change the way you think about the current situation; perhaps you need to re-examine your limiting patterns of beliefs, thoughts, and behavior; perhaps there is specific action you can take to rectify the situation; perhaps you need to clear up matters with others; or perhaps you need to develop a new strategy for dealing with whatever is provoking your response.

You are your own best detective, since you know yourself better than anyone else; and, let's face it, you're probably more concerned with your own well-being than anyone else. So take advantage of the opportunity your emotional responses afford you. You will be well rewarded for your efforts. Viewed this way, life will continue to unfold as an adventure, offering continuing opportunities for learning, personal evolution, and greater joy.

IN CONCLUSION

In your journey of healing and recovery from amputation of a limb, you are bound to find yourself on a roller coaster of emotions. Remember that emotions are valuable in adding texture, dimension, and richness to your life. All of your emotions are valuable. They offer you the information and feedback you need to take positive steps in your life and to enhance the quality of your experiences. When you enlist your emotions as allies, they become tools to better your life. Rather than allowing your emotions to rule you, you can effectively learn to take charge of them.

I wholeheartedly encourage you to apply the concepts and suggestions presented in this chapter as aids in working through painful, difficult, puzzling, or challenging emotional responses. By actively taking charge of your responses, you empower yourself and may even find yourself enjoying the ride.

8

MOURNING YOUR LOSS

Loss is a natural part of the ebb and flow of life and the cyclical rhythm of nature. From a seed, a tree grows; eventually the tree dies, and from its seeds new life springs forth. Seasons change; death follows life; day gives way to night, which gives way to day again.

No one is immune to loss. It is an unavoidable part of life—the death of a loved one, a divorce, the loss of a job, a move to a new location, the loss of youth, etc. Loss, however, opens the door to new beginnings.

Amputation of a limb is a great loss—a part of you is permanently gone, your life is irreversibly altered. In many ways, losing a limb is similar to the death of a loved one. You must work through various stages of grieving in order to recover. Grieving provides opportunities for healing, renewal, growth, and spiritual development.

A PROFOUND LOSS

I don't know anyone who has said to himself, "When I grow up, I'm going to lose a limb." People assume, unless they are born with a congenital abnormality, that they will go through life with their limbs intact.

If you face amputation, you will undoubtedly feel that the "rug" has been pulled out from under you. Basic assumptions about who you are and the course of your life will be irrevocably altered. Dreams for the future, based on those assumptions, may be radically impacted; the very fabric of those dreams may be torn asunder. The underpinning of your well-being may come undone. The shock, confusion, and resulting pain can be devastating. Some people attempt consolation by trying to convince themselves that, "It's only a limb. It's not such a big deal." The truth is that amputation of a limb or limbs is a very big deal; it is a profound loss.

While investigating the intensity of the grieving process, a researcher named C.M. Parkes conducted a fascinating study in which he compared the emotional reactions to the loss of limb with the reactions to the death of a spouse. He assessed the psychosocial changes in two groups—one group included people with amputation, the other included widows.

In both groups, the initial experience of grief was very similar. Both groups reported a numbness that was followed by an uneasy fixation and preoccupation with the object of loss. This preoccupation included visual memory and a sense of presence. Denial of the loss was common to both groups.

In the period shortly after the loss, the widows were more demonstrative in their distress than were those who had undergone amputation. By the following year, the symptoms of distress had greatly diminished in the group of widows, while the intensity of the grief response in those who had experienced amputation was virtually unchanged from that of the first year! This finding clearly demonstrates the deep nature of the loss sustained due to amputation.

Common Physical Responses

While you are engaged in the grieving process, your body may register and reflect your emotional state in a number of ways. You may find yourself having difficulties with normal sleep patterns or notice changes in your eating patterns or sex drive. You might experience periods of confusion and disorientation, as well as feelings of emptiness, helplessness, hopelessness, restlessness, uneasiness, or numbness. You may feel fatigued and unable to continue your usual routines. It is not uncommon to get caught in self-destructive behaviors, including substance abuse and withdrawal from others. You may find yourself becoming argumentative and irritable, with a very short fuse that easily ignites into anger.

Common Myths on Dealing with Loss

We live in a society in which "more is better." The media focuses on youth and beauty, and the acquisition of material goods and external status. We are, therefore, groomed to value "more" and associate it with material goods and goals. Loss, on the other hand is accociated with "less." As a society, we are generally mentally and emotionally ill-equipped to cope with loss.

As John W. James and Frank Cherry point out in *The Grief Recovery Workbook* (New York: Harper and Row, 1988), we are often taught myths about grieving that do not promote our recovery. Some of these myths are summarized as follows:

• **It is better to deny or bury true feelings than it is to express them.** When dealing with a loss, how often have you been told not to feel bad? This is an encouragement to discount your authentic responses.

• **You can replace the loss.** Even though this is clearly impossible, it is something we are taught to believe. For example, when a child's pet dies, he may be told, "That's all right, we'll get you another."

- **You need to grieve alone.** Society, uncomfortable with loss, does not prepare us to gain comfort from others.
- **Time cures all.** This concept can cause further pain to those who mourn past "socially acceptable" limits.

In addition to these common myths, loss may cause us to regret the past. We wish it could have been "different, better, more." Many people fall into the trap of holding onto memories and enshrining the past. (Perhaps you know of someone who has kept their loved one's room untouched for years after that person's death.) We are also taught not to trust. By closing their hearts and minds, the holders of this belief hope to eliminate the potential for pain by not taking any risks.

These myths and harmful messages are often a part of what our parents or society has taught us. We simply do not question them; we assume them to be true. This is why conscious awareness of our beliefs and assumptions is so critical for optimizing our internal healing.

THE STAGES OF GRIEVING

Loss of limb impacts you on many levels. Some reasons to grieve are readily apparent, while others are more subtle. You may find yourself not only grieving for the lost limb itself, but for the many things connected with that loss. Grieving stretches out in all directions on the time continuum of your life: You grieve for what you had in the past, what you believe you lack in the present, and for what "might have been" in your future. Loss is difficult to cope with even once you have acknowledged it as part of the flow of life. Grieve at your own pace, but do your best to complete the process. Unfinished grieving can interfere with other aspects of enjoying life.

Dr. Elizabeth Kübler-Ross, in her book *On Death and Dying* (New York: MacMillan Publishing, 1969), has outlined five stages of the grieving process that occur in conjunction with dying. These stages, which parallel the grieving that occurs with loss of a limb, are:

1. **Denial and Isolation.** "This is impossible. It's not really happening! I feel nothing at all."
2. **Anger.** "Why is this happening to me? I'm enraged! God is unjust!"
3. **Bargaining.** "If I promise to do such-and-such, then maybe I'll get my old life back."
4. **Depression.** "I feel hopeless. Everything is beyond my control. Why bother trying? I give up."
5. **Acceptance.** "I don't like it, but the amputation is a reality. I'll find ways to make the best of it and go on."

In your experience, these stages may not occur in the order presented, nor do you have to experience all of them for a successful recovery. They do, however, provide a useful overview of the grieving process.

INITIAL EMOTIONAL RESPONSES

What follows is a more in-depth discussion of some common emotional responses that many people experience following amputation. These feelings may overlap, or they may come and go at various times during your recovery process. All are normal and are to be expected. But, just like a physical injury, emotional pain must be tended to or it may fester and worsen.

As you learned in Chapter 7, the way out of grieving is by going through it. In other words, allow yourself to fully experience the range of your emotional responses with as little suppression as possible. In this way, these painful emotions will play themselves out.

Remember, it is work to go through the grieving process; and as such, it requires your conscious commitment and participation. You will need perseverance, patience, self-tolerance, self-compassion, a sense of humor, and forgiveness. The greater and more meaningful your loss, the more intense your grieving process is apt to be. Most experts suggest that you should not try to go through it alone. Get support by sharing your process with those who care or by seeking professional help.

Denial

We live in a society that tends to ignore or deny the reality of death and loss. We are rarely taught how to deal with this subject. I know a physician who had been on the staff of a large hospital during the time that Dr. Elizabeth Kübler-Ross first offered to give lectures on the subject of death and dying. The hospital administrators turned down her offer, telling Dr. Kübler-Ross that there was no need for such information. Imagine that—a hospital where no one needed information on death and loss!

Desire to deny the reality of your amputation is understandable, especially right after the amputation. (Denial is a natural defense to help buffer the shock.) Although denial may be useful at first to give you time to recover physically and help shield you from the many real challenges that you will have to face, eventually, you must deal with the realities.

Denial will not alter reality as much as you might want it to. The problem with being stuck in a state of denial is that you will not be able to marshall the strength and creative decision-making capabilities that are necessary to address the reality of your physical condition and its impact on so many areas of your life. If you cannot admit that amputation has impacted your life, then you will not be able to deal with the very real changes that have occurred. The result—a prolonged adjustment period. If you continue to deny the reality of your limb loss, its acceptance and integration into your life will be very difficult.

Confusion and Disorientation

As you emerge from the shock, numbness, and denial of your amputation, it is natural to feel confused and disoriented. The amputation has brought on many changes. You may find yourself feeling that nothing in your life makes sense anymore; life may seem like an illusion; you may not know what to do next; you may become temporarily forgetful; tasks that you normally took for granted may seem impossible to complete. All of these experiences are an expected part of your transition.

You have been thrown into a situation filled with many firsts—looking at your residual limb, using crutches or a walker, walking with a prosthesis, and needing physical therapy. It is the first time you have to deal with the comments made by others. In the face of all of these new experiences, confusion and disorientation are perfectly normal.

Why Me?

A universal question that arises with personal misfortune is, "Why did this happen to me?" Depending upon individual beliefs, you might find yourself asking additional questions such as "Am I being punished?" "Did I do something to bring this on myself?" "Why is this my fate?" "Is God angry with me?" "Is there no justice and fairness in this world?"

Your belief system can either help or hinder your recovery. If, for example, you believe your limb loss is part of God's plan, you might find comfort and the courage to move on more easily than if you tell yourself that you are being punished for some reason. If you look upon you limb loss as only one aspect of your being, rather than the central one, you will have an easier time learning to cope with the inevitable changes.

"Having cancer is hard. It's scary. The fact that you are going through it doesn't make you a bad person, so disengage your self-esteem from what is happening to you. It's not that you are being punished. These things just happen; it's very democratic. Try to stay optimistic."

—Marcy

Asking yourself, "Why me?" is a natural part of the healing and recovery process. You will know you are making progress when you stop agonizing over this question. Although releasing feelings of guilt and blame will not automatically give you total peace and acceptance of your loss, it will enable you to move on emotionally in your healing process.

Sadness

"I still feel sad once in awhile and feel the need to cry. People must allow you to do that. I did a lot of crying during the period that directly followed my surgery, but it did recede as time went on. This is your reality. You can't undo it."

—Leslie

Sadness is inevitable following limb loss, and there is great value in being able to express this sadness. Many adults are out of touch with their ability to release sadness through tears. They have been taught that "big girls don't cry" or that crying isn't manly. Many believe it is a sign of weakness to express vulnerability through tears. As a little kid, can you remember how good it felt to cry when you were upset? Tears provide a great cleansing, a release of emotion.

Guilt

Guilt results from feeling responsibility and remorse for some wrong you have committed; it causes you to feel painfully culpable whether the offense is real or imagined. The positive purpose of guilt is to motivate you to change your behavior either by redressing the wrong or by taking new action to prevent this wrong from recurring.

Many people feel responsible for their amputation. Some believe it is a punishment for past bad deeds or due to a lack of good physical self-care. Others feel their situation is somehow the result of their own lack of character. It is a natural human response to torment yourself by wondering if the necessity for amputation might be partially your fault. Do you believe you are being punished for your behavior? Do you believe you could have prevented the trauma or illness that necessitated the amputation? (Children are especially vulnerable in thinking that whatever "bad thing" has happened is somehow their fault, particularly if, in anger, they wished that something rotten would happen to someone else.)

If your amputation is the result of a medical problem, your physician can probably reassure you that nothing you could have done would have prevented the need for surgery. If you suffer guilt by believing your amputation is a punishment for past deeds or because you are a "bad person," a professional counselor or spiritual advisor can help you work through these feelings.

Following your amputation, you must take care of your own health-care needs and tend to your emotional recovery. While you are taking care of yourself, your family's need for you will not go away, and you must juggle the competing demands of self-care with the needs of others. This can be the perfect setup for guilt in which you find yourself taking on obligations that are not in your best interest. If you overemphasize pleasing and tending to others, you will set yourself up for guilt and resentment.

The following suggestions can help you alleviate guilt you may be feeling as the result of your amputation.

Let Yourself Off the Hook

If your amputation was due to medical causes, and you did everything possible to halt the underlying disorder, give yourself a break. If an accident has occurred that you could not have prevented, go easy on yourself. Even if you unwittingly took (or didn't take) actions that may have contributed to your need for amputation, prolonged guilt will do nothing to change the situation. Hindsight always makes it easier to say, "If only . . . if only . . ." This "if-only syndrome" promotes remorse, self-recrimination, and other forms of blame; it does nothing to promote healing.

Self-forgiveness can do wonders in terms of allowing you to get on with your life. Forgiving others can be equally liberating. When you hold onto thoughts of revenge, resentment, and bitterness, who do you think is actually being hurt? You or the other person? Think about it.

Holding onto guilt will not only continue to hurt you, it can inhibit a healthy relationship with those who care for you. Guilt keeps you stuck in the past, preventing you from participating in the present. It serves as a distorting filter that limits your objectivity and influences your actions in unhealthy ways.

Don't Wallow in Misery

Wallowing in the muck is fun for pigs but miserable for humans. It is healthy to allow yourself to acknowledge your true feelings and experience them in their fullness; but, if you find yourself wallowing in misery and are unable to let go of the guilt after a reasonable period of time, you will be further injuring yourself. As with other hurtful emotions, trying to repress or deny the guilt allows it to ferment and decay your sense of well-being. On the other hand, if you sink into the quagmire of your guilt and do not come up for air, your sense of well-being can be smothered. The pain of guilt can be staggering.

What has happened cannot be changed. Have some compassion and, if necessary, forgiveness for yourself and others. Compassion and forgiveness are healing in and of themselves; they permit you to progress in your recovery process.

A misguided sense of justice causes many people to believe that they must experience great internal suffering before they deserve to forgive themselves or be forgiven by others. If you are one of these people, I encourage you to let go of this false and destructive belief, fast! It will not permit you to enjoy the life you deserve to live. Once you have heard the message of your guilt, stop wallowing in it. Let it go.

Deal with the Guilt

Guilt is very real and very painful; however, it can motivate you toward positive action. Through modification of the beliefs or expectations that prompted your guilt, you may prevent a recurrence of similar situations.

Once you have learned your guilt's lesson, let that guilt go! Give up the misguided notion that you must torture yourself with endless remorse and self-recrimination. Commit yourself to whatever changes are necessary to avoid similar situations in the future. Once you have made this commitment, holding onto the guilt serves no further purpose, so let it go and move on in your life. Self-compassion and self-forgiveness will help you "wipe the slate clean" and allow you to experience inner peace.

You can prevent the occurrence of guilt by establishing healthy, realistic responsibilities for yourself. Give up the idea that you must do everything perfectly and fulfill all roles ideally. What can you realistically do for yourself, your family, and friends? Be honest when assessing what you can offer your community and workplace. Know that you do not have to please others all the time. Your self-worth is not dependent upon the opinions of others.

Free yourself from the burden of guilt that you may associate with your amputation. Letting go of guilt will lighten your spirit and allow you to live more fully in the present, which will aid in your recovery process.

Shame

Like other emotions, shame, in itself, is neither good nor bad. It is simply a normal human emotion. However, shame usually causes us to feel that there is something fundamentally wrong with us, that we are flawed or defective as human beings. Considering ourselves this way also causes us to feel vulnerable, afraid that others will discover and expose our "hideous truths." In turn, this vulnerablility causes us to take defensive measures so that others will not be able to discover any of our shameful secrets.

When you lose a limb, you may feel shame that your body is no longer whole. An underlying medical condition, such as cancer or diabetes, can compound your shame if you believe that living with a disease means there is something "wrong" with who you are.

You may feel shame in your intimate relationships, and consider your body repulsive and unacceptable to your partner. You may also feel shame if you can no longer fulfill roles in your family, at work, or in your community in the same ways you did before your amputation. To protect yourself from the fear of rejection and feelings of unworthiness, you might withdraw from social interactions or give up pursuing your goals and dreams.

Shame can certainly undermine your well-being, and must, therefore, be addressed. To deal with shame you must admit your feelings and acknowledge your humanness. Part of being human is being imperfect—

we have flaws, we make mistakes, we are not always exactly how we would like to be. It is important for you to find ways in which you can be happy with yourself and accept who you are. Learn to be honest with your feelings and share them with others who care about you.

Learn to identify with those aspects of yourself that are beyond the superficial. Your worth is not determined by your appearance, your health status, or your physical ability. I encourage you to make peace with who you are, as you are. To do this, you must develop compassion, forgiveness, and acceptance of yourself. Most of the chapters in Parts II and III will assist you in doing this.

It takes courage and commitment to your healing to expose your vulnerable areas. It is like opening a festering wound—once exposed to the purifying rays of the sun, your healing will accelerate.

Isolation, Alienation, and Loneliness

Following my initial trauma and amputation, I often felt alone. Nobody else could have known what I was going through as I struggled to stay alive; no one else could have experienced the myriad of changes wrought by my amputation. No one could have gone through my surgeries or the grueling physical therapy sessions for me. No one could have relearned to walk for me, or make the emotional adjustments that I needed to get on with my life. Despite the fact that I was blessed with a loving family and friends who rooted for me and encouraged me, I felt isolated, burdened, and very much alone.

These feelings of isolation cause you to feel cut off from fellow human beings and those who care for you. Help yourself through this period of isolation by doing the following:

• Recognize destructive self-talk. What are you telling yourself about the "way things are" that is causing you to feel alienated from others? You may, for example, be distorting reality—making things worse than they really are. Correct yourself, then replace the negative self-talk with more positive thoughts and encouragement.

• Recognize your human need for connection with others and reach out. Examine what you feel you are lacking—friendship, someone to care about you, intimacy, etc. Let your friends and family know what it is you need. Spend time with loved ones and those who care for you. Even if they do not know exactly what you are experiencing, their love and caring should nurture your spirit.

• Join an amputee support group; the people in such groups can truly empathize with you. Contact with others who have limb loss can greatly decrease your feelings of isolation and provide invaluable support.

• Do what nurtures you. You know what best soothes your soul. Stay active. Laugh. Play. Get plenty of rest. Do something to contribute to others.

• Get support through professional counseling, if necessary.

While it is true that no one can step inside you and experience exactly what you are going through following the trauma of amputation, you need not feel alone. Chapter 17, "Developing Your Support System" offers many additional suggestions to aid in building yourself a newtwork of support. By opening yourself to the empathy and compassion of others, you will feel nurtured during this difficult time. So reach out to others, and allow them to reach out to you.

WELL-MEANING FAMILY AND FRIENDS

"I know just how you feel." "You just need time, and you'll get over it." "You were fortunate to keep your limbs as long as you did." "At least you weren't paralyzed, or left blind or mentally retarded." "You've been tested by God." "You'll be stronger for this, it will build your character." "Just keep busy and your pain will pass."

Although they are well-meaning, generally, friends and loved ones will not know how to comfort you adequately. They themselves may not know how to adequately cope with loss in their own lives; so, they cannot possibly offer insights that they do not have. This becomes apparent in both their verbal and nonverbal behavior:

• Uncomfortable with their own feelings, they may avoid you.

• Their own sense of immortality has been threatened, and they may project their fears onto you.

• They may not be in touch with their own feelings, leaving them unable to help you deal with yours.

• They may intellectualize and encourage you to do the same (stay "in your head" rather than feel the genuine emotions in your heart and gut). This will not aid in your emotional recovery.

• They may be hesitant to invade your privacy by bringing up what they deem to be an intimate, highly personal issue.

These types of responses may leave you feeling alone and misunderstood. Your feelings may be invalidated or discounted, so that you feel alienated and isolated in your mourning; you may feel judged for the experiences you are having. It is no wonder that when someone asks how you are, you might mechanically reply, "I'm doing really well. I'm getting on with life."

The question: How can the well-meaning people in your life help you if they do not know how? The answer: You have to help guide them. Remember, this is a new experience for them as well as it is for you. Let them know that their loving presence can, in itself, be a comfort and support. Offering advice or trying to "fix" your situation is not necessary. What they can do is offer an empathetic ear when you wish to express yourself. This will help you validate your feelings. Their acceptance of your amputation can be tremendously reaffirming when you discover that they treat you as the same person you were before your limb loss.

You must be vocal in letting others know what they can do to be supportive. Perhaps you would like more quiet time for yourself, or a hand with some household responsibilities. Maybe you would like to get away from your routine for a few hours or even days—a good friend can be an enjoyable companion. Perhaps you would like someone to accompany you on your medical appointments.

Whatever your desires—and they will be different for each individual—be sure to express them. Your friends and family will welcome your guidance in telling them how they can help.

HOW LONG IS THE GRIEVING PROCESS?

There is no single timetable for how long it takes to go through the process of grieving. You will experience differing degrees of emotional intensity at different times. The process may seem to progress in "waves." You may be on an even keel for a while and then some incident or memory will launch you back into your pain.

Special days or events such as birthdays, holidays, and the anniversary of your amputation may serve as potent triggers to your pain. Over time, the intensity of your emotional response will diminish. For instance, in my own experience, I find I now recall many of my former activities, such as hiking and involvement in the martial arts, with a certain poignancy rather than with heart-wrenching pain and overwhelming sense of loss.

There is no way to force the mourning process to its conclusion prematurely. It takes its own time and has its own pulses and rhythms. On the other hand, trying to repress the mourning process, by pretending the loss does not hurt or that nothing in your life has changed as a result of your amputation, does not work, either. Repressed emotions take their toll. When you least expect it, these emotions will emerge in new forms, such as an illness or a numbing of true feelings. You can be cut off from a full emotional life, and instead experience loss of "aliveness" and zest for life.

When is Enough, Enough?

In retrospect, my own emotional recovery took several years. Since I had sustained serious trauma to many parts of my body, my rehabilitation included multiple surgeries. There was difficulty in fitting my prosthesis. A lawsuit connected to the original auto accident settled one day shy of seven years from the date of my original trauma! All of these factors served to keep my limb loss central in my awareness for a prolonged period of time. Once these issues were settled, my limb loss was finally able to recede into the background, rather than occupy the foreground of my life.

My recovery time is in sharp contrast to others who describe making peace with their limb loss in a matter of weeks or months. Your timetable for recovery is, thus, very individual. It depends on your emotional and personal make-up, medical circumstances, and other external factors that impact the grieving process.

Your body will "speak" to you, giving you information about your healing process. Notice if your body reacts with a heaviness or ache in your heart, or a catch in your throat. These "messages" are telling you that you have more grieving to do. Recognizing the factors that prompted your body's response will provide clues to these areas that still require healing.

While it is important that you fully experience your emotions in order to transmute them in the healing process, eventually you must move on in your life. How do you know when enough is enough? If you find yourself wallowing in the same emotions for months or years, or if you simply cannot accept or enjoy the life you now have, you can probably benefit from some professional assistance.

Help Yourself Through Your Grief

Your grieving is uniquely personal. You need to reach deep inside your heart and find the faith and perseverance to believe that things will work out. You must believe that you will get through this difficult period and go on to have a satisfying life in which you will not only survive, but thrive. You need to know that you can lead a fulfilled life even with your amputation; it is possible to be happy.

Ultimately, it is you yourself who must do what is necessary to recover. The pace and style of recovery will be uniquely your own. You must take an active role. Make a commitment to yourself to do whatever it takes to truly nurture and support yourself in your healing process. This investment in yourself is well worth it; your reward will be inner peace and the ability to experience joy and freedom in your life.

I encourage you to draw on any available resources that support your mourning process. Take the following concrete actions to help you through your grief.

Be Good to Yourself

Now is not the time to adhere to a busy, productive schedule. Give yourself permission to take some time to adjust to your new realities. If your emotional pain is severe, concentrate on doing what is necessary to make it through each day. Have compassion for yourself; be gentle and kind. If a young child were experiencing a difficult time, you would probably know how to comfort that child; apply those same concepts to yourself.

Oftentimes, persons in the grieving process are especially fatigued and require much rest and sleep. Take naps, and go to bed early. At the same time, try to find a balance between activity and your need to rest and recuperate.

Follow the suggestions in Chapter 12, "Stress." Engage in restorative activities such as meditating and exercising. Follow a sensible diet. Work with your imagination. Turn to spiritual guidance.

Do whatever nourishes and heals you. Perhaps being outdoors—at the beach or in a park—will bring you pleasure. Maybe participating in a hobby you love will allow you a creative outlet. It might be useful for you to keep a journal to explore the process you are undergoing and help provide new perspectives and clarity to your situation. At times, you may just need quiet moments to meditate and reflect; this will help you sort out, assimilate, and make peace with the changes in your life.

Nourish Yourself with Healing Relationships

Perhaps you know someone—a friend, family member, or member of the clergy—whose presence you find especially comforting. It is important that these people allow you to just "be" where you are in your recovery process. Their acceptance of your physical and emotional situation is healing in and of itself.

Sharing your grieving process with another person is extremely helpful for your recovery. Speaking about your grief and getting feedback will help you assimilate the experience and move through it. Ask your "support people" ahead of time if you can call on them when you are going through emotional turmoil. Have them promise to be honest with you when you call on them; they must feel comfortable in letting you know if they are too tired, too busy, or simply not in the mood.

In addition to a personal friend, a professional counselor or a member of an amputee support group can also provide an open ear and an understanding heart. Being surrounded by innocent life can also be healing. Young children or a pet dog or cat can remind you that joy and a sense of wonder are still an integral part of life.

Seek Out Others with Amputation

A person of a similar age who has an amputation that is comparable to yours is an invaluable resource. Knowing someone like this will immediately keep you from feeling isolated. You will see someone in your situation who is leading a full, satisfying life; someone who knows the pain you feel and is capable of true empathy.

This connection will make you feel better understood, while providing hope and inspiration. Further information concerning the benefits of peer support can be found in Chapter 17, "Developing Your Support System."

Nourish Yourself Spiritually

If you are a person who draws strength from your spirituality, now is an excellent time to reconnect with whatever form your worship takes—be it through traditional religion in a community of others, or through solitary prayer, meditation, and reflection.

Often, when people experience a profound loss, their hearts are especially open, and they deeply question their values and purpose. This state of being provides a fertile ground for internal deepening, healing, and growth.

Care for Yourself Physically

During this period of stress, it is essential for you to take care of your physical health to keep up the level of vitality and well-being that is necessary to support your recovery. The danger exists that you may focus too much energy and attention on your amputation, and neglect other aspects of your health care. So keep in touch with your regular physician and attend to your overall care.

Fully Experience Your Feelings

Give yourself permission to fully acknowledge and experience the sense of loss you feel, as well as other related emotions such as sadness, anger, resentment, and frustration. Be honest with yourself. When you allow yourself to fully experience your emotions, you will notice that they do not last indefinitely. Eventually you will recover your equilibrium and equanimity.

Allow yourself to be with your feelings. This will allow you to work through them. The simple fact that you are having these responses demonstrates that you are a living, breathing, feeling person who is capable of responding to life.

There is a temptation to detach yourself from painful feelings so you will not have to experience them. This is useful to a point; but, eventually the feelings must be dealt with. What you do not deal with will persist, emerging from time to time until you have faced it.

Know that all feelings are okay. There are no taboos. Perhaps you are railing at God, "Why did this happen to me?" The truth is that you are angry, and you must allow yourself to express that anger honestly in order to work through it.

Let Go of "How Life Should Be"

Acknowledge your dreams and fantasies. Gently, and with compassion for yourself, let go of your ideas about "how life should be." The truth is, as someone who has recently experienced amputation, you do not really know what is possible for you in the future. Remember, the loss of a limb is only that. Most adults and children with amputations or limb abnormalities lead full, rich, rewarding lives. Some say the experience, although difficult, has caused them to be strong and self-reliant, to recognize what is really important in life, and to reorder their priorities in a meaningful way.

Letting go does not mean that you must let go of your dreams, your memories, or your spiritual beliefs. It means letting go of *how it was*, and embracing *how it is now*.

Focus on discovering what you can do now to make the most of your life. Try using the power of your imagination to visualize the life you might like for yourself, based upon your current reality. Take a few minutes and try the following visualization exercise:

Using all of your senses—smell, touch, taste, hearing, sight—imagine yourself enjoying your life, revelling in your aliveness, enjoying the moment. What is it that you are doing? What are you telling yourself about how you feel? Are you imagining new hobbies, new interests? Are you traveling or maybe doing some enjoyable volunteer work?

Now, think about what you can do to make this enjoyment happen. Whatever it is, do it! Take a risk. Be adventurous. First, play out the scene in your imagination and see what happens. If your imaginary actions result in something that you would choose to actualize for yourself, then align your actions to fulfill those goals. And remember that there is no such thing as "failure." Your environment or the people around you will let you know when what you are doing isn't working. Take that feedback and use it to readjust your actions to be in closer alignment with your goals.

Accept Your Limb Loss

It is important to understand that there is a difference between acceptance of your amputation and approval of it. *It is possible to accept that your amputated limb is permanently gone, and still not like or approve of that reality.* Some persons never fully accept their limb loss. This denial is their method of coping with an undesirable reality. While their life does indeed go on, they may lack inner serenity.

You will have easy days and hard days as you progress on the path to recovery; you must be flexible, creative, and willing to make adjustments to meet the challenges you will face. A sense of humor will lighten your heart. Denial of your loss is like building your future on a foundation of sand; accepting the reality of your amputation allows you to build your future on a solid foundation.

Develop a Sense of Closure

Closure is the act of tying up internal "loose ends." By developing a sense of closure, you will experience greater peace of mind. Without it, "unfinished business" can easily turn into preoccupation, a source of anxiety and malaise. Once closure is achieved, you are free to move on in your life.

There are a variety of ways to establish closure within yourself or with others. For example, it helps to have any questions you may have answered by your physician, prosthetist, or members of an amputation support group. You may feel a bit funny mentioning some of your concerns, but by doing so, you will help yourself achieve a sense of completion, which will speed your emotional recovery. For example, it is very important to ask your surgeon if everything possible had been done to save your limb. You may have questions about how the actual surgery was performed, or where your limb was taken once it was amputated. Getting the answers to these and other questions can provide you with a sense of control and inner peace.

If you feel unresolved about what has transpired between you and your physician, take a risk, and share your thoughts and feelings with him or her. Get over any shyness or embarrassment. Have your questions answered, and share unexpressed thoughts and feelings. You will release an internal sigh of relief when you have achieved that sense of completion.

Allow yourself to let go of the idea that your life should have been different, or that you did not fully utilize your limbs while you had them—"I could have been a ballerina, a baseball player, a concert pianist, a gymnast . . ." Perhaps you are idealizing how your life was before amputation—"I had everything. I had it all. My life was perfect. I'll never be happy and content again. I didn't appreciate what I had. If only . . ." We need to let go of what might have been—"I had plans to . . . One day I was going to . . ."

There are a number of exercises you can perform to facilitate closure in your recovery process. The exercises here are examples of what a counselor might initiate during a session or assign as "homework." The idea is to complete that which feels unfinished, or express what you couldn't at the time of an emotionally charged incident.

1. Write a letter to your limb. Admittedly, this might sound silly or even a bit weird, yet by expressing what your limb meant to you, you might be able to discharge pent-up emotions that are retarding your healing

process. You may want to tell your limb how it has served you and how you have appreciated its role in your life. If a diseased limb was the cause of your amputation, you might want explore your feelings of anger or disappointment toward it.

2. Have a dialogue with any aspect of yourself that you feel needs completion. For example, you might have a talk with your "dreams of what might have been." Role play those dreams and have a dialogue with them. It may be useful to place two chairs facing each other for the dialogue, and switch chairs as you switch parts. Instead of using the chair method, you may opt to write out the dialogue.

   Dialogue exercises allow you to sort out conflicting thoughts and feelings by expressing emotions that have been kept inside. Such exercises can make you aware of new insights, and help you develop increased clarity and an expanded sense of well-being.

   Your limb loss may have resulted in unfinished business with others—loved ones, doctors, children, and colleagues. The dialogue technique is helpful here, too. You can express emotions that have been kept inside, own up to your own responsibility for any current or past conflict, and offer yourself (or the other) compassion and forgiveness for what has transpired. In order for you to develop closure with another through this technique, the other person does not necessarily have to be present. It is not always possible for the person to meet with you, or you may feel that your emotions are so intense, it is not wise to share them face to face. The other person may be uninterested, unwilling, or unable to "hear" you. Since the conflicting emotions that plague you originate within you, it is here where you must create inner peace. You can come to internal resolution by working alone in this way.

3. Create ritual. Develop a personal ritual that lets you symbolically release the past, allowing you to live in the present. For example, you may choose to have a brief ceremony for yourself in which you give away physical reminders of "how it was." In my case, I gave away my high-heeled shoes, which I could no longer wear. They had been sitting in my closet, reminding me of my old life quite long enough. Giving them away helped me tie up a loose end and put the past behind.

No matter what you choose to do to facilitate closure, try to give thanks for your survival and feel an appreciation for how far you have come since your surgery. You must look within and create an experience that will serve you best.

WHEN TO SEEK PROFESSIONAL HELP

When is it time to seek professional assistance? In his book *Life After Loss:*

A Personal Guide to Dealing With Death, Divorce, Job Change, and Relocation (Tucson, AZ: Fisher Books, 1988), Bob Deits recommends you call in professional help when your grief has become destructive. The following symptoms are tip-offs that you require assistance as soon as possible:

1. **Persistent thoughts of self-destruction.** You feel desperate and suicidal, and have thought of specific ways to end your life.
2. **Failure to provide for your basic recovery needs.** You fail to take care of your health, stay withdrawn from others, or persist in being nonfunctional in everyday life.
3. **Persistence of one particular reaction to grief.** You experience overwhelming, persistent depression, or your continued denial prohibits you from coping with the demands of daily living.
4. **Emergence of substance abuse.** You rely on prescription drugs, alcohol, or street drugs; there are radical changes in your food intake (symptoms of bulimia/anorexia).
5. **Recurrence of mental illness.** You experience persistent anxiety, hallucinations, thought distortions, or inability to function.

For detailed information and suggestions on how and when to seek professional assistance, refer to Chapter 16, "Seeking Professional Counseling."

HOW TO KNOW WHEN YOU HAVE RECOVERED

You will know that you have made a large shift forward in your recovery when you find that you have stopped asking, "Why did this happen to me?" and start to ask, "Since this has happened, what can I do to transform the experience into one that is life embracing?" Your amputation will have taken on new meaning, and you will have given your life a higher sense of purpose and order. Here are some other ways you will know that you have recovered:

• You feel better! Rather than ruminating on the past, you are able to enjoy living in the present.

• You demonstrate an active interest in life—renew friendships, develop hobbies, and cultivate new experiences.

• You are either back at work or involved in some other meaningful activity.

• While acknowledging that your limb loss is tragic, you go on with your life. You are able to enjoy memories of your life before your amputation without those memories triggering painful associations laced with sadness, remorse, or guilt.

• You laugh more and find joy in being alive.

• You feel better about yourself; you have regained your equanimity.

• You find it easier to concentrate.

• You are less self-involved and more interested in life around you.

• You feel strengthened and more confident that you can handle your life and what it brings; you know that you have survived, and that you will continue on as an evolving, vital person.

• You discover creative outlets for self-expression.

• You take charge of your life, rather than allowing external circumstances to control your responses.

• You may find yourself assisting others who are going through their own grieving process in response to loss.

Most people recover from their grief; you will too. Grieving is a process with a natural progression. Your healing will have its ups and downs, and starts and stops, but be assured that it will progress.

When you notice that your life is no longer revolving around the fact that you've undergone amputation, you might want to mark the progress in your recovery with a gathering of family and friends. Special toasts of appreciation for those who have been of support can be a way to formally recognize, for yourself and others, that you have made significant improvement in your recovery. The act of marking such a milestone, especially in the company of friends, can be a way to add weight to the occasion, and give you additional momentum towards living an enjoyable, well-adjusted life.

9

FRUSTRATION AND ANGER

An inevitable consequence of amputation is repeated frustration. When you cannot live your life as spontaneously (physically) as you would like, or when medical complications or prosthetic problems arise, frustration is bound to rear its head. When repeated experiences of frustration occur, anger is likely to follow at its heels. For most of us, experiencing anger is, at the very least, uncomfortable. Anger is a highly charged, intense emotion; many of us are afraid we will be swept away by it, and do or say things while under its influence that we will later regret.

In this chapter, the frustration and anger you are likely to experience as a result of your limb loss is discussed. Coping strategies are presented to assist you in dealing with these unpleasant emotions.

FRUSTRATION

Some days your amputation will seem like a minor inconvenience, and other times (especially early in your recovery) its requirements will seem to consume most of your time, as well as your physical and emotional energy. The impact of amputation on a daily basis can be insidious, infiltrating areas you might never have imagined.

Sometimes for me, just having to be extra aware of the terrain beneath my feet, or driving around looking for a close parking space, or spending hours at the prosthetist's office can provoke frustration that puts a dent in my sense of well-being.

While frustration may seem to be a relatively minor discomfort, the bothersome, irritating feelings that accompany it can gradually build and erode your sense of well-being and enjoyment of life. It is, therefore, important to come up with strategies to address frustration. By simply becoming aware of the areas that have frustrated others with limb loss, you will be less surprised and better able to cope with these situations when they arise.

Initially, one of the most common sources of frustration is the time-consuming follow-up medical care following amputation surgery; another is the lengthy process of being fitted with an artificial limb. Lack of adequate information on the best prosthetic devices and options is another common source of frustration.

One man's experience with his first prosthetist is presented below. (This example also illustrates the importance of making it your business to investigate available options.)

"He [prosthetist] knew that a more modern device was out there, but he never even told me about it. Instead, he gave me a wooden leg. I would have been hobbling around on it the rest of my life if I hadn't spoken to this other guy [a new prosthetist]."

—Darrel

The most common source of frustration mentioned by those coping with limb loss involves problems with mobility and the consequent difficulties in daily living. Recovery and rehabilitation can be very draining, and many individuals report that it takes a long while for their energy level to return to where it was before the surgery. Often, the simplest of daily activities takes longer to perform than usual, and requires more energy due to the nature of the prosthesis and/or the severity of the limb loss:

"That's probably the biggest thing—it gets frustrating. You want to advance faster than what you're capable of. You think, 'Well, I'll go do this this afternoon,' but by the afternoon maybe you've done too much and you're too sore and you can't do what you had planned on doing. You have to space out your day. You can't just get up and go from morning till night."

—Rob

For many individuals, a debilitating source of frustration is the inability to be physically spontaneous:

"I get frustrated by not being able to do spur-of-the-moment things with my kids, like getting out and throwing around the football or having a catch. Sometimes it seems like all the spontaneity is gone from my life. Even the simple act of getting dressed has to be planned. You put pants on the prosthesis first, then the sock and shoe. You can't do things impulsively any more."

—Mort

Here is a similar theme sounded by another individual:

"Little things that never mattered before my amputation matter now, and I have to take everything into consideration. Every day is a challenge. Even the simplest tasks must be planned out. Sometimes it takes enormous effort just getting through a day."

—Dent

For some individuals the frustration comes from not being able to do simple tasks that they once took for granted:

"I used to love to mow the lawn. I've done it since my operation, but now it takes me forever. This frustrates me."

—Dale

Dealing with Frustration

The following suggestions are provided to help you deal with the frustration you will likely experience after your amputation.

• Learn to accept the inevitability that living with amputation is bound to include some daily frustration.

• Recognize the source(s) of your frustration. Determine which of these sources can be alleviated. For instance, if there is something about your prosthetic limb that bothers you, you may be able to have the limb adjusted to relieve the problem. On the other hand, you may have to learn to live with some other unavoidable frustrations. For example, you may have to accept the fact that it will usually take you a bit longer to perform certain routine tasks.

• Find physical outlets to discharge your pent-up frustration. Participate in some form of vigorous physical activity, have a good cry, or scream into a pillow at the top of your lungs.

• Be aware of other ways to relieve frustration, including self-hypnosis, visualization, and involvement in a hobby or other interest. Additional ideas are presented in Chapter 12, "Stress."

• Prioritize what must be done in a day and let the other stuff go. Make time for yourself to relax or engage in other pleasurable activities.

• Work on your attitude. Learn not to "sweat the small stuff." Accept your limits as a human being. Tolerance, patience, self-compassion, and a good sense of humor are priceless.

It is important to deal with your frustrations and keep them from building up. Pent-up frustration can easily escalate into anger or even rage.

ANGER

You will likely feel anger many times during your recovery process. If you perceive that the amputation was somehow your fault, you may rail at yourself. You may feel anger toward your physician if, for instance, you believe it was his fault for not halting the disease that led to your limb loss. You may lash out at your loved ones, and somehow shift the blame for your amputation onto them. You may just lash out at life or at God—"Why did this have to happen to me? Life stinks!"

Anger is often the result of frustration that has built up over time until it reaches a breaking point. Personally, I can remember becoming very frustrated over the amount of hours I spent in physical therapy, at the doctor's office, and with my prosthetist. It seemed that tending to my rehabilitation was consuming all of my time and energy. While, logically, I knew there was no one else but me who could ultimately bear responsibility for my recovery, every once in a while I would become sick and tired of the whole process. I would occasionally explode with venomous rage because of the sense of helplessness and powerlessness engendered by my situation.

Anger can often serve as a cover-up for other emotions that are too painful to acknowledge, such as helplessness or anxiety. One of the primary responses that anger often camouflages is that of fear. You may unconsciously use anger to avoid facing the very real fears that are connected with your recent amputation, such as how your limb loss is going to affect your relationships or your vocation. Perhaps the underlying medical condition that prompted your limb loss has forced you to consider your own mortality. Your fear has been elicited in response to a real (or imaginary) threat to your physical or psychological survival. The issues you face can be very frightening.

Range of Anger and Physical Responses

The intensity of emotions and their physical responses escalate as you move further along on the anger scale. Mild displeasure or *annoyance* builds up over time. When you do not allow yourself to vent these feelings, you may harbor resentment, which can gradually wear down your sense of well-being and lead to *frustration*. After your amputation, your new physical limitations and other realities will likely result in frustration (especially if your new physical reality is worse than you had expected it would be). It is important to deal with your frustrations to keep them from escalating into *anger*. When you feel anger, the resulting physical tension begs to be released. Strong feelings of displeasure are aroused. Adrenaline courses through your body, and you have an irresistible impulse to retaliate at what you perceive to be the injustice, wrong, or injury. Hot-blooded anger may, in turn, give way to violent, explosive *rage*. During moments of rage, reason flies out the window, and may result in regrettable actions.

"Seething with anger," "seeing red," "blinded by rage," "boiling mad," "ready to explode". . . . These graphic descriptions point to the changes in the body's physiology that occur in response to anger. When you are angry, your body's survival instincts kick into motion to prepare your body for rapid response to perceived dangers. This "fight or flight" response, originated in primitive times. When early man was confronted with a wild animal or some other danger, a surge of adrenalin shot through his body, causing him to either stay and fight the danger, or turn and flee from it.

The fight-or-flight response, which is triggered by the stimulation of your sympathetic nervous system, causes the release of adrenaline, a hormone that affects you in a number of ways. With the release of adrenaline, your body's metabolism (the overall rate of the physical and chemical changes within the body) speeds up; your blood pressure rises; you become mentally alert; there is an increase in your heart rate; you feel heat; you sweat; and your blood sugar level rises. All of these reactions prepare you for a burst of activity. Hopefully, you will choose to take some kind of action that is not destructive to yourself or others!

Choosing a physical outlet can be an excellent way to expend the adrenaline response caused by your anger. Vigorous exercise, a fast run, hitting a punching bag, or whacking a tennis ball—any activity that allows you to dissipate your body's reaction—will help you return to a more even keel.

Withholding Your Anger

Since anger is an unpleasant, sometimes frightening emotion, many people tend to "keep a lid" on their angry feelings. Those who are especially vulnerable to the opinion of others, or those who have invested in a social mask that projects an image of being cool, calm, and collected may not want to shatter that image by venting their anger. Although repressing anger may work in the short run, that anger will continue to churn inside and can explode at an inopportune time. If you perpetually squash your responses without a compensating physical outlet, you may find your body chooses unwelcome means to express itself. This internalization of responses can result in ulcers, hypertension, headaches, and/or emotional problems.

Consider the fact that by honestly expressing your feelings to others, even if you consider those feelings to be "negative," you are letting others know you are a fully human being; they will recognize that you are capable of expressing genuine responses, rather than wearing a false ("everything is just fine") social mask. Allowing yourself to be viewed authentically, vulnerabilities and all, then finding out that you are still accepted for who you are is a powerfully healing experience. It is also a vast relief!

Some people are afraid to express their anger because they are terrified at the prospect of losing control and acting in a harmful way. To prevent destructive unleashing of your anger, it is helpful to become adept at managing your feelings, so they do not build to a great intensity in the first place. Both managing your feelings and discharging the tension in your body will help dissipate your fear of losing control.

Constructive Use of Anger

Anger is a flashing red light. Its message may be that your needs are not being met, that you are being violated in some way, or that your personal boundaries have been crossed.

Anger creates explosive energy that pushes to express itself outwardly. The act of expressing anger liberates a certain vitality, and can actually be energizing. You can use anger constructively as a fuel to propel you into positive action, or to power your survival through tough times. If properly expressed, anger can enhance your self-esteem if you have been violated in some way; it is an appropriate form of self-care.

Generally, however, anger is not a favored or welcomed emotion. We are taught from childhood that it is not "good" to be angry, and we learn to repress our angry responses. This becomes so ingrained that it is often difficult for us to be in touch with our feelings of anger. We may fear our own anger and that of others because it is anxiety provoking, threatening, and often implies that action must be taken to right a difficult situation.

We must first be honest with ourselves—we feel what we feel. To deny our true feelings is to lie to ourselves. There is nothing inherently right or wrong with our natural responses and feelings. Once we have acknowledged our anger, the question naturally arises, "What useful measures can I take to work with this anger?"

Like every other emotion, anger in moderation is okay. It is a healthy response in certain situations, such as when you are angry at some type of injustice and express your indignation. Anger may even serve to help you mobilize your inner resources to redress a wrong. However, when anger becomes a permanent state of being, or occurs so often that it stands in the way of your healing process or lashes out to hurt others, it becomes both detrimental and destructive.

It is what you tell yourself about events that determines how you will respond. As was discussed in Chapter 7, "Coping with Your Emotions," no one can make you angry; in fact, no one can make you feel any emotion. Somewhere between observing an event and acting out your emotions lies your interpretation of what that event means to you. You then respond, based upon your interpretation of an event, rather than to the event itself. When you realize this truth, you regain your power, placing responsibility for your responses where it belongs—within yourself.

The much quoted Serenity Prayer, *God, grant me the serenity to accept the things I cannot change, the courage to change the things I can, and the wisdom to know the difference*, contains valuable insight that can be applied to dealing with anger. It is helpful to step back and discover whether or not the event that provoked your anger was something within your control. If it was beyond your control, you will recognize there was nothing you could have done to affect the outcome. This being true, you might as well vent your feelings and then relax.

Handling Your Anger

You will find the following suggestions useful in helping you deal with your anger. I encourage you to experiment with them and discover what works best for you.

• **Discover the cause of your anger.** Sometimes the cause of your anger will be very real and apparent; other times, if the anger is a cover-up for another emotion, its cause may not be as obvious. You may need to step back from the drama of your life and ask yourself, "What's really going on here? What's causing my anger? Is the anger I am feeling just a cover-up to keep me from feeling scared or hurt?"

Use your awareness to monitor your internal talk, so you can examine any distortions of thought and/or destructive belief patterns that might be contributing to your current feelings. (Refer to Chapter 11, "Depression," for a more in-depth discussion of cognitive distortions and harmful belief systems.) Once you identify and adjust these thoughts and beliefs, you will find yourself defusing angry feelings and experiencing emotional relief.

• **Lower the intensity of your anger.** First, honestly assess the intensity of your feelings. If your anger is highly charged and heated, or if you are enraged, it is obviously not the best time to confront others. You must do something to lower your boiling point. Vigorous physical activity is an excellent way to expend some of your body's adrenaline response and lower your emotional temperature. You can physically "act out" your anger in a way that won't actually harm anyone—scream into a pillow, sit in the car with the windows rolled up and scream at the top of your lungs, or punch a pillow until you have depleted some of your aggression.

When you actively discharge the physical energy associated with anger, you will discover that you have lowered the intensity of your angry feelings. This will help prevent you from taking actions that can be physically or emotionally destructive to yourself or others.

• **Do not attack or blame others.** You will not achieve constructive results when you attack, blame, or judge someone else. That person's defenses will spring up, and he won't be able to hear you. You have a much better chance of getting your message across when the other person feels accepted and respected, rather than rejected by your accusations, judgment, and blame. If you can make a distinction between the person himself and his action, it is more likely that he will listen to you. After all, it is easier for someone to hear that he has made a mistake, than it is to hear that he's a horrible person.

To follow this suggestion, first, describe the specific event or behavior that has stimulated your anger; then, present your emotional response beginning with an "I statement." For instance, say, "When such and such happens, I feel..." Own up to any responsibility you might have had in contributing to the anger-inducing event. Welcome the other person's input on how to resolve the problem. Find common ground and common goals, then work towards resolution from there.

• **Do not surrender to your anger or rage.** You will know your anger has gotten out of hand when it has become destructive to you or others. If you let anger take over your actions, you have surrendered your power to your emotions. If you have allowed your anger to rule you, and you respond by lashing out, it is likely that you will regret your actions and their results. When this happens, your task becomes threefold. First, you must heal the damage wrought by your actions; second, you must learn new patterns of preventive thought and behavior; and third, you must have compassion and forgiveness for yourself in order to let yourself move on.

IN CONCLUSION

During the ups and downs of the recovery and healing process following your amputation, feelings of frustration and anger are inevitable from time to time. While frustration is a relatively minor discomfort when compared with the intensity of anger or rage, it can still erode your sense of well-being; so, it is important to come up with strategies to address it.

When you find yourself experiencing anger you are faced with choices. You can repress or deny the anger, act it out, channel the energy, or rationally confront others who triggered your reaction. You can turn your anger into an ally by recognizing its constructive possibilities. When evoked, anger can serve as a signal to take action. You can allow it to energize you and propel you into taking positive steps to achieve your desired results.

10

ANXIETY AND FEAR

Amputation. . . . I don't know about you, but before my limb loss the very word conjured up dread, fear, and images of mutilation. When you first learned you needed an amputation (or discovered you had just undergone one), the concept was probably enough to trigger considerable anxiety and fear in you, too. It is normal to fear the unknown—and your amputation has cast you into a world that is filled with unknowns. The uncertainties of what your limb loss will mean to your daily living and your future can be cause for great anxiety. The far-reaching effects of limb loss on your self-concept, your relationships, your vocation, and most other arenas of your life are yet to be seen. This chapter presents a discussion on anxiety and fear, and offers strategies for coping with them.

DISTINGUISHING BETWEEN ANXIETY AND FEAR

Anxiety is often perceived as a vague mixture of malaise, apprehension, dread, and agitation that arises when we feel there is some threat to our well-being. We may be uncomfortable and anxious when dealing with uncertainty. Not expressing our feelings can leave us uneasy and contribute to our malaise. Often when we experience these unpleasant feelings associated with anxiety, we find that our energy level is low or our actions are paralyzed.

Fear tends to differ from anxiety in that it is usually linked to a specific situation, while anxiety is more of a diffuse, generalized state. We may not know the exact cause of our anxiety, but we are often aware of the source of our fears. When we are afraid, we face danger that threatens our survival in some way. The cause of our fear or anxiety may be founded in reality or simply imagined. In either case, the resulting feelings and bodily responses we experience are real. Physiologically, when we feel either anxiety or fear, our survival instinct kicks in and our body responds with the fight-or-flight response (described on page 125). Since fear is so closely linked with our survival instinct, it is inevitable that we have known fear many times in our lives.

UNCERTAINTY

The more uncertain or ambiguous a situation is, the more anxious you are likely to become as you approach it. Not knowing what to expect in a given situation can be unnerving; many times, you may tend to imagine the worst possible outcome. When you lose a limb, you are suddenly cast into a whole new world that is fraught with new challenges and first-time experiences. You are plunged into a multitude of new and, therefore, uncertain situations. Your life's experience to this point may or may not have prepared you to handle the circumstances you now face.

Depending on the reason for your amputation, many unanswerable questions may arise. What will happen to my health? Will any underlying disorders progress? What will the effects be on my personal relationships? Will I find anyone to love me? How will my work be impacted?

People respond to uncertainty in different ways. Some individuals launch a "preemptive strike" and give up or revise their goals, rather than deal with the uncertainties inherent in their situation. Others surrender their will to an outside authority, such as their physician, and give up all decision-making ("Whatever you say, Doc. Just tell me what to do. I can't handle making any more decisions.") Not knowing what the future holds for their physical well-being, some people experience a kind of emotional paralysis. They find it hard to make long-range plans about such things as their finances, vocation, and retirement.

Learning to Live with Uncertainty

One of the very best ways to reduce the anxiety of uncertainty is with information. The more you know about a situation, the better you can prepare yourself to deal with it. Knowledge will cause a drop in your anxiety level. Therefore, do all that you can to gain information.

Make use of the expertise from members of your rehabilitation team— speak with your physician about your medical concerns, talk to your social worker about available community resources, discuss ways to return to optimal strength with your physical therapist. Speak with others who have coped successfully with amputation and are enjoying their lives. They will be able to address your practical concerns, while serving as models of how life goes on after limb loss.

The greater your tolerance for uncertainty, the easier time you'll have. Acknowledge and accept that your immediate future inevitably will entail many situations that are new and different for you, and that uncertainty is bound to be present.

Live your life as fully as you can in the moment. The quality of your "being" (living in the present, rather than worrying about an uncertain future) contributes to the richness of your life. Use this as an opportunity to reorder your priorities, so that you have little remorse or regrets about what might have been. Don't sweat the small stuff. Make a contribution to others, perhaps through some form of volunteer work. By serving others you may transcend your own difficulties and feel better about yourself. You can find your own way to decrease your anxiety and to enjoy your life even when uncertainty exists.

FEAR

Fear can range in intensity from simple apprehension and dread to sheer terror. Everyone lives with fears of one kind or another. Common among humans is a fear of the unknown. With recent amputation, this may mean fearing the unknown effects of limb loss on your relationships, your vocation, and your physical abilities. You may fear living life as a disabled person, or becoming dependent on others. Depending on the cause of your amputation, you may fear death, as well.

Fear plays a crucial role in our survival; it provides an invaluable service. Fear lets us know when we face danger, and spurs us to take some kind of action to preserve ourselves or others from a perilous situation. In this respect, like anger, fear can serve as a great motivator.

CONQUERING YOUR FEARS

As with other painful emotions, people tend to respond to fear in a variety of ways. If you surrender to or deny your fears, or if you are unwilling to deal with the realities that threaten you, there is no way you can take the actions necessary for self-preservation. *As a result, you will suffer the consequences of the threat that underlies your fear.*

However, when you meet your fears head on and address their causes, you demonstrate a powerful combination—courage and the ability to take action. You may find yourself internally strengthened by the experience, no matter what the outcome. In this way, facing your fears is self-affirming. Overcoming fear takes a positive frame of mind and a willingness to put forth some necessary effort.

Discover What is Really Bothering You

Knowing what is really bothering you is a key factor in meeting and conquering your fears. If you take time to probe deep within yourself and examine what truly frightens you about living with amputation, you will probably discover one basic fear—*the fear that you will not be able to cope successfully with the physical, emotional, and/or spiritual challenges that confront you.* This underlying fear serves as the foundation for other fears.

I urge you to take in this concept. Digest it. Contemplate it. Assimilate it. (If you're a sci-fi fan, "grok it.") When you realize that doubting your ability to successfully deal with what confronts you is your main fear, you can turn your efforts from the fear itself to the strategies necessary to strengthen your confidence.

When you feel that you can successfully handle whatever comes your way, you will have the confidence needed to cross through your fear. What follows are some strategies to help you reduce your fears by bolstering your confidence.

Recognize and Acknowledge Your Fear

It is very hard to take action to combat a fear without first recognizing specifically what the fear is. That's why it can be more difficult to deal with vague anxiety than with fear. Thus, the first step in coping with fear is to become clear about what you are afraid of—what is it *specifically* that you feel you cannot handle? When answering this question, be as honest and exact as possible.

For example, instead of telling yourself, "I'm afraid to go out in public," be more specific about that fear. Rather admit, "I'm afraid I won't be able to handle the responses of others—their stares, their cruel and insensitive comments, their rejection . . ." Once you have zeroed in on specific fears, you can more easily come up with strategies to help you handle them.

Naming your fear is the first step to help you gain a sense of control. When fear is generalized, there is no direct target to attack, no way to construct a strategy to guide your actions.

Realize You Have Mastered Past Fears

Recognize all the times in your life in which you have demonstrated courage and worked through your fears. Each of us has had this experience innumerable times as we have grown from children to adults. Perhaps you can remember experiencing fear of the dark, of monsters, or of the school bully. Perhaps you experienced a fear of going out on that first date. Can you remember feeling fear during a job interview? Somehow or other, you developed successful strategies that enabled you to work through those old fears. Knowing that you did so in the past can give you the confidence to do so again.

To help you rekindle the qualities that enabled you to surmount past fears, try the following technique: Close your eyes and take a few deep breaths. Relax, and allow the tension to flow out of your body. Take time to fully remember a specific instance in which you took action and overcame a fear. Use your senses to recall how you felt and what you saw as you mastered your fear. Listen to what you told yourself about the experience, and notice how you felt about your self-worth and your ability to surmount the obstacle. Try to remember how wonderfully energized and uplifted you felt when you conquered that fear. Repeat the sequence using at least two more examples, remembering to use all of your senses when doing so. Now, carry all of those positive, empowering feelings forward with you, and imagine yourself meeting your current fear with all that internal strength and confidence intact. Imagine yourself taking successful action and conquering your fear. You'll discover that when you act "as if" you are fully confident of your ability to conquer your fear, it is easier to manifest that ability.

Use Positive Affirmations and Visualization

Strengthen your confidence to successfully meet challenges and work through your fears through the use of positive affirmations, visualizations, and self-hypnosis.

One of the ways we tend to generate anxiety and fear is by anticipating the worst. We may tell ourselves such things as, "I won't be able to deal with . . ." "I'll fall apart if . . ." or "I can't handle . . ." If you tell yourself these kinds of statements over and over, they are likely to become self-ful- filling prophecies. When you repeatedly visualize the worst possible out- come, you are actually giving yourself a series of hypnotic suggestions.

In Chapter 13, "Self-Esteem," you will learn to recognize and counter this type of negative self-talk of the internal critic. You will also learn to tell yourself realistic, affirming statements, such as, "I will get though this," "I can relax and trust my inner wisdom to guide me," and "No matter what happens, ultimately, I will be okay."

Be aware of the power of language (detailed in Chapter 15, "Making Meaning of Your Amputation"). For example, notice the difference in your self-concept when you consider yourself an amputee, rather than "a person with amputation." Notice the difference in your responses when you consider difficulties in your life as "challenges," or crises as "opportuni- ties." Instead of telling yourself, "I don't know how I'll ever meet this fear," rather say, "I don't know which strategy is best to meet this fear *yet.*"

Meet Your Fears Head On

Honestly acknowledge your fear, and then put it into proper perspective— the totality of who you are is much greater than that of your fear. Imagine what would happen if your fear were fully realized. You would probably find a way to make the best of the situation, and then move on. It's been said that if you are willing to accept the "worst," then you are ready to accept the "best." After interviewing many people for this book, and counseling a wide variety of individuals who have survived physical and/or emotional abuse as children or adults, I am convinced that we, as human beings, have great resiliency. We have the capability to conquer our fears, the capacity to heal, and the ability to prosper.

By addressing the topics discussed in other chapters in this section, (managing stress, coping with emotions, enhancing self-esteem, etc.), you will build a strong foundation to help provide you with the strength, self-confidence, and courage to triumph over your fears.

Adjust your attitude and beliefs. Become aware of areas in which you are distorting reality through faulty thinking, then correct those distortions. Replace negative self-talk with encouraging, affirming statements. Do what you can to manage your stress and to relax. Draw on your strengths. If you are spiritually inclined, draw on the strength of a higher power to aid you.

Use the many resources that are available to help you through your fears. Speak with or read about others who have conquered similar fears, and find out how they did it. Work with a professional counselor who can help you name your fears, correct distorted or destructive thinking patterns, and teach you strategies to make your coping process easier. Visit the self-help section of your local bookstore or library. There are a number of valuable books and audio tapes available to assist you in developing strategies to help you surmount your fears. Once you decide on the best strategies, you can take action.

TAKE RISKS

What is it that you truly want in your life? A satisfying relationship? Material success? Meaningful work? To be able to express your creativity? To make a contribution to others? To live in alignment with your highest spiritual aspirations? Whatever goals and dreams you set for yourself are worthwhile; realizing them involves taking risks. When you reach out and take action to make your visions a reality, you must be willing to "stick your neck out," "put yourself on the line," "go for it," and "just do it." These very expressions imply that living your life fully, attempting to realize your dreams and goals, is risky business. Risk involves fear in that you are extending yourself beyond your normal comfort zone to try something new.

What happens if you take a risk, attempt something new, and then fail? You can use the results to provide information on how to readjust your actions to achieve your desired result. An integral part of the learning process is trial and error. So try one approach; if it doesn't work out to your satisfaction, either adjust it or try something different. Remember, there is no such thing as failure—just feedback.

You must be willing to risk the possibility of being uncomfortable and vulnerable while attempting new ways of thinking, feeling, or behaving. You must be willing to act, even when you are uncertain of the outcome. When you are not willing to take risks, you "risk" staying stuck in a familiar, narrow world. Most things worth having, doing, or being involve risk; you cannot grow without it.

TAKE ACTION

Fear produces energy. Use this energy as a catalyst to move through the fear. Channel that intense feeling into sharp focus, then concentrate your efforts to take action.

Fear can be converted into power. To illustrate this notion, let me share a personal story with you. At one point during my recovery I completed a "firewalk." I successfully traversed a path of burning coals, alternating steps over those blazing embers with my bare foot and my prosthetic one. (Hey, I'm from California, what did you expect?) Seriously, although I don't advocate firewalks for everyone, it was a positive experience for me. (Certainly, this is not something to try on your own! I carefully prepared for my firewalk under the guidance of an expert, and during my walk I was carefully monitored by a skilled facilitator. If I had not been fully ready for the firewalk, I would have been stopped before I stepped.)

What was the point of my adventure? What was the point of risking my only foot? The goal of a firewalk is to convert fear into power—it involves consciously acknowledging the fear, developing a strategy to meet that fear head on, then taking action to pass through it. It is an empowering experience. You can bet the experience of walking over a bed of hot coals (without even raising a blister) served to reinforce my belief that I can cross through my own fears and find power and self-mastery on the other side.

Every day, all types of people successfully complete their own versions of firewalks—perhaps by mastering a fear of heights, taking risks in a relationship, asking their boss for a raise, going out in public for the first time with their amputation visible, or taking their first steps with a prosthesis. These "personal firewalks" include acknowledging a fear, developing a strategy to get through that fear, and then taking whatever action is necessary to get to the other side. They are thus empowered. If others can do it, you can, too.

IN CONCLUSION

Fear and uncertainty are a part of living. Unlike reading a novel, you can't jump ahead to discover the outcome of future events. The story of your life is written as you live it. Uncertainty actually contributes to the excitement and suspense of living. Realize that you can still enjoy your life without having all the answers. Once you understand this, you can relax a bit, recognizing one thing that is certain—uncertainty is to be expected.

Fears are bound to arise when you undergo the trauma of limb loss. It is what you do once you have acknowledged your fear that allows you to use it as a catalyst for empowerment. Keep in mind the role fear plays in your survival; it lets you know when you face danger and must take action. Acknowledge and specifically "name" your fear. Develop strategies to increase your ability to master it, and then take action. When you let your fear motivate you to draw more deeply on your inner resources, and then act accordingly, you come away strengthened by your experience. While it requires courage to meet you fears head on, the risks are well worth it. In approaching your fears in this way, you will grow. You will demonstrate the strength, perseverance, and courage, through which to realize your goals and dreams. The rewards of mastering your fears include the exhilaration of internal freedom and self-mastery, as well as the peace and confidence that comes from the realization that you can cope successfully with whatever life brings your way.

11

DEPRESSION

At one time or another, most of us have experienced bouts of feeling "blue," "down in the dumps," "disillusioned," or "down and out." Occasional feelings of depression are a natural part of life, as are feelings of great joy and quiet contentment. When you add the stress of amputation to the usual pressures of life, it is not surprising that you might have some difficulty maintaining your equilibrium and feel depressed from time to time.

Depression following limb loss is perfectly normal, and to be expected at times as you adjust to your new physical reality. Bouts with depression may be brief or extended and may come and go as you progress through your own unique path of healing. Let's face it, losing a limb and readjusting to life is no picnic.

Depression has been called "anger turned inward." Following amputation, your anger may be due to the realization that limb loss is irreversible, and you are powerless to change that fact. You may experience feelings of helplessness and hopelessness over your new-found circumstances—having to undergo medical treatment and physical therapy, possibly having to deal with an underlying medical condition, and having to go through the process of being fitted for a prosthesis. Concern about the effects of your limb loss on your personal relationships, work, and lifestyle; fear of becoming dependent on others for physical assistance; and worry that your situation will never improve significantly can all take a toll on your well-being and understandably put a damper on your *joi de vivre*.

This chapter presents information to help you understand what depression is and what causes it. It suggests steps you can take to diminish the hold depression may have on you and to prevent it from recurring.

EXACTLY WHAT IS DEPRESSION?

There are many misconceptions about what depression is. Sadness, fatigue, and feeling blue, although often confused with depression, are actually natural reactions to loss. However, when these symptoms persist beyond a reasonable time and are coupled with other symptoms (presented below), then you have a chronic condition, which psychologists term as an *affective disorder.* This may be diagnosed as clinical depression, and you deserve some assistance in treating it.

According to the American Psychiatric Association, depression includes a variety of physical and psychological symptoms, although all do not have to be present to make the diagnosis. And depending on the severity of the symptoms, depression can be classified as mild, moderate, or severe. Symptoms of depression include:

• Depressed mood most of the day, nearly every day.

• Markedly diminished interest or pleasure in all, or almost all, activities most of the day; signs of apathy.

• Significant changes in normal appetite with weight gain or weight loss.

• Changes in sleep patterns, such as increased sleeping or insomnia.

• Slowed speech or body movements.

• Signs of increased physical agitation, such as the inability to stay still.

• Diminished ability to think or concentrate; indecisiveness.

• Fatigue or loss of energy, nearly every day.

• Feelings of worthlessness or excessive guilt.

• Recurrent thoughts of death or suicide.

These symptoms represent a marked change from usual levels of functioning and are relatively persistent. There is some degree of interference with the activities of everyday living in areas such as vocation and interactions with others.

You, yourself, will most likely know when you have become truly depressed; others who are close to you may also notice and point it out to you. If life is "without flavor," if you just don't seem to find any pleasure in living, or if you don't seem to care about improving the quality of your life—you may be depressed. If you give in to feeling helpless, hopeless, and/or disillusioned, or if you display symptoms from the list above—you may well be depressed. It is important to be sure that your symptoms are not due to an underlying physical condition or illness, or the result of medication. These can cause symptoms that mimic depression. Therefore, a thorough physical evaluation by your physician is advisable.

Depression is painful! Often people who are depressed will do whatever they can to deaden themselves, so as not to feel the pain. Some people may find themselves withdrawing from their usual circle of friends and family, or from activities they used to enjoy. It is as if they have made a decision to curl up into a little ball and form a self-protective cocoon to block out the exterior world. Normal zest for life and the motivation to be actively involved in living is diminished.

Other individuals turn to drugs and/or alcohol to mask painful feelings and to avoid facing reality. In addition to the obvious threat of addiction, another problem with this approach is that the underlying cause(s) of the depression is not treated, so the depression will persist.

In a very small percentage of individuals, the severe depression that follows amputation can have the most serious of emotional consequences—suicide may seem like the only way to put an end to their pain. These people do not want to die but can see no other alternative to end their suffering. They are without hope for their future. When the pain you are experiencing is unbearable, you may have thoughts that you might be better off dead, no longer a burden to yourself or others. You may feel that things will never get any better, or that your life has lost all value without your limb. Although such thoughts may creep into your mind, know that they will usually pass. And remember that suicide is a "permanent solution to a temporary problem." If you succeed in ending your life, there is no second chance.

If you are severely depressed and feeling desperate, and you contemplate "ending it all," *seek professional help immediately!* If necessary, get assistance from a loved one, a friend, or a health-care provider to find immediate professional help. If you are feeling absolutely desperate, pick up the phone and dial the operator. Explain that it is an emergency and ask to be connected with a suicide hotline. You have nothing to lose and everything to gain by getting professional assistance. Know that there is help for you.

It is crucial for you to believe that you can make it through this painful time and enjoy your life again. For more information on this topic, see Chapter 16, "Seeking Professional Counseling."

TREATING DEPRESSION

The good news is that while depression is a common by-product of the stresses and challenges brought on by amputation, it is generally temporary in duration and very amenable to treatment. This is particularly true when your depression has much of its origin in patterns of thought and beliefs that are destructive to your well-being. Life-long patterns of destructive thinking, feeling, or behaving have set you up for depression, so when the crisis of amputation came along, depression followed. You can, however, learn to interrupt these negative patterns and feel good about yourself again.

It is often difficult for people who are depressed to talk about their feelings and seek professional help. It may help motivate you to know that, fortunately, depression is very responsive to treatment that involves psychological counseling, or a combination of drug treatment and counseling.

Nobody wants to feel the pain and despair of depression. The problem is that most people don't know how to change their condition. You can help yourself combat depression by developing positive ways of thinking, feeling, and behaving. In order to support a lifestyle in which you feel good, you may need to establish a new balance in all dimensions of your being—physical, mental, emotional, and spiritual. The approaches presented in this chapter are for treating depression on all of these levels.

In addition to the approaches discussed in this chapter, addressing the topics in other chapters in this section (managing stress, enhancing self-esteem, coping with emotions, etc.) will also help combat depression. Any combination of these approaches may work for you. Just as more than one tool can be used to accomplish a given job, the more tools in your belt, the more options you will have. Having options results in a greater degree of flexibility and allows you to free yourself from destructive thoughts, beliefs, and behavior patterns. Since you are a unique individual, what works for you may be different from what might work for someone else.

Psychological Treatment

When symptoms of depression persist and are ruining the quality of your life, it is definitely time to seek help from a professional psychological counselor. It is also important to obtain an evaluation from your physician to uncover a possible underlying physical disorder that may be contributing to your depressed state, such as a biochemical imbalance that can be treated with medication.

People may have misconceptions about what it means if they seek counseling, or what will happen during counseling sessions. They may wonder what type of counselor or counseling might work best for them. For detailed information on this topic, see Chapter 16, "Seeking Professional Counseling."

Physical Exercise

Participating in regular physical exercise and other physical activities can be a valuable tool to help promote emotional well-being, as well as physical health. Due to the interconnection of body and mind, your physical state can effect your emotional/mental state, and vice versa.

Perhaps you have noticed some of the physical signs associated with depression—slumped shoulders, shallow breathing, shuffling feet, etc. Often, you can change how you are feeling emotionally by changing your physical state. In addition, when your depression is due in part to repressed, painful feelings, such as anger and deep frustration, it is especially useful to discharge that pent-up energy through vigorous activity. You will feel more energized and at peace when you do so.

Sometimes depression seems to suck your vitality dry, so the very thought of exercise can be depressing in itself. (As my father has said on occasion, "Whenever I get the urge to exercise, I sit down until the urge goes away.") Yet, vigorous exercise may serve to snap you out of a stuck place. Changing your physiology might not in itself "cure" depression, but it can permit you to feel good enough to approach what is underlying your depression with a bit more energy and vitality. Aside from its physical health benefits, participating in a regular exercise routine can also help prevent a re-emergence of the blues.

Drug Treatment

If your depression has been long-lived or is very severe, you might not feel motivated or well enough to participate in therapy. Drug treatment can be very effective in combating the symptoms of depression. Sometimes antidepressants can raise your feelings of well-being so that you can participate in therapy. It is my opinion that drug therapy alone is not a good idea, because the underlying issues that have triggered the depressed state are not addressed.

The only counseling professionals who can prescribe drug treatment are psychiatrists, since they are also medical doctors. Many times, other types of counselors have a working relationship with a psychiatrist and can refer you for an evaluation for drug therapy.

Some researchers believe that certain individuals experience depression due to a biochemical imbalance. In some cases, drug treatment may help restore normal body function, causing the depression to cease. When undergoing drug therapy, it is important to be under the careful supervision of a doctor. However, even in these cases, destructive thoughts and behavior may also contribute to depression. Therefore, for maximum well-being, it is helpful to learn to modify one's thinking and actions.

WORKING WITH YOUR EMOTIONS

One of the most effective ways to help work through your depression is to allow yourself to acknowledge and express your feelings. It may be that you have repressed feelings such as anger, sadness, or despair, which may have seemed too scary, too painful, or too overwhelming to express.

Sweeping platitudes made by others, such as, "Everything will be just fine," or "You'll get over this," or the guilt-instilling, "You've got to get over this for the family," do not match the reality you are encountering. Such statements may leave you feeling that your emotions are not valid, and that it is not okay to feel depressed. Nonsense! It would be very unusual indeed to lose a limb and not feel down about it at times. While it is important to accurately acknowledge your feelings, it is not a good idea to allow your negative feelings to rule you and your actions. This will keep you depressed. Try to maintain balance by placing value on your rational thoughts. Use the information that your thoughts and feelings provide to guide you in changing any destructive thought patterns or beliefs; this will help to disperse your depressed state.

What follows is a discussion of some common emotions that may contribute to depression. Other emotions that may help to generate depression, as well as coping strategies for dealing with them, are detailed in other chapters in Part II.

Disappointment

As ecstatic as you may feel to finally be home from the hospital after your surgery, it is also likely that you will feel a bit let down after the first few weeks or months. You may notice that you have fallen out of the limelight, you are no longer the focus of attention. Eventually, friends and family will stop their frequent visits. You may find yourself suddenly alone, surrounded by time and solitude to confront the life-altering changes you have been through. Disappointment may set in.

Going home can be daunting and, perhaps, depressing in that you have returned to your old familiar surroundings with an altered body. You have undergone personal trauma and must learn to adapt; you must not only survive, but, hopefully, thrive.

When you are disappointed, you feel your expectations or desires have not been fulfilled. You may thus feel thwarted, frustrated, and perhaps even sad and defeated. Since you may conclude that your expectations will never be realized, you may tend to stay stuck in your disappointment.

Rather than letting your disappointment puncture your dreams and goals, thereby immobilizing your efforts, I encourage you to use your disappointment as an opportunity to revise your goals and develop new strategies to achieve them. This is an excellent time to really reconsider what it is you wish to achieve. In devising new goals, you need to remember that your desired objectives may take time to achieve, so your timetable must be realistic. Develop an optimistic outlook, and stay focused on your life-affirming goals and visions.

Feeling Overwhelmed

Life surges ahead on many planes simultaneously. Following your amputation surgery, you are thrust into a relatively new world in which it seems you must attend to many concerns at once. Your immediate physical and medical needs, your emotional adjustment, and your family all call out for your attention. During this time, you are encountering many firsts, such as the first time coping with the responses of others, and the first time attempting a task one-handed, or from a wheelchair, or while wearing a prosthesis. Since the process of your recovery is not linear, your attention and focus may be pulled in several directions at once. No wonder you might, at times, feel overwhelmed by it all. If you attempt to take in everything at once, you will likely succumb to feeling overwhelmed. Also, if you don't view items separately, it will be difficult for you to attend to them one at a time in a manageable way.

Feeling overwhelmed can contribute to depression, since it causes you to feel as if you are drowning emotionally and can't get your head above water. You may lose sight of your priorities, and surrender by letting everything go and no longer attending to your needs.

Feelings of inadequacy often exist concurrently with feelings of being overwhelmed. You may fear that you do not have the personal resources necessary to meet the tasks at hand. With the many challenges you must face, particularly those immediately following amputation, it's no wonder that from time to time, you might find yourself feeling inadequate to meet these challenges.

I don't know many people who can give wholehearted focus and attention to more than one challenging issue at a time, no matter how much of a Superman or Wonder Woman they are! It is no surprise that people can lapse into anxiety, despair, and feelings of being overwhelmed when they attempt to deal with too many issues at once!

The following suggestions are designed to keep you from becoming overwhelmed with the many challenges you must address:

• **Prioritize the issues you must deal with.** "I'll attend to this now. That can wait until later." It is simply much easier and more efficient to deal with one issue at a time, rather than several at once.

• **Recognize areas in which your efforts will be for naught.** "There is nothing I can do about that, so I'm going to let it go."

• **Be specific with your goals.** Know exactly what you want and where you want to go. Define for yourself some measurable criteria that will let you know when you have achieved your objective.

• **When you are feeling inadequate, get outside assistance.** An expert in the area in which you need improvement can help you learn new skills and/or develop a new approach. By actively engaging in learning new skills, you are telling yourself that you are capable of learning and growing. In this way, you empower yourself.

• **If necessary, shift your perspective of yourself.** If you have been judging yourself too harshly and demanding an unreasonable performance (given your current skill level or physical health), have some compassion for yourself. Readjust your standards to be more realistic. Remember, you can modify your standards again when you learn new skills as your recovery progresses.

Life is complex. Its multidimensionality adds depth and richness to our experience of living. Following the suggestions just presented will assist you in regaining your confidence and equanimity, as well as a sense of mastery over the challenges you face.

Feeling Loss of Control

One way we survive as human beings is by imposing order in our lives through controlling ourselves and our environment; this helps us make sense of our reality and rule our destiny. We seek control so that our world will be predictable. Based on that predictability, we are able to make decisions and assign meaning to our lives. When you undergo amputation, often predictability is thrown out the window; you are forced into a new realm in which your body, medical and prosthetic care, and the responses of others seem outside your control.

When you feel as if you have lost control over your life, you may also experience feelings of anxiety, helplessness, frustration, anger, and/or resignation. Feeling overwhelmed is almost inevitable. When events in life seem to dominate and dictate your responses and behaviors, you have "given up your power" to these exterior events. When you feel at a loss to rule your own destiny, depression may result.

It is vital to learn to make the distinction between what you can control in your life, and what is outside the boundaries of your control. When you try to exercise your power and influence without first making that distinction, you may be setting yourself up for frustration, disappointment, anger, resentment, and ultimately, depression.

In *Free Yourself from Depression* (Emmaus, PA: Rodale Press, 1992), Dr. Michael Yapko presents two common distorted beliefs about control that are actually opposite of each other—one is the belief that *you have no control over a situation in which you actually do have influence;* the second is the belief that *you do have control over a situation in which you actually have no power.* The natural result of either belief is a sense of powerlessness and helplessness. Believing you have no control creates passivity in the face of obstacles that can be overcome with the right strategy; on the other hand, believing you can control a situation that, in actuality, you can't, results in feelings of impotence and ineffectiveness. Thus, it is important to your well-being to develop a realistic view of what can and cannot be controlled in your life.

The following suggestions are provided to help you maintain a realistic sense of control over the situations you face in life:

• **Realistically evaluate what you can and cannot control.** Think about it, you have no or very little control over many aspects of your world, such as the weather or world politics. You cannot control other people—you cannot make them like you or force them to have the same value system that you have.

Therefore, it is crucial for you to evaluate a given situation or problem realistically, and recognize how much control is reasonable for you to exert. By doing so, you will save time and emotional energy in situations that are bound to turn out differently from how you would like them to.

So approach problems and situations with realistic and specific strategies. You will likely get better results when the steps you take are within your sphere of influence.

• **Be an active participant in your life.** Assert appropriate control when you can realistically influence the outcome of a situation. Whenever possible, make conscious choices about your actions, attitudes, and responses. Seek answers to questions you might have, and gather any information that might assist you. If needed, enlist the aid of others. Even when something seems beyond your control, ask yourself, "What can I do to influence the outcome of this event?" Any small aspect of influence can permit you to feel more in control, less directed by outer circumstances.

Be an active participant in your life, rather than a passive bystander; be someone who lives life, rather than someone who life happens to. Objectively analyze events, your goals, and your dreams, and discover what part you can play in influencing their outcome. By actively participating in your life, you will regain a sense of control over your circumstances. You will feel that your health care and recovery are not happening *to* you, but *with* your conscious involvement. Your self-esteem will be enhanced and you will feel empowered.

• **Work with your own responses to those events that are beyond your control.** When a situation is actually beyond your intervention, work with your responses to it. You can have direct control over your responses; this is an area in which you can greatly impact your level of internal equilibrium. Examine you feelings; look for destructive or nonproductive beliefs underlying your responses. Work on yourself to change your attitudes, beliefs, and assumptions.

Be gentle and compassionate with yourself. When you've done all you can to affect an outcome, tell yourself you've given it your all, and make peace with that outcome. If you feel you might have handled the situation differently, note specifically how you might have done so; consider it a learning experience, and to the best of your ability, let go of your remorses, your "what ifs," and your "if onlys." Let go of the past—live fully in the present, while sowing the seeds for a positive future.

WORKING WITH YOUR THOUGHTS AND BELIEFS

Ups and downs are a natural part of living. Along with the profound joys that are part and parcel of our lives as human beings, sooner or later we all face times of crisis and sorrow. Why do some of us seem to sail through the choppiest waters, while others flounder and sink? In part, the answer lies with each person's thoughts, beliefs, and ways of interpreting reality. Your thoughts and beliefs have a profound influence on your well-being. When you act as if your thoughts and beliefs are an accurate description of reality, or the only possible interpretation of reality, a "self-fulfilling prophecy" may ensue. You will tend to materialize the fruits of these thoughts and beliefs through your actions and interpretations of events. For example, if you are depressed and tell yourself the worst things about your life, you will interpret events and act in ways to reconfirm your negative feelings; your downward spiral will continue. If you tell yourself you are no longer a "whole" person due to your limb loss, you will act in ways which demonstrate that you no longer feel "worthy" and are no longer of equal value with others.

The meaning you make of the events in your life is highly personal. No two human beings have exactly the same value system or interpret circumstances in exactly the same way. We each have own distinctly individual filters through which we evaluate our life's experiences. These filters are based on such things as the influence of past events on our lives, our biological make-up, our thinking style and values, and our social environment. We interpret both outer and inner circumstances through these filters, causing us to project subjective meaning onto the events in our lives.

Thus, when you act as if the meaning you assign an event is the Truth (with a capital T)—as if it were handed down from on High, etched in stone—you may be setting yourself up for disappointment. This can lead to frustration, anger, and eventually, depression. For more detailed information on this topic, refer to Chapter 15, "Making Meaning of Your Amputation."

Destructive Beliefs

How do limiting thoughts, attitudes, and beliefs arise? While growing up, you learned them from such sources as your parents and other family members, your peers, the media, as well as society in general. You were influenced by the actions that others took or didn't take, by what they said or didn't say.

Many of these beliefs are so ingrained in our minds that we don't even recognize them as beliefs at all; instead, we assume they are truths that reflect reality. "I shouldn't express anger. It's a sign of being out of control," and "I should always act nice, no matter how I feel," are examples of common beliefs that are mistakenly considered truths. Such beliefs cause us to limit our actions and narrow our options.

Let's take a look at a few simple examples of how distorted beliefs can contribute to self-limitation:

• Suppose your mother taught you that it was rude to ask for anything that wasn't offered to you. (Are you likely to ask for what you need in life?)

• Suppose your father had the attitude that children are to be seen and not heard. (Are you likely to speak your mind easily?)

• Suppose your grandfather believed that it was time for him to die when he could no longer drive, hear, or walk. (How are you likely to handle physical limitations?)

While these examples may not fit you exactly, you will likely find other obvious examples from your own life. When you see how negative beliefs can limit and hinder you, you can begin to imagine how other negative beliefs and attitudes can block your happiness and well-being.

How We Distort Reality

We distort reality by imposing our own subjective feelings and perceptions onto what objectively exists. Richard Bandler and John Grinder, in *The Structure of Magic* (Palo Alto, CA: Science and Behavior Books, Inc., 1975) detail how this alteration of reality occurs. We do this through the use of *deletion, distortion,* and *generalization*.

When you *delete* reality, you leave out portions of information that are important in obtaining a complete objective view. For example, a person with diabetes swears his physician never told him the consequences of not following a careful diet, when, in fact, these consequences were discussed in depth on several occasions.

When you *distort* reality, you alter the facts so that things appear to be better, worse, or otherwise different from objective reality. For example, suppose that because of a physical limitation due to your limb loss, you fantasize yourself as hopeless and dependent on others for the rest of your life. Such a distortion may cause you to give up hope without a fight.

When you *generalize,* you make broad sweeping statements about the way things always are, even when there may be many exceptions to prove you wrong. For example, suppose you fall once while learning to walk with your prosthetic leg. As a result, you tell yourself that you will *never* learn to master walking with a prosthesis, so you give up trying. (Notice when you use such absolute words as "always" and "never." They are clues that you might be generalizing.)

It is easy to understand how through the use of deletion, distortion, and generalization, you can quite effectively launch yourself into the depths of despair, and then keep yourself there. Any thoughts, attitudes, and beliefs that fail to recognize simply "what really is" are are actually distortions of reality. They are impediments to your well-being if they prevent you from living happily and productively.

There are concrete steps you can take to prevent distorted, and therefore, limiting, thoughts and beliefs. Consider the following suggestions:

• **Become aware. Learn to recognize limiting thoughts and beliefs.** When you find yourself feeling emotionally constricted, depressed, or having a strong negative reaction to the events in your life, take time to become aware of your thoughts and beliefs; analyze them, challenge their objectivity. Are your thoughts and beliefs based upon a distorted interpretation of objective reality? If you're not sure, ask the opinion of a trusted friend, family member, or professional counselor.

• **Rule your thoughts and beliefs, rather than be ruled by them.** It is within your power to consciously choose how you interpret the events in your life. Through awareness, you can learn to catch yourself in patterns of distorted thinking, and negative thoughts and beliefs, and then transform them into beliefs that are life-affirming. By using your awareness, you can shift what you choose to tell yourself and believe about reality.

Learning to do this is a new skill for many people. Just as with time and practice you learned how to recite the alphabet, how to read, and how to ride a bicycle, you can master the skills necessary to lift yourself out of the habitual patterns of negative, distorted thinking.

• **Become aware of your "inner critic" and diffuse its power.** Listen to the running commentary you make in your mind about what is happening in your life. How often do you criticize or judge yourself negatively, and then draw conclusions about such areas as your worth, loveability, attractiveness, and competency? The problem with the inner critic is that the conclusions it draws often are not based on objective reality. If you act as if these conclusions are real, you may end up very depressed, overwhelmed by your life, frustrated by your own "inadequacies," and burdened with a negative self-image. For further information on this topic, see Chapter 13, "Self-Esteem."

• **Discover the benefits of a positive belief system.** Just as distorted beliefs can be extraordinarily limiting, beliefs based on the assumption that you are worthy and will have a positive future can be expansive and freeing. Take a moment and ask yourself, "What goals would I set for myself in my life, if I knew I would succeed?" "What talents would I like to express?" "If I had confidence and felt great about myself, what risks would I be willing to take?" "How might my life be different?" "If I believe myself to be worthy, deserving, loveable, and fully capable, how would it affect my life and sense of well-being?"

Take time to shift your focus away from your immediate concerns and develop a vision of how you would like your life to be; clearly define your dreams and goals. Where are you heading? Imagine your life in six months—in a year. How do you envision yourself most positively? What concrete steps can you take to draw yourself closer to your goals? Realign your self-talk and your actions to be consistent with your vision.

As you make progress toward realizing your goals, take the time to acknowledge your successes, whether large or small. This will reinforce your sense of competency and well-being, enabling you to progress toward a positive future.

• **Be flexible.** A person with behavioral flexibility is well equipped to move through the changing currents of life. This flexibility is especially helpful when responding to depression. While a tree that is supple and able to bend in many directions will do so in the winds of a storm, a tree with a rigid trunk or branches will break. When you free yourself from limiting thoughts and beliefs, you will find that you have the ability to make conscious choices about your beliefs and actions. Knowing that you have choices and can respond flexibly and creatively to the events in your life is both effective and empowering.

You have the ability to greatly enhance your well-being by becoming aware of your thoughts and beliefs, and challenging those that do not serve you. Instill ones that do. This ability has nothing to do with the number of limbs you have or your physical condition. I encourage you to discover the constraints of your mental limitations and lift the lid off them. The reward for doing so will be self-empowerment and internal freedom.

Is Your Glass Half Empty or Half Full?

One way in which your thoughts and beliefs influence your well-being is through your level of optimism. If you tell yourself, "There is no hope. Why should I bother trying? My efforts won't amount to anything," you have provided reasons to give up. While this attitude may protect you from failure and disappointment, you will never get a chance to find out what is truly possible when you meet life's challenges head on. Therefore, you are not only limiting your potential for failure, you are also limiting your potential for success.

The state of disillusionment is like looking at your life through mud-colored glasses. Each negative assessment of your reality adds more mud to the lenses, so you feel further trapped in powerlessness and despair; in this state, it is hard to summon the energy and enthusiasm to believe that any of your efforts will make a difference. There is a danger that you will be drawn to "self-medicating" with drugs and/or alcohol to numb your sense of hopelessness.

Your beliefs and attitudes have profound impact on your actions, motivations, and the way you feel about yourself. Since the same event can be interpreted in totally different ways (depending upon your point of view), it is obviously more useful to be an optimist than a pessimist. Optimism generally allows you to enjoy your life more.

Considering it objectively, a glass that is half full holds the same amount of liquid as a glass that is half empty. Since you have the choice, why not choose to view the glass as half full?

IN CONCLUSION

The good news is that while depression is often a by-product of the stresses and challenges brought on by amputation, it is generally temporary in duration and very amenable to treatment. You can learn to handle depression and prevent its recurrence by understanding what it is, and by employing some of the many concrete steps and strategies to combat it. It has been said that every adversity contains within it the seeds for growth and improved quality of living. Depression can provide just such an opportunity. The price is self-effort and commitment, but the result is definitely worth the cost. Whether you work on your own or with the help of a professional, do something today! Life is too precious to waste.

12

STRESS

Stress is defined as:

—a physical pressure, pull, or other force exerted on one thing by another.
—any stimulus, as fear or pain, that disturbs or interferes with the normal physiological equilibrium of an organism.
—physical, mental, or emotional strain or tension.

In a way, these definitions are superfluous—given that you are alive, you already know what stress is, since it is an inherent part of daily living. Who hasn't felt some degree of stress when sitting in rush hour traffic or stuck in a never-ending line at the Department of Motor Vehicles? Who, at times, hasn't experienced some pressure over a job, a relationship, or over paying the bills?

Having undergone an amputation, you know what "major league" stress is. You are bound to be exposed to a wide variety of stressors—the surgery; the process of recovery and rehabilitation; the inevitable changes in lifestyle, relationships, and, possibly, vocation; and the necessary modification of self-concept and body image.

Stress intensifies whatever process you are going through. And stress can be either useful or harmful. Useful stress enables you to mobilize your inner resources for action; harmful stress, due to its intensity and/or duration, can deplete your internal physical and emotional resources, and overwhelm your ability to cope.

How you handle stress depends upon your overall make-up and general coping abilities. The toll stress takes on you is determined by a number of factors, some of which include: how many stressful events you have experienced in the past; how frequently you face stress; how well you generally adapt to it; and what conscious measures you take to counteract the triggers of stress.

If you do not expect to face stressful events in your life, you will likely become upset when things do not go your way. On the other hand, by *accepting* the fact that stress-invoking situations will inevitably crop up a the most unexpected times and places, you will be more relaxed, better humored, and more capable of responding flexibly to situations.

Accepting the realities of life includes the recognition that we are not perfect, we have strengths and frailties. When we can accept ourselves for who we are, "warts and all," a great deal of internally generated stress is diminished. We have taken ourselves off the hook of having to be perfect. A more detailed discussion of self-acceptance is presented in Chapter 13, "Self-Esteem."

HOW STRESS SERVES US

In the chapter "Learning to Cope with External and Internal Stressors" from *Learning to Live Well with Diabetes* (Minneapolis, MN: DCI Publishing, 1991), Randi S. Birk, M.A., L.P. says:

> Each of us is like the strings on a violin—if there is no tension on those strings, there will be no music. Similarly, if we have no stress—no challenge—in our lives, we may become bored or even ill. Yet, if we keep tightening the pegs on that violin, the strings will surely snap. And if we keep adding more and more stress to our life, at some point we will "snap" in the sense that we may experience a physical or emotional problem. . . . try to identify the right level of stress for you—the level at which you can "play well" and yet not be overwhelmed.

Not only is stress an inherent part of life, but taken in the proper balance, it can actually serve us. Consider the following examples of people who thrive on stress—the athlete who uses the pressure he feels to help him surpass his personal best or compete with others; the businessperson who uses the excitement of a sales contest to motivate her to do her best work; the actor who transforms his "stage fright" into an electrifying performance.

These examples illustrate a principle that you can apply to your life, no matter what the activity. Simply facing a change in your life or trying to make a change produces stress. Sometimes stress takes the form of a psychological friction that is provoked by the tension between what you currently have and what you want for yourself in the future.

Just as an athlete uses the stress of an upcoming competition to provide motivation and focus for his training, you can use stress to help move you toward your goals. In any area of your life where you feel stress, you can interpret that stress as a message to do the following: stay calm and relaxed, keep very clear about what it is that you want for yourself, become very efficient in your efforts, and be determined to create the outcome you truly desire.

A moderate degree of stress, when kept in balance with other factors in your life that nourish and support you, can be a powerful factor to move you forward to a life of greater fulfillment.

CAUSES OF STRESS

The causes of stress can be both external and internal. External stressors are outer events (inclement weather, environmental disasters, your job, world politics, illness, the actions or reactions of others, etc.) that place a strain or demand on you. Internal causes of stress are generated by your internal responses to outer events. In other words, your thoughts, feelings, and interpretations about the significance of outer events will determine whether or not you experience stress in response to them. You can serve as your own source of stress when you feel emotions such as anxiety, fear, and shame, or harbor judgmental thoughts about your worth or adequacy.

Books and articles that discuss stress typically present a scale of the relative intensity of various stressors. The death of a spouse tops the list. As discussed in Chapter 8, "Mourning Your Loss," the results of a study showed that the grieving associated with limb loss may be qualitatively as great as that experienced by recent widows. The grief over limb loss may persist at the initial level of intensity even a year after surgery. Amputation—talk about a stressor!

Since you often cannot affect external stressors or prevent them from occurring, it is far more productive to focus your attention on managing your internal responses to external events. Individual responses to external circumstances vary widely. What one person may find stressful, another might find pleasurable. One person may enjoy speaking in public, while another finds it unnerving. Skiing down a snowy mountain at seventy miles an hour can be exhilarating for one person, but terrifying for another.

If you blame your stress on external factors (such as your job, your mother, or the weather), you are doing yourself a great disservice. You are "giving your power" to that person or circumstance by allowing it to determine your internal state of well-being. In truth, it is your reaction to or your interpretation of that event that determines if it is stressful for you. I'd like to stress the following point (pun intended)! *You can choose either to empower the external circumstances that provoke your stress, or retain that power for yourself.*

You may place demands on yourself that can be as stressful as those exerted by outer events and individuals. Do you believe that you need to be Superman or Wonder Woman? Do you feel the need to be all things to all people—an excellent parent, spouse, and employee? Are you hooked on pleasing others, yet neglect your own self-care?

Become aware of unrealistic demands you place on yourself. Maybe you have created an unreasonable self-imposed timetable on how quickly you should physically and emotionally recover from your amputation. It's important that you modify such unreasonable expectations. When you do, you will free yourself from the unnecessary burden of self-generated stress.

THE BODY/MIND CONNECTION

The way your *body* responds to stress largely depends on how your *mind* responds to the stress-triggering event. And in turn, the way your mind responds to stress is influenced by how well you have learned to relax.

Psychosomatic theory says that the body and mind constantly influence each other. Our bodies literally "em-body" our thoughts and emotions. Thus, stressful thoughts, emotions, attitudes, and beliefs are known to contribute to conditions such as asthma, ulcers, migraine headaches, and high blood pressure.

There is a great deal of language that refers to our bodies, and often accurately registers the effects of stress. We say that we "bear the weight of the world on our shoulders," "clench our jaws with tension," or have "a pain in the neck." When we receive an emotional blow we may "tighten our guts." When you withhold expression of your thoughts and emotions, or fail to "get it off your chest," you may internalize those responses and end up with chest pain or a related ailment.

When you are under stress, your body may also respond with a rush of adrenaline (see the fight-or-flight response described on page 125). Obviously, it is useful to remove the underlying trigger of the stress whenever possible. It is also important to find a physical outlet, such as vigorous exercise, through which you can work off increased adrenaline, or you will be left feeling agitated and irritable.

Your physical condition influences your mental health in many ways. Fatigue, lack of exercise, a poor diet, and/or partaking in recreational drugs can cause you to be prone to the effects of stress, and result in physical illness. You may also tend to be irritable, emotionally volatile, and easily provoked.

MANAGING STRESS

Since stress is an integral part of living, you will never be able to eliminate it completely. You can, however, learn to manage stress—decrease it, control it, and even prevent it to some degree.

Learning how to decrease some of your stress can help you "take a load off" your shoulders and be more relaxed. Whenever possible, remove or decrease external stressors from your life. For example, if there is a health-care professional who repeatedly irritates you by failing to understand and provide for your needs, it may be time to find a new provider. If you live in a house or apartment with structural impediments that make it difficult or dangerous to deal with, you might consider remodeling these problem areas.

You have far more control over your internal responses to life's circumstances than over the circumstances themselves. It is also easier to learn to alter your responses by adjusting your attitude, than it is to alter outer circumstances or other people. For instance, if there is someone who reacts to you insensitively or rudely, remind yourself that his or her response is a reflection of ignorance, not a statement about you.

Allow the events that trigger stress to serve as warning lights that draw attention to areas in which you should take action. In this way, stress provides invaluable feedback. When you perceive stress as your ally, the very process of managing your stress can serve as a powerful catalyst for growth. As you take action and address the message that your stress is sending, you will feel empowered and more in control. Thus, each stressful situation houses within it the seeds for growth, which can be activated by your attitude and actions.

To consciously take action to manage stress, begin with awareness—recognize when you are indeed experiencing stress, and whenever possible, pinpoint the cause or causes of that stress. When you find yourself experiencing emotional turbulence, tune into your body. Do you feel a tightening in your gut or butterflies in your stomach? Do you have a tension headache? If so, pay close attention to the external circumstances in your life—your relationships, job, health, etc.—to help you better figure the source of your stress.

Once you are aware of the presence of stress, there are four avenues you can take to better manage it:

1. Learn and use techniques for deep relaxation.
2. Develop a lifestyle of self-care.
3. Take care of your physical health.
4. Maintain dynamic balance in your life.

In the discussion that follows, let's take a closer look at these effective ways of controlling stress.

Deep-Relaxation Techniques

Deep-relaxation techniques are antidotes to stress; they can revitalize and replenish both body and mind. Conscious deep relaxation, practiced regularly, can have profound positive effects on your health and overall state of well-being.

By learning to relax deeply at will, you can decrease the effects of stress that are already present and prevent the build-up of new stress. You will begin to experience benefits to your physical health, especially in disorders that are influenced by your mind (high blood pressure, headaches, asthma, ulcers, etc.). An abundance of "calm energy" will be available to enhance your physical activity, emotional responses, and mental acuity in terms of memory, focus, and concentration. You will feel refreshed and revitalized. Your increased sense of well-being will aid in your productivity. When you are physically relaxed, emotionally balanced, and mentally clear, you will be able to handle greater challenges by responding calmly and flexibly.

While learning the martial art of T'ai Chi, students are reminded that a rigid tree will break in a strong wind, while a blade of grass is flexible and will just bend. This is true both literally and figuratively. If your body is tight or tense, it is more liable to be injured if you should happen to fall. (How many times have you seen a child walk away from a fall that would have incapacitated an adult, simply because the child has not yet learned to be tense?) When your body is tight or tense, your emotions are likely to be the same; like the tree in the stiff wind, you may "break" under pressure.

This principle is far more than just a pleasant metaphor. It underscores the importance of understanding the role that your physical body plays in your emotional, mental, and spiritual well-being. The many wonderful benefits that are provided through the practice of deep physical relaxation cannot be over-stressed (okay, another bad pun).

Some effective relaxation techniques include meditation, progressive muscle relaxation, massage, visualization, and yoga. They are all excellent ways to relax and revitalize. These techniques, which are briefly introduced in this chapter, can be practiced effectively by just about anyone, regardless of physical condition. They require no special equipment and cost nothing. So, why not discover their benefits for yourself?

Meditation

In his book *The Relaxation Response* (New York: William Morrow & Co., 1975), Herbert Benson, M.D. describes the effects of the deep relaxation produced by simple meditation as the "relaxation response." These effects are a physiological counter to those produced by stress, and are noticeably different from those provided by sleep. The relaxation response has been found to change several bodily functions including a decrease in heart rate, respiratory rate, blood pressure, metabolic rate, and oxygen consumption; and an increase in alpha-wave activity in the brain, skin resistance, and the ability for analytical thinking. All of these physiological changes are antidotes for countering stress.

The state of meditation has been referred to as "restful alertness." During this state, the mind is calm and quiet yet alert; it is not focused on anything in particular. Although the Western world has seen a dramatic increase in the practice of meditation since the 1960s, there is still much confusion over what exactly constitutes meditation. There is a wide variety of types of meditations with very different goals for the practitioner. In general, it may be said that any type of practice that shifts one's awareness from the external world to the interior can be considered meditation.

Thus, it is possible to meditate on the breath, a sound, a picture, a thought, or even a movement, as any one of these can transfer our attention toward our internal being. When we are able to withdraw our focus from the dizzying cyclone of the outside world, a sense of peace and calm rises almost automatically.

It is beyond the scope of this book to go into great detail about the various meditation techniques. For more detailed information on meditation, check your local library and bookstores. The "Further Information" section, beginning on page 327, offers titles on this subject.

Progressive Muscle Relaxation

It is fairly simple to release some of the accumulated tension from your body through a technique known as progressive muscle relaxation; this relaxes your mind, as well as your body. Begin by loosening constricting clothing, then lie down or sit comfortably. Imagine your body warm, heavy, and relaxed. Give yourself a series of gentle suggestions that are intended to relax different parts of your body. You can either tape the instructions or silently give them to yourself.

A sample of your instructions might be as follows:

1. Toes, relax . . .
2. Feet, relax . . .
3. Ankles, relax . . .
4. Shins, relax . . .
5. Slowly continue to move up toward your head, instructing each body part along the way to relax. Really feel the tension melt from each body part before moving on to the next. Continue to relax each body part until your entire body is calm.

When giving instructions, be as specific or general as you want. For example, you might prefer giving separate relaxation instructions to each finger, one hand at a time, while another person might choose to instruct both hands to relax at the same time. Regardless of the instructions, the outcome should be the same—a relaxed, tension-free body and mind.

Massage

Who hasn't enjoyed a good back rub at the end of a stressful day? Massage feels wonderful and is a great way to relieve both physical and emotional stress. Beyond this, touch can be healing. Pleasurable touch can serve to counterbalance the trauma of amputation and the uncomfortable procedures associated with your physical recovery. Massage by a family member or friend can convey comfort and empathy. Caring, loving touch can also promote self-acceptance of your physical body.

Chronic musculo-skeletal tension and imbalances are sometimes best released by someone who is trained in the therapeutic use of massage. Such a professional understands the function of each muscle and knows various methods to release deep tension, increase circulation, and help realign your posture.

I have found that postural realignment by my massage therapist has been invaluable in helping to relieve the stress throughout my body caused by the imbalances in my gait. Before my amputation, I thought of massage as a luxury; now, professional massage therapy has become an integral part of my ongoing care. After a good massage, you will feel relaxed yet energized. Treat yourself to a massage—it feels wonderful.

Visualization

Visualization (sometimes referred to as guided imagery) is an effective, potent tool that can help you manage stress, increase your confidence and self-esteem, improve your health and physical skills, and heighten your creative abilities. It can also help you achieve goals, heal emotional wounds, and get in touch with your inner wisdom. If you could benefit from enhancement in any of these areas (and who couldn't?) learning to tap into the power of visualization is worthwhile for you. Do you see what I mean? (Please forgive another bad pun.)

What is visualization? It is the technique of using your mind and imagination to tap into your inner resources in order to optimize a successful outcome to a chosen situation.

Why does visualization work? It has been suggested that our powerful subconscious does not make a distinction between actual experiences and imagined ones. So your mind and body will respond to vivid imagery in much the same way as they would to "real life" events.

For example, if a basketball player visualizes himself executing a shot perfectly and sees the ball dropping into the basket, his game may well improve. If you visualize yourself as confident and relaxed in an upcoming challenging situation, such as a job interview, you have ingrained that experience of confidence into your subconscious, and your actual experience will be enhanced. If you visualize yourself as profoundly relaxed and calm, your body will respond by lowering your blood pressure, decreasing your metabolic rate, and showing other signs of decreased physical stress. Visualization has even been shown to strengthen the immune system enough to slow or even reverse the course of diseases such as cancer.

The keys to effective visualization include:

• Being in a very relaxed state of mind and body.

• Vividly using your imagination—include all of your senses—to make your mental images as alive and multidimensional as possible.

• Visualizing a successful outcome of a situation and your response to that outcome.

You can find excellent audio tapes on visualization and other relaxation techniques at most bookstores and libraries. What is great about these tapes is that you can kick back, relax, and let the tapes guide you to deeper and deeper states of relaxation without having to memorize instructions or refer back to a printed page. After using this type of tape for a short while, you may find you have internalized the instructions, and can lead yourself to the relaxed state without the external aid.

Yoga

Yoga is a term that best translates as "union." The many different practices of yoga aim at producing a state of union with the Divine, whether this is done through focus on the physical body, the emotions, the mind, or the spirit.

When most people hear the word yoga, they probably think of Hatha yoga, a branch of yoga that builds health through a number of exercises that stretch and relax the physical body. In Hatha yoga, you generally place your body in a position that gently stretches a group of muscles. You then hold the position while breathing deeply and slowly, imagining that the breath itself is stretching the muscle and releasing any tension. Because many of the positions taken in yoga are on the ground, it may be particularly suited for those with lower-limb amputation. Of course, as with the undertaking of any new type of physical activity, it is wise to discuss with your physician the effects of such exercise on your physical condition.

Most schools of yoga also teach breathing and meditation exercises. Bookstores and libraries are filled with information on this subject. If you do a little investigating, you may find that yoga classes are offered in your local area. If you are interested, why not try it out? Many places offer free introductory classes.

DEVELOP A LIFESTYLE OF SELF-CARE

Another way to control your stress level is by developing a lifestyle of self-care. As you build a lifestyle that supports your recovery and promotes your well-being, it can be helpful to develop a daily routine. There is comfort in the familiar, and the familiarity of a daily routine can reduce stress. Knowing what to expect in a given part of the day can be comforting, and, in itself, a relief (especially when you are challenged by so much due to losing a limb.)

In addition to the basic routines of daily living, set aside some time for special practices. Such practices can include exercising, meditating, and/or expressing your creativity through such outlets as writing, painting, or playing an instrument. You can choose to perform these routines a few days a week or all seven. It's up to you. At first, your practices may require conscious effort. With time, however, your routines will probably become a matter of habit, and will be sorely missed when they are not performed. For instance, when practiced joggers miss a day of running, they find themselves missing that exhiliration and infusion of energy that their running provides. This is the same with any activity that, when practiced regularly, promotes health and well-being.

If you think about it, for optimum performance your car needs regular maintenance. And the human machine is a far more delicate mechanism; it works best when treated to regular preventive maintenance. When your self-care routine becomes regular, your state of health and well-being will move to a plateau of greater peace, satisfaction, and enhanced vitality.

Keeping yourself surrounded by the familiar is also a soothing source of comfort. Now is not a good time to move, change jobs, or make radical changes in close relationships. It is helpful to have the support of old friends and colleagues.

TAKE CARE OF YOUR PHYSICAL HEALTH

Taking care of your overall health is another major key to successful stress management. When you undergo amputation, you might be so focused on your orthopedic needs that you may neglect taking care of your general physical health. The following suggestions are part of a program for well-balanced self-care.

Nutrition

It is important to follow a sensible, nutritionally sound, well-balanced diet. You may elect to decrease or eliminate your intake of caffeine; sugar; and fried, fatty, and processed foods. Drink plenty of fluids so you do not become dehydrated. Consider taking a multivitamin and mineral supplement to help compensate for any dietary deficiencies. Prolonged stress has been known to strip the body of important nutrients and weaken the immune system. Vitamins B and C help offset the effects of stress and should be taken in appropriate amounts. Your physician, a qualified nutritionist, or a dietician can answer your questions and prepare an optimal nutritional dietary plan for you to follow.

Recharge with Sufficient Sleep and Rest

Adequate sleep and rest will help keep you energized and prevent fatigue. Fatigue can take a toll on both your physical and emotional health. When you are recovering from amputation surgery, your body will naturally let you know you need extra rest. Once you have recovered, it is still a good idea to break up your day with brief periods of rest. This will leave you feeling restored and refreshed, and can revive flagging concentration and focus.

Physical Exercise

Do something physical. Swim. Run. Exercise. Do anything that allows you to discharge stress and pent-up physical energy, and to increase your oxygen flow. You'll feel better. Exercise on a regular basis is good medicine for us all.

You may not be sure how to exercise with your physical limitations. Set up an appointment with a physical, occupational, or recreational therapist, who can suggest various ways to be safely active and stay in shape. Working out with certain exercise equipment or participating in a special sports program that is specifically designed for those with physical limitations may open up new dimensions for you.

Exercise serves several purposes. It gives you a break from everyday worries and stress-provoking situations, while it revs up your energy level, tones your body, and promotes health.

Pace Yourself

If there are certain times when you find yourself feeling physically and mentally drained, pay attention to those areas in which you expend excessive amounts of energy. Do you over-stimulate yourself with a barrage of activity? Can your activities be performed in a different time frame or pace than the one you assume is necessary? Are there small tasks and obligations from which you can extricate yourself? Do you need to be active every minute of the day? Can you allow for more quiet time, if that is what recharges you?

Just as a long-distance runner must learn to pace himself in order to finish the race, you will be much more effective in reaching your goals for health and well-being if you learn to pace yourself. Remember the valuable lesson from Aesop's fable "The Tortoise and the Hare"—*slow and steady wins the race.* If you have a hard time pacing the activities in your life, display this motto on your bathroom mirror, where it will serve as your daily reminder.

MAINTAIN A DYNAMIC BALANCE IN YOUR LIFE

By learning to maintain a dynamic balance in your life, you will provide yourself with a healthy balance between harmful and useful stress. Some of the ways you can establish such a balance are presented below.

Establish Priorities

Realistically speaking, you cannot always do all the things you would like —there may not be enough time in the day, or you may not have the energy or the resources. Therefore, learning to separate what *must* be done from what *might* be done is crucial for decreasing your level of stress. Are there tasks you can let go of entirely or delegate to others? What are you doing that really is not necessary? Are you trying to fulfill others' expectations of you? Are you being too much of a perfectionist about your accomplishments? It's up to you to establish priorities about how you spend your time and energy.

Experimenting with a "things to do" list is a simple way of organizing and prioritizing the tasks you wish to accomplish. At the beginning of each week, make a list of things that you would like to accomplish. Next, pick those tasks that are the most pressing or the most time-sensitive. Each time you accomplish one of your goals, scratch it off the list. Even accomplishing seemingly insignificant tasks can provide a sense of satisfaction and can give you the momentum to successfully complete other goals.

Balance Work and Play

When we play, we take ourselves out of our ordinary circumstances and away from our responsibilities. Play is refreshing and revitalizing and necessary for our well-being. We give ourselves a break. We are spontaneous and creative. Play is fun.

I can vividly recall a time in graduate school when I was involved in an intense program in pediatrics. There were not enough hours in the day to accomplish all that my demanding study load required. For a lark, I went to see an old woman, who was reputedly a gifted psychic. She made a cup of tea, then dumped it out and studied the leaves. She said to me, "Here is a figure of you, sitting at a desk. She has been there too long. Here is a butterfly at her shoulder. She thinks she cannot afford to take the time to play—the truth is she cannot afford *not* to!" I was duly impressed. I took her words to heart and began taking time out from my studies to enjoy some leisure activities. I found my stress level dropping and my state of well-being growing.

You know what activities best nourish you on a deep level. When you make the time for yourself to enjoy these activities, you are really taking care of yourself. What is enjoyable for you? Seeing a film? Shopping?

Working on a favorite hobby? Reading a book while sitting on a secluded beach or in a beautiful park? Rebuilding a carburetor? Spending time with friends? Playing, singing, or listening to music? Working with wood? Painting? Gardening? Involving yourself in a sport?

You owe it to yourself to do whatever appeals to you. No matter how old you are, there is a child within you who can suffer from an excess of seriousness and responsibility. Learn to keep your inner child happy by giving him or her plenty of opportunities to play. Your entire life will be more vibrant and enjoyable.

Contribute to Others

An excellent way to get away from the narrow focus of your everyday concerns is to devote some time and energy to others. Whether you volunteer to work in a neighborhood soup kitchen, hospital, or nursing home, or pay peer visits to those who have recently lost a limb, you will find that by contributing to others, you will also recharge yourself.

Be True to Yourself

You face numerous pressures in your daily life to please other individuals. No matter how well you are loved and supported by family and friends, no matter what your job or career responsibilities, no matter what opportunities life drops in your path, it is vitally important that you always remember to be true to yourself.

You have an inner sense that tells you just what it is you truly desire in order to be satisfied with yourself and your life. When you ignore your own inner voice, or act or say things to the contrary, you will likely feel a loss of integrity, which, in turn, can easily produce stress.

This is not to suggest that you become an egomaniac, and seek to have the outside world kowtow to your whims and wishes. Rather, you should learn to recognize what makes you feel good about yourself—what allows you to go to sleep each night with a sense of accomplishment and a clear conscience. No one can tell you what is true for you, not your mother, father, boss, lover, priest, or rabbi. You are the only one who knows what is good for you.

How can you tell if you are being true to yourself? When you act with integrity, you will discover that your heart (emotions), head (intellect), guts (intuition), and spirit (beliefs) are in alignment. When you are internally aligned, you are energized and focused; your whole being says, "Yes!"

Keep a Sense of Humor

But seriously folks, did you hear the one about the Dalai Lama, who said to the hot dog vendor, "Make me One, with everything" ? It has been said that humor is the best medicine. Laughter can lift your spirits and give you a new perspective on life at the same time. So, why not discover what inspires your sense of humor? For instance, there are a few television shows that keep me laughing, so I watch them regularly. The antics of my dog and cat inspire laughter. My husband's unique point of view often cracks me up, and we laugh a lot together.

Try to make those things that provoke your laughter and help you view life with a lighter perspective a regular part of your life. Remember, not only is laughter the best medicine, it doesn't require a doctor's prescription, and it's free!

IN CONCLUSION

Stress is an inherent part of life. You can no more remove stress from your life than you can dispense with the need to breathe. While it is impossible (and also undesirable) to remove all stress from your life, it is important to understand it and keep it well-managed. In this chapter, a number of approaches have been presented to help you manage stress in your life. Now, it's up to you to put this information into action. Reading alone isn't enough. Tune into yourself and decide which of the suggestions appeal to you most. Try a few, experiment with them, and finally develop your own personal action-oriented program to deal with the stress in your life.

13

SELF-ESTEEM

No matter how successful you appear to the world, how financially secure you are, how handsome or beautiful you look, or how healthy and fit your body is—without a positive self-concept, you will never be at peace with yourself or fully enjoy your life. You can have fame, fortune, and the approval of others; but, if you don't feel good about yourself from the inside out, you will feel emptiness deep within.

When you undergo amputation, your self-concept may be badly shaken. You may find yourself wondering if you are still "the same person" you were before your limb loss; you may question your worth. Your self-confidence may have been dealt a severe blow.

If you had a good, healthy sense of self before your amputation, there is a good chance the foundation of your self-esteem will still be in place after the surgery. And even if you are not one of the individuals blessed with a strong, positive self-concept, have hope. You can still learn the elements of self-esteem and apply them with a little effort. Enhancing your sense of self will enable you to better enjoy your life.

WHAT IS SELF-ESTEEM?

Self-esteem is a way of thinking, feeling, and acting that implies that you accept, respect, trust and believe in yourself. When you accept yourself, you can live comfortably with both your personal strengths and weaknesses without undue criticism. When you respect yourself, you acknowledge your own dignity and value as a unique human being. You treat yourself well in much the same way you would treat someone else you respect. Self-trust means your behaviors and feelings are consistent enough to give you an inner sense of continuity and coherence despite changes and challenges in your external circumstances. To believe in yourself means that you feel you deserve to have the good things in life. It also means you have the confidence that you can fulfill your deepest personal needs, aspirations, and goals.

E.J.Bourne, Ph. D.
The Anxiety and Phobia Workbook

From where does self-esteem come? From within. Its roots are found in childhood experiences. When you were little, you relied on your parents or other primary caretakers as your first teachers. Through their overt and covert behavior (what they said and did, as well as what they didn't say and do) you gradually formed your self-concept. If, as a child, it was communicated that you were a worthwhile, deserving individual, who was capable, loveable, and worthy of dignity and respect, you internalized these messages and developed a positive self-concept based on acceptance and love.

The High Price of Low Self-Esteem

Through my psychotherapy practice, it has been my experience that the most common reason individuals seek professional counseling assistance is due to low self-esteem. Feeling somehow unworthy and undeserving, unloveable and unloved, these people lose their sense of well-being when responding to the ups and downs of life's challenges.

The price you pay when you suffer from low self-esteem is inestimable in terms of its impact on the quality of your life. A negative self-concept may surface behaviorally in a number of ways—an over-dependence on others, hostility, depression, emotional withdrawal, emotional volatility, and either timidity or inflated self-confidence. In contrast, a positive self-concept may be expressed as self-assurance, independence, even-temperedness, and a sense of well-being.

Often, when people don't feel good about themselves, they are aware of a lack of something in their lives. To compensate, they may try to fill this void in detrimental ways, such as through excessive use of alcohol or recreational drugs, physical overexertion, overeating, or overworking. While these compensations may temporarily mask the pain generated by a poor self-concept, they do nothing to address the underlying causes, and eventually, the feelings of dissatisfaction are bound to resurface. This void in one's life can be compared to a weed—it is relatively simple to snip off the top of a dandelion with a weed-whacker, but unless you use the proper tool to dig down and get to the root, you can bet your calluses that the weed (like the void in your life) will reappear.

Acceptance

As human beings, we have limitations and frailties, we make mistakes; this is a natural part of who we are. On the other hand, we also have the strength and capacity to transcend our limitations.

Self-criticism, judgment, blame, and rejection will diminish your level of contentment and inner peace. If you hold yourself to unrealistic goals and ideals, you will disappoint yourself when you don't live up to them. Feelings of guilt, resentment, and remorse for having failed yourself will result. You must learn to accept yourself as a human being, with all the frailties and strengths inherent in human nature.

When you do not accept yourself in your entirety, you set yourself up for the emotional pain and deprivation that accompanies a constricted experience of living. You give up reaching for your dreams if you feel you don't deserve them or are incapable of achieving them. You take fewer risks in your work. You are less willing to let others get to know the "real you" if you don't like or approve of who you have judged yourself to be.

There is often confusion about the notion of acceptance. You can accept yourself and still not like or approve of all of the aspects of yourself. When you accept yourself as you are, you can still actively work on those areas that you would like see grow. If you were going to remodel a building, you would first objectively assess the foundation. You wouldn't reject the entire structure if you discovered a few weaknesses; you would correct the weaknesses and build up from there. Rather than starting from a place of self-rejection, self-acceptance allows you to work on self-improvement by first honestly embracing who you are.

Self-acceptance can provide emotional release and dramatic relief. Some of the many ways you can nurture your self-acceptance are explored in this chapter. With a little effort, this nurturing will do much to aid in your confidence and personal growth.

Your Sense of Self-Worth

There is a tendency to define self-worth based on cultural, social, family and personal values. For some, self-worth is related to wealth, accomplishments, and social status. Others measure their own worth by the amount of love in their lives, or some other intangible standard. If you place standards on your behavior or state of being, so that when you fail to live up to these standards you deem yourself not worthy, you are setting yourself up for self-imposed rejection.

Throw out arbitrary measures of self-worth, and recognize that we are all, each and every one of us, worthy and deserving. As our birthright, we have intrinsic self-worth; this is not dependent upon our family's origin, our role in society, or any other external standards. Is a doctor worth more than a young child? A business executive worth more than a chef? Is an "able-bodied" person worth more than a person with limb loss? Not one of us has a golden measure with which to judge another's worth.

Think about people who meet the prevailing social criteria of "having it all" yet don't feel good about themselves. What you think of yourself is what is most crucial to your emotional well-being. It is what matters most.

If you don't honestly assess your strengths and weaknesses and accept yourself for who you are, you cannot expect to change for the better (since you are denying reality as it is). Your self-rejection and its associated guilt will do nothing to promote positive change. You may fall into the circular trap of blaming or judging yourself for your guilt and self-blame. You may even consider yourself somehow less worthy than others, as did these individuals following their amputation:

"I felt like I was worthless, totally different from everyone."

"My ego was crushed. I wasn't the person that I used to be. People told me that I was still the same person on the inside, and I believed that people still saw me that way . . . but I had a much lesser physical image of myself than I used to."

"I didn't think I was a whole person. I felt like I couldn't have fun anymore."

In order to break out of this vicious cycle of self-blame and rejection, you must first accept yourself as you are. Do not allow someone or something outside yourself to define your sense of self-esteem. Be honest with yourself. If you find you have reliquished your power to an outside control, you must disengage yourself from it and regain mastery of your well-being. Realize that it is within your conscious control to affect how you are influenced by outside forces. You can then become anchored in an internal sense of confidence and peace, which does not fluctuate with the vagaries of external events.

Read the following sense of relief experienced by Melvin, when he recognized that he did not have to be a slave to outside forces or opinions:

"My amputation made me a stronger person, mentally. It has also made me a lot more aware of the frailties of life. . . . I think people look at me and accept me more for being myself, rather than for what they thought I was. Also, the accident allowed me to be me. My personality changed. I wasn't trying to tell people what I was like. It was, 'Okay, this is me, whether you like it or not.' There is no grand illusion."

SELF-TALK

What you tell yourself about external and internal circumstances often determines your emotional reactions and state of well-being. Your "self-talk," that internal monologue that runs continuously, has a great deal of influence on your feelings of self-worth. You are the star in the melodramas of your life. Sometimes the film is a tragedy, and other times it is a horror film; sometimes it is poignant and inspirational, while other times it can be a comedy.

You run a commentary inside your head, a narration that interprets external and internal events. It is the nature of your mind to run this commentary. It is up to you to believe and act on what your mind tells you. When you realize you can be in charge of your responses, you become empowered. You are responsible for your well-being, independent of external circumstances.

The Internal Critic

The voice within you gives critical feedback that can be helpful at times. Perhaps you can recall being in school and using literary criticism to clarify your expression or elaborate your thoughts. In a similar way, self-critique can provide useful feedback to help you stay on task. It can also help realign your behavior to be consistent with your values, set high goals for yourself, and motivate you to do your best.

The "internal critic," however, is different from the inner voice in that it judges, belittles, and demeans us. The internal critic takes a heavy toll on our self-esteem through repetitive negative comments and reproaches. This inner critic is judge and jury—comparing us to others or setting impossible standards for us to achieve. This is the voice that finds us guilty, unworthy, and woefully inadequate.

The following is an example of the internal critic at work:

"Since my amputation, I feel like half a man. I can't perform anything that I used to. I can't take care of the yard work, can't work at a job and provide for the family. . . . got a little boy that is just starting to play sports and needs to be shown what to do, and I can't go out and show him. I have problems—I can't function and do things for myself."

—Denny

Your self-talk can be so automatic and rapid that you may find yourself engaged in a highly emotional reaction without even knowing how you got there. Self-talk tends to be robotic—your internal critic runs a monologue "on automatic," playing the same old destructive "tapes" that eventually erode your well-being. You've probably heard the statement, "Tell someone a lie often enough and they'll start to believe it." By constantly repeating negative beliefs, you can actually brainwash yourself into believing them.

The following examples show how the internal critic can undermine your confidence and self-esteem:

• In order to prevent you from "failure," the internal critic undermines your self-confidence to the point where you take less risks in your life, or you give up your aspirations and dreams. ("You're an amputee, how could you ever expect to . . .")

• In a personal relationship, your internal critic causes you to stage a "preemptive strike" and you reject the other person, rather than wait for him or her to reject you. You either withdraw from a relationship or fail to pursue it in the first place.

• The internal critic is a master at instilling guilt. If you feel guilty enough for your thoughts, feelings, and/or behavior, the critic may also make you believe that you can make amends through suffering.

It is obvious that the actions of your internal critic can erode your well-being and rob you of the richness that life has to offer. It is critical for your well-being to disarm this destructive inner voice.

Disarming the Internal Critic

An interesting phenomenon is that people tend to believe whatever their self-talk tells them (the good as well as the bad). Critical self-talk eats away, bite-by-bite, at the very fabric of your well-being. The rules, the expectations, the judgments, and the comparisons are all areas from which the inner critic draws its ammunition. It may remind you of your shortcomings by dredging up memories of scenes in which you did not live up to expectation, or it may cause you to reassess unpleasant feelings in your current situation and connect them to negative past experiences.

The good news is that you can disarm your critic and prevent its repetitive negative programming from impacting your well-being. In order to disarm your internal critic, the first thing you must do is listen to what it is telling you. Once you are aware of what the critic is saying, question those statements. Shut the critic up by putting it in its place. By doing so, your self-esteem will be left intact.

Note the two very different responses given by people regarding their limb loss:

- *"My body is grotesque. No one will ever find me attractive again. I'm destined to stay single because of my amputation."*

This person has rejected himself before he has even tried interacting with others. He is obviously not at peace with his amputation. This person is likely to influence social interactions in such a way to elicit responses of rejection.

- *"I don't find my residual limb particularly attractive, but it is just a small part of who I am. I know I'll meet someone who will see beyond my exterior and who will love and accept me for who I am."*

This individual is more accepting of his altered body. He doesn't find it beautiful, yet he has found a way to accept it. This person will exude that self-acceptance, which will make it easier for others to be accepting of him.

Remember, you tend to believe what your self-talk tells you. The keys for countering destructive self-talk are listed below.

1. **Begin with awareness.** Catch yourself in the act. Monitor what it is you are telling yourself. Notice your own put-downs, self-judgements, comparisons, and tendencies for self-blame. Notice your uncomfortable emotional responses or negative internal imagery.

Like other skills, your ability to monitor your internal monologue will improve with practice. It takes conscious effort to stay with the monitoring process. You may realize your internal critic has spoken after the fact. If so, review your internal monologue. Trace it back to the point that triggered the critic's response. What were you telling yourself at that point?

Since negative self-talk is often the product of habit, know that you can break its repetitive nature. Just as you might modify your eating or smoking habits, you can modify your thought patterns so they become affirming rather than destructive. Once again, it takes commitment, practice, awareness, self-compassion, and a sense of humor.

2. **Answer some important questions objectively.** "Do I deserve to be put down in this situation?" "Is this criticism harming my sense of well-being?" "Is my internal critic running on automatic, voicing habitual, robotic put-downs that are not based on reality?" To defuse the power of the critic, discover where its message is coming from. Is its message based on reality, or does it come from "shoulds," rules, comparisons, or expectations from others?

3. **Refute destructive messages.** If the talk of your internal critic is simply mechanical, rooted in the past without any positive intentions, directly address the critic and refute its message. Tell it, "You're wrong. That's bullshit. I'm not willing to listen to your harmful lies any more!"

    Counter destructive self-talk by correcting distortions in the message. Ask yourself, "Is this an objective truth, or is it something I was taught to believe without questioning? Is this statement *always* the truth, or is it true only in certain situations? And even if this were true, what is the worst possible outcome as a result of this statement?

4. **Try to discover positive intentions in a critical message.** When your self-talk is harmful to your self-esteem, ask yourself if there are any positive intentions hidden in the seemingly negative message. For example, let's say, at the urging of some friends, you decide to participate in a basketball game at the local gym. Still unsteady on your new prosthesis, while attempting a basket, you lose your balance and end up on the floor. Your internal critic tells you, "Boy, you really messed up that time!" resulting in a negative blow to your self-esteem. But, think about it. Is there a useful message underlying this put-down? It isn't difficult to see that behind this negative judgment is another voice telling you to find a way to improve your performance for the next time.

    Deciphering the good intentions behind negative messages will help you stay focused on the positive and keep your self-esteem strong and intact. Once you have found the positive intentions, ask yourself, "Are there other creative, constructive ways I can satisfy that intention and strengthen my sense of well-being without putting myself down?" Explore means to improve on your performance next time without being so harsh on yourself. In this way, you'll feel good about yourself.

5. **Use your awareness to acknowledge your successes.** In other words, catch yourself being good. Feed positive messages into your internal computer. Remind yourself that although you have lost a limb, you are still worthwhile, whole, capable, and attractive. Self-compassion, acceptance, and forgiveness are avenues toward healing.

You *can* change the habitual, robotic tapes your critic plays over and over in your mind. You *can* stop the repetitive loop and change the destructive messages to ones that empower you. With awareness, you will discover the internal critic is like a big bag of wind—once caught in distortions and falsehoods, the bag is punctured and your internal critic loses the power to interfere with your well-being.

REBUILDING SELF-TRUST

"When it really comes down to the nitty-gritty, the core of my emotional support comes from me. My therapist and my girlfriends have all helped me in many ways, but when it has really come down to rock bottom, I have resolved emotional difficulties by myself. It is a wonderful feeling—the feeling that I can trust myself. I can trust myself with other people, with my emotions."

—Marcy

To rebuild self-esteem, you must gradually build a new relationship with yourself. You need to re-establish a sense of trust in your decision-making abilities and in the ways you take care of yourself. As you do this, you will find a gradual increase in your self-confidence and self-worth, as well as your self-acceptance and self-respect.

You can learn to develop compassion for yourself, forgive yourself for the past, and accept yourself in your entirety. You can learn to change the destructive ways you may think or feel about yourself into constructive ones.

"I spend less time thinking about what my body looks like and more about how I come across to people with my personality, in my accomplishments, or through my work. I have convinced myself that I am all right as a person."

—Leslie

You can't always have control over external circumstances and events in your life; however, you can control your responses to these external factors. You can control the meaning (interpretation) of these circumstances. Control over your mind is one of the single most powerful ways you can affect your well-being at a very fundamental level.

"My amputation sets me apart and makes me unique. It has given me something that I have had to confront, and challenge, and overcome—something that other people haven't. It has given me a reservoir of self-confidence. . . .

Rather than dwelling on the things you can't do, you've got to go ahead and search out those things you can do, and start doing them well. Your self-confidence will gradually pervade other areas of your life."

—Mickey

VITAL ELEMENTS OF SELF-CARE

Vital elements of self-care that enhance self-esteem include knowing how to set up and negotiate personal boundaries with others, knowing how to be appropriately assertive, and having the ability to say "no."

Set Boundaries

Setting personal boundaries is one way to maintain your integrity as an individual. A boundary establishes limits; it demarcates one territory from another and gives it definition. When applied to relationships, personal boundaries give you a sense of your own integrity and independence. Through boundaries, you know your limits and are able to separate your well-being and sense of self from that of others. Boundaries keep you from using others to define who you are or what you are worth. (Examples of limiting self-definitions include statements like, "I'm Fred's wife." "I'm the mother of Joan and Mary." "I'm the husband of an alcoholic." "I'm the father of a child with limb differences.")

If your life revolves around caring for or rescuing another (an aged parent, a chronically sick child, an alcoholic spouse, etc.) at the expense of caring for your own needs, your relationship is a *co-dependent* one. If you are trapped in such a situation, get professional and/or peer support to emancipate yourself. Groups such as Co-Dependents Anonymous and Al-Anon can help. Refer to your yellow pages for phone contacts of local chapters.

You must let go of any roles you are using to define your self-worth, and face any underlying insecurities or fears rooted in your past that have set you up for co-dependency. You need to learn to center your welfare around taking care of yourself in a balanced, healthy way, rather than entwining your well-being with another. In this way, you reclaim yourself.

Know your own boundaries and respect the boundaries of others. Allowing others to live their own lives, even when you believe they are making mistakes, is a sign of respect for their personal growth. They may need to face the consequences of their actions before they make an internal commitment to let go of destructive behavior. Making yourself responsible for their life choices is unrealistic and will likely be self-defeating, especially if you hook up your own self-worth to their behavior. There is a fine line between caring for the welfare of others and making yourself responsible for it.

Demonstrate Assertiveness

"My personality has changed. I'm more verbal. I have more spunk now. I know I have to speak up for myself or get trampled over. I don't want others to think of me as a poor little crippled person in a wheelchair, who doesn't have self-worth."

—Molly

Knowing how to be assertive is extremely important for your self-esteem. When you are appropriately assertive you are truly taking care of yourself. You know what you need and make sure you get it. Some people wrongly associate assertiveness with pushiness, egocentricity, or aggression. Being assertive means doing what has to be done in order to assure your rights; this can be done without resorting to heavy-handed tactics.

Since you have become physically challenged, you have probably found yourself in awkward situations at times due to society's ignorance. It is especially important for you to learn how to stand up for yourself. By standing up for your rights, you demonstrate self-respect. You can say "no" to requests that you don't choose to fulfill, you can express honest feelings, and you can ask for what you need.

Being assertive was not always easy for me, especially during the time immediately following my amputation. Let me share an experience I had with you. There is a law in California that allows handicapped people to display a special placard in their car windows. This placard permits them to have their gas pumped at "self-serve" islands by an attendant. One day, I requested help at one of these pumps (at the time, I was using a walker and was physically weak). The attendant growled at me, "Lady, pump it yourself!" I burst into tears. Although I considered leaving the station, I didn't. Instead, I regained control and told the attendant that I had a disabled placard and he was required by law to assist me. He apologized profusely, told me he hadn't seen the placard, and explained he had been having a bad day. Here's the point—even though it had been difficult for me to assert myself to the attendant that day, I did it. And guess what. It made it easier for me to assert myself in the future.

Assert yourself! You are the only one who knows your needs and desires, who recognizes when your rights are being violated. You must be the guardian of your own integrity.

Be Able to Say "No"

A part of maintaining your personal boundaries and asserting yourself is being able to say "no." By saying no, you set limits. While I was a patient in a teaching hospital I was asked by a student if I would permit him to practice bronchoscopy on me. Since this meant letting him push a tube down my windpipe into my lungs to look around, I was appalled. In this case, it was very easy for me to say "No!" with total conviction. Until you learn to set your boundaries by saying "no" at the appropriate times, you will likely face a multitude of people who want to perform equally distasteful activities upon you or your wallet. If you really want to let them have their way with you, fine; however, if what they are suggesting trespasses your boundaries, just say "no!"

Ways to Maintain Boundaries, Be Assertive, and Say "No"

When you acknowledge your right to maintain boundaries, be assertive, and say "no," this shows you consider yourself, your needs, and your wishes to be worthy. You recognize that you deserve to be true to yourself. The following suggestions will help you.

• Know that you can learn to handle the responses you will receive when you take care of yourself. If someone responds to you negatively, accept the response as feedback, not an assault. The responses you receive are reflections of the other person, not of you or your self-worth.

• If you feel you must assert yourself and request something from another person in order to fulfill a need, take the following steps:

1. Know precisely what it is you want or need.
2. Be sure the other person makes time to hear your request.
3. In a straightforward, nonjudgmental fashion, describe how your needs are not being met. Express how this directly and/or indirectly affects you. Be respectful of the person with whom you are speaking.
4. Request precisely what it is you would like that person to do or stop doing.

Others will respect you for speaking your mind and taking care of yourself.

• Just as practicing a skill helps you become good at it, it may also be helpful for you to practice being assertive, maintaining boundaries, and saying "no." One way to do this is by recalling past experiences in which you successfully stood up for yourself. Try to recall specific times when you were appropriately assertive; remember as vividly as possible all the strengthening feelings and positive thoughts associated with those times.

Next, carry those good feelings and positive thoughts forward and imagine them in different situations in which you currently need to be assertive. Then go ahead and try out new behaviors. You will discover that as you practice letting others know your true feelings and desires, you will feel internally strengthened. You will experience enhanced self-respect, and you will gain the respect of others.

• For a particularly emotionally charged situation, ask a friend to practice role-playing the difficult situation with you. You can take turns being you (the one asking to have needs met), and the person who is transgressing your boundaries or discounting your rights or needs. In addition to having an opportunity to practice standing up for yourself, you may be surprised at what you might discover by putting yourself in the other person's position.

Maintaining personal boundaries, having the ability to say "no," and knowing how to be appropriately assertive are all vital components of self-care. As you master these elements, you will find yourself internally strengthened by the confidence that comes from acting on your own behalf.

NEGATIVE PARENTING AND YOUR INNER CHILD

What is your "inner child"? It is that part of you that is playful, spontaneous, and impressionable. The inner child is shaped by the messages it receives, especially during impressible childhood years.

Any time a parent gives the message to a child that he is somehow not okay exactly the way he is, or that he is not worthwhile, loveable, capable, or valued as an individual, that child's sense of self-worth may become damaged. Repeated over time, hundreds of these messages will take their toll; the child will internalize these messages and believe them.

Some examples of negative parenting are obvious, while others are more subtle. If a child is physically or sexually abused, he is likely to feel that the world is an unsafe place and no one is trustworthy. He may feel inadequate, powerless, like an object to be hurt or used, and he may carry all of these feelings with him through his life.

While less obvious than physical abuse, words that tell a child how stupid or insignificant he is can hurt just as much and can produce similar outcomes. A child who is or who has been verbally abused may experience a host of negative feelings, including guilt, inferiority, and unworthiness.

Parents who are unwavering perfectionists or overly critical, can undermine a child's confidence in himself. Imagine what happens to a child's self-worth when nothing he ever does seems to be good enough to meet parental standards.

At the other end of the spectrum, there exist parents who do too much for their children. Their children can do no wrong and are praised whether or not they deserve to be. These children are coddled; they are not allowed to take on age-appropriate responsibilities or risks. They cannot learn from their mistakes because they are never in a situation to make any. These children grow up with an exaggerated sense of their own abilities. Often, when they finally come to live on their own in "the real world," they are unprepared for the realities they must face, and their sense of self-worth may come crashing down.

Some parents abandon their children through divorce, death, or simple desertion; these children are often left feeling like the abandonment is somehow their fault. Another kind of abandonment occurs when a parent is still physically present in the home, yet has emotionally deserted the child by not attending to his physical, emotional, intellectual, and spiritual needs. The child, once again, will tend to internalize the situation and blame himself for his parent's lack of care. He may tell himself that he is unwanted because he is unloveable and undeserving of better treatment. These problems are more complicated when there is drug or alcohol abuse present; the family may lie about what is going on, and give the child mixed messages, which are confusing and will teach the child to doubt his own perceptions.

Healing Your Inner Child

If your childhood needs were not met (as just described), your emotional growth was probably arrested in certain areas. You also may have developed certain coping methods and psychological defense mechanisms that helped you to adapt and survive in your family, but no longer continue to serve you as an adult. When situations arise in your current life that are consciously or unconsciously reminiscent of childhood circumstances, these same coping and defense mechanisms may be triggered. Although they may have worked in your family, they may be unproductive or even harmful now. When you were a child, you depended on others to take care of your needs. Part of the benefit of being an adult is that you have a lot more conscious control over your well-being. Learn to "re-parent" yourself. You can learn to become aware of old methods of coping that no longer serve you, and consciously choose your responses to troubling situations. Use your adult awareness to notice when you communicate to yourself that you are undeserving of love and respect. If you catch yourself feeling "less than" others because of your amputation, correct such misconceptions in the same way a loving parent would reassure a child that he or she is loveable and worthy.

Let go of self-criticism and disapproval; you can give yourself what you should have received as a child. And guess what. Once you learn to take care of yourself in this very essential way, you won't need to rely on the approval of others to feel good about yourself. Like an appliance that plugs in and recharges its own batteries, you will become self-recharging and self-regenerating. What freedom!

There are a number of good books available that go into more depth about healing your inner child. If this is a topic you would like more information on, check the "Self Help" section of any large bookstore. Many therapists are also skilled in working with the inner child. Sometimes it is very helpful to work with a skilled counselor, especially when you become stuck in an area. Outside expertise can help you move forward.

THE "SHOULDS"

"You should do this." "You ought to do that." "You have to . . ." "You must always . . ." Sound familiar? We adopt and then internalize beliefs, values, expectations, and rules from our parents and society at large. We may then have the expectation that we, as well as others, must live up to these obligatory standards.

Often, these "shoulds" are not based on objective standards, but rather on narrow, limiting beliefs that have never been fully questioned or examined. These internal injunctions may be applicable to some situations, but not others. If you generalize these rules and apply them to every situation, you will become inflexible and unadaptable.

When you don't live up to these standards you may find yourself feeling guilt, resentment, anger, shame, and remorse, which are all detrimental to good self-esteem. Being human, it is simply impossible to live up to rigid, high standards every moment of your life. If you judge and blame yourself for your "lapses," it will be hard to feel good about yourself.

Since the "shoulds" are often based on family, social, or cultural attitudes, they may not be objective. If you feel the need to rigidly follow the "shoulds," you will feel terrible self-recrimination and poor self-regard when you fail to live up to them.

So, it is important to examine the conscious and unconscious rules you use to govern your actions. Of course, the validity of some rules, such as "Don't take candy from strangers," is readily apparent. Other rules that you may have modeled from your parents or society may not always be in your best interest—"You must always be polite" and "Don't let your feelings show."

When you use words like "must," "always," and "never," you are generalizing and can lock yourself into an inflexible position that won't serve your highest good. You can induce anxiety, guilt, shame, and a sense of failure when you expect yourself to rigidly adhere to unrealistic standards.

Don't "should" on yourself! Notice if any of the following statements apply to you. Can you think of others?

• "I should put on a brave front about how I feel about my amputation."

- "I should give up my goals since they aren't realistic."
- "I should keep my negative feelings in and express only positive ones."
- "Big girls/boys should not cry."
- "I should be able to handle my amputation on my own. I shouldn't have to rely on anyone else."

Values and beliefs that are flexible and based on your own conscious evaluation will serve you infinitely better than those that are swallowed without question. If you blindly follow beliefs and rules that are not your own, you are not being true to yourself and will suffer as a result. But if you follow beliefs that you have examined and have found to be congruent with your heart, head, guts, and spirit, you will know these beliefs are truly your own. They will bring integrity and satisfaction to all of your actions that proceed from them.

Letting Go of the Need to be Perfect

Part of what makes us human is that we have both strengths and weaknesses. There are areas in which we excel, and areas in which we fall short of being perfect. If you are a perfectionist, amputation is bound to throw you for a loop. Things that you once did in a matter-of-fact way now require your full attention and considerably more effort to accomplish. It is unreasonable to expect that you will be able to excel at everything you did before amputation surgery. It is important to face reality, and recognize that your external circumstances have changed. Your body will have some limitations. When attempting to overcome those limitations, you are apt to make mistakes, experience shortcomings, and even seem to fail at times. There may be simple everyday activities that you cannot perform as well as others can.

Although it is understandable that you might want to do everything perfectly for self-approval and the approval of others, this strive for perfection can also be a trap that can set you up for self-recrimination, frustration, and depression. This is not to recommend that you give up on having standards of performance that make you proud of your efforts; this is only to suggest that while learning to live with loss of limb, you maintain a "kinder, gentler" attitude with yourself than you might have taken before your amputation.

One of the wonderful qualities of being human is our willingness to explore, to take risks, "to boldly go" where we have not gone before. Any time you explore new territory or learn new skills, you are bound to make mistakes. It is important to remember that as long as you approach life as a continuous learning experience, there can be no failures—only feedback. If you look for the feedback that your mistakes and shortcomings provide, you can grow from your life experiences.

Perfectionism may be all right for those people who practice a limited range of skills over and over in order to perform them—a concert pianist, a downhill skier, or a gourmet chef. Anyone else who is involved in learning new skills, or interacting with a constantly changing external environment, is wise to approach their process as a learning experience, rather than a performance.

There is a great measure of peace to be gained in the recognition that you do not have to be perfect. It is liberating to accept yourself with your flaws and imperfections.

COMPARING YOURSELF WITH OTHERS

Sound the alarm bells! Flash the warning lights! Comparing yourself with others is a trap that is apt to cast you into the waters of despair! This trap of comparing your physical appearance or abilities with others can be just as "crippling" (or even more so) as your actual physical condition.

Your comparisons may be based on fallacies. For example, you might assume that because someone looks as if "they've got it made," your assumption is true. Haven't we all been shocked by the suicides or other self-destructive behaviors of famous men and women who seemed to possess all the world had to offer—fame, physical beauty, wealth?

While some people begrudge the good fortune of others, if your heart is open, you will celebrate their happiness and good fortune. You belittle yourself when you begrudge the successes of others.

When you fall short of self-imposed measurements that are based on comparisons with others, you have set yourself up for misery and depression. For how will you ever be content with yourself if you have set standards of perfection that are impossible to achieve?

A variation of this trap occurs when you negatively compare your current life with your life before amputation. If your physical freedom has been somewhat curtailed and your body irrevocably changed, how can you possibly expect life to be exactly as it was before? It simply isn't. Nevertheless, your life can still be rich and beautiful. To achieve this realization, you might have to do some inner maturing. Like it or not, when you lose a limb, you are given a dramatic opportunity to re-envision who you think you are, and what is important in life. The payoff for this inner growth is an enriched experience of self.

"Basically, my personality hasn't changed since my amputations. Fortunately, I have always been an upbeat, outgoing person. I have had to learn to do some things over again, and do other things more slowly than I used to. I have more patience than I used to have; and that is an advantage—especially at work or when dealing with my kids. I am more realistic in my expectations of how long it takes to do

things. Sometimes, I overlook things that I can't do, like keeping the house as clean as I might like or chasing the kids down. I am just a little bit more mellow."

—Leslie

"I'm definitely a better person now than I ever was before I lost my leg. I am a lot more confident now. Before I lost my leg I had no ambitions. I had gotten a lot of my confidence from competitive sports. Suddenly, I realized I couldn't rely on sports anymore, and I turned to myself to find confidence in other ways. I had to find something within me that was worthwhile. For the first time in my life, I began developing my mind. As a result I really developed myself, which I honestly don't believe would have happened the way it did had I not become an amputee."

—Margaret

IN CONCLUSION

How you feel about yourself permeates and affects every aspect of your life. Good self-esteem is vital for your emotional recovery following amputation. Some of the varied elements that go into maintaining good self-esteem and building a positive self-concept have been presented in this chapter. Many of the topics discussed in other chapters address aspects of self-care and other concepts that will also contribute to feeling good about yourself.

When you have good self-esteem it is easier to keep on an even keel amidst life's storms. Since your good feelings are self-generated regardless of the vagaries of external circumstances, you have the ability to go deep within to your "center" to maintain your sense of well-being and self-confidence. Good self-esteem is at the very core of your well-being.

Wherever you go in life, whatever you do—you take yourself along. There you are! The quality of your experiences and your interactions with others will depend to a large extent on your self-esteem—the way you feel about yourself and how you treat yourself. The world that you see is a reflection of you, the observer. When you love and accept yourself, the outside world looks beautiful and fascinating. Improve your self-esteem, and it is like giving yourself a new set of glasses with which to positively view yourself and the world.

14

BODY IMAGE

Beauty, youth, vigor, and health are extolled in our society. It is impossible to watch television, view a film, or read a magazine without seeing ideal-looking models or actors portraying the way we are "supposed" to look. Advertising is geared to create increased desire for "the good life," which includes looking and dressing the right way, and owning the right things. In short, we are taught that outer appearances are everything. By having enough of the right material stuff (body, clothes, car, home, job, etc.) we will be happy, successful, and fulfilled. The emphasis is on *having* rather than on *being*.

Therefore, the physical reality of losing a limb can be especially difficult to integrate. No matter what you achieve in terms of physical recovery, the simple fact is that your limb is still gone. For the rest of your life, you will have to live with this physical reality. Society's ideals of physical perfection are now clearly impossible to achieve.

Thus, amputation of a limb may understandably deal a devastating blow to your body image. This chapter discusses the effects of amputation on body image with the hope of assisting you to be more comfortable and accepting of the body you now have.

ELEMENTS OF BODY IMAGE

Body image is your internal concept of how you appear on the exterior. This image is based upon more than just physical characteristics; it also reflects your subjective perception of your outer self. Since perceptions are generated in the mind, your personal experiences will contribute to the concept you have of your physical self.

Body image is based on emotional, psychological, and socially influenced considerations according to Rita Freedman, Ph.D. in her book *Bodylove: Learning to Like Our Looks—and Ourselves* (New York: Harper and Row, 1988). According to Dr. Freedman, some of these considerations include:

• Your appearance (visual concept).

• What you think about the way you look (mental concept).

• How you feel about your appearance (emotional concept).

• How you sense and control your body (kinesthetic concept).

• Your life experience of living with your particular body (historical concept).

Normally, body image includes having all four limbs; it may also include external objects that you associate with yourself. For example, you may generally picture yourself wearing clothes, rather than being in the buff. When driving, you may include your automobile as a part of your body image. Body image is not static. It changes with your age, the current fashions, how you feel about yourself, your state of health, and how you are seen by others.

Accuracy of How You View Your Body

Your body image is affected by many subjective factors. The judgments you make about whether or not you like or approve of your appearance can impact your well-being. When you view your body positively, you will tend to feel better about yourself. When you don't like what you see, you will tend to feel bad.

You assign your perceptions personal value, which may not correlate with objective reality. To illustrate this concept of faulty perceptions, consider the person with anorexia. Although she may be emaciated, she *perceives* herself as fat (therefore, unattractive) so she continues to starve herself.

Sometimes, individuals with (or without) physical impairments become obsessed with a particular body part that they believe ruins their appearance. There are others who are not happy with their overall size or body contours. They tend to ignore the rest of their bodies, which may be very attractive on the whole.

In a similar way, body image may be distorted in some persons with limb loss, especially if their amputation was recent. Studies suggest some of these individuals view their bodies as if they are segmented, not whole.

Physical State or State of Mind?

Most of us know plain-looking individuals who carry themselves as if they are attractive. We also know people who are attractive yet very insecure about their looks.

I grew up with a dear friend who was bright, witty, and a lot of fun. Unfortunately, her nose, which was large and a little crooked, was the bane of her existence! When we reached our teenage years, she became especially self-conscious of it. Eventually, she got a nose job, and she looked great! Yet, even after her nose fit society's concept of beauty, she still acted as if she were not good-looking. She did not project the self-assurance that is usually radiated when people are at ease with themselves and confident in their attractiveness. Although my friend's physical body had changed, she had not correspondingly altered her body image. What follows is the experience of Leslie, a woman who lost both legs and one arm. Shortly after her surgery, she realized that she needed to be more confident in her appearance, and she had to project that confidence to others:

"After months of existing in the same old T-shirts and shorts, I can remember my orthopedist saying to me,'Leslie, you have to start getting dressed up and making yourself look better.' He was right. I needed to take the time to care more about how I looked. I began to realize that I was like everyone else—I had to get dressed up and project myself a little bit. Soon, I found myself saying things like, 'I've got a waist! I've got to put a belt on so people can see that I've really got a waist.'"

Cultural Standards of Beauty

Although standards of beauty vary from culture to culture, within any given culture most people tend to agree when judging who is physically attractive. Beauty standards are generally tougher for women, and women themselves tend to be more critical of their own appearance than men are of theirs.

Simply turn on the television, flip through a magazine, or go to a movie to witness our culture's obsession with body image. It is no wonder that so many people are not content with their bodies. With social emphasis on ridiculous standards such a being skeletally thin and always looking youthful, no matter what your chronological age, it is no wonder that having a body that has undergone amputation can be extremely distressful. It is also harder to camouflage loss of an upper-limb than a lower one, since arms cannot be as effectively covered up by clothing as can legs. This may prove harder for females than males because of societal standards of perfection.

Being "Different" in the Eyes of Others

As someone who has had a limb removed, you have no doubt already discovered that being physically different has social consequences. The effects of your limb loss must be considered not only in terms of you, yourself, but also in terms of your interaction with others. One of the most "handicapping" aspects of losing a limb stems from the common attitude that those who are physically different are somehow special, set apart from so-called normal people. This attitude can impact your body image and self-concept.

Behavior of "able-bodied" persons has been shown to change in the presence of those who are physically different. These people are often less comfortable and less spontaneous when interacting with those who have physical limitations. In turn, those with physical differences may be self-conscious and extremely sensitive to the reactions of others. These interactions can prove awkward, even in the simplest at-home situations:

"Whenever I get ready to take a shower and relax at the end of the day, I remove my prosthetic leg and get around on crutches. If my son has a friend over, it means I have to walk around on crutches in front of his friend, and I really don't like to do that. I'm very self-conscious of my stump, and I don't want people seeing me without my prosthesis. When I take off my leg, I don't feel like a whole person and I don't like the feeling."

—Rob

As an individual with limb loss, you will gradually find your own way of dealing with the self-consciousness that may arise in your interactions with others. Not allowing the reactions of others to interfere with your well-being or choice of activities is a sign of inner strength and self-confidence. Read the following experience of a woman who had one of her legs removed:

"I am very conscious of my body (mostly because of the way our society is). I am also very aware of my amputation. Because I have always liked staying in shape, I still try to keep physically fit in spite of my missing leg. I am an avid swimmer and weight-lifter.

I've never been a shy person. After I go swimming, I hit the showers before heading home. Of course, I usually get stared at (especially by those who haven't seen me before). In spite of the stares, I don't hesitate taking off my bathing suit and showering. Sometimes kids start shouting, 'Mommy, Mommy, she's got one leg!' But that's all right. I'm still going to take my shower; I am not going to hide. I would be embarrassed to hide. I feel as if I am educating the public."

—Marcy

Know that you are not alone. Every person with visible differences has experienced a wide variety of obnoxious reactions from others, which include staring, rude questions, insensitive comments, and thoughtless actions. It is important for you not to take any of this behavior personally. Recognize that it says far more about the ignorance and social ineptitude of the "offender," than anything about you.

EFFECTS OF AMPUTATION ON BODY IMAGE

Very young children may not be concerned about how they appear to others, but as they age they tend to become more self-conscious. This is greatly heightened in the teenage years, as adolescents become more aware of their changing bodies and those of the opposite sex. Adults can be just as self-conscious. When you lose a limb, your appearance is inalterably changed, both in how you view your own body and in how you are viewed by others. When you don't match up to social or personal standards, it may be hard to accept yourself or to be accepted by others.

Amputation inevitably reminds us of our mortality. For anyone, a change in body image produces anxiety. The psychological impact of amputation greatly heightens this anxiety, since loss of limb is a permanent condition. As a person living with amputation, you must redefine your self-concept as well as your body image. This is in addition to the fact that your trauma must be considered in terms of general health, disability, and disruption of your normal lifestyle. Reforming your sexuality and dealing with society's responses are additional factors with which you will have to deal. Nobody said adjusting to loss of a limb would be easy!

If you have recently lost a limb, your entire life probably revolves around the physical impairment. Due to the many medical and prosthetic requirements that follow amputation (and sometimes an underlying medical condition) this makes sense. You may not have met anyone else who has lost a limb, so you have no realistic idea of the ways in which your life will be impacted and the ways it will remain the same. All these factors can contribute to difficulty in accepting your change in appearance.

Over time, your limb loss should gradually recede in importance and become just one aspect of your life. Although they are never happy about it, most individuals learn take their limb loss in stride. They accept the reality of their altered body and move on:

"My body is my body. Having one leg makes a difference, but I don't think any less of my body. I wish I had a broader chest—but I don't. I'd like to have two legs—but I don't. That's just the way it is."

—Mark

Impact of Prosthesis on Body Image

Often the most significant event for a person, after the amputation surgery itself, is the fitting of the first prosthesis. Your acceptance of and attitude toward your artificial limb are central to your sense of well-being and sense of self. Use of a prosthesis not only helps you regain physical mastery and freedom, it can lead to many emotional advantages as well. Greater acceptance of your physical impairment, feelings of social equality and enhanced independence, and a sense of security may all result from prosthetic use.

Most persons with amputation will incorporate their prosthesis into their body image. In fact, many will say they feel incomplete when not wearing it. If you are someone who does not wish your limb loss to be apparent, an artificial limb is a satisfactory solution. The cosmetic appearance of your prosthesis may be important to your sense of well-being.

On the other hand, you may be perfectly at ease with your obvious physical differences whether you choose to wear a prosthesis or not. For a variety of reasons, it may not make sense for you to use one (see Chapter 3, "Prosthetics"). Your own comfort level is a highly individual matter. Wearing an artificial limb is not necessarily better or worse, nor is it an indication of your emotional adjustment.

Note the differences in the attitudes of these two well-adjusted men:

"I regard my prosthesis as 'my leg.' I am a little self-conscious just as everybody is. I'm sensitive about the cosmetic appearance of my leg. Some people don't even know I'm an amputee. Sometimes, out of the clear blue sky someone will ask, 'Did you hurt your ankle? I notice you are limping a little today.' A few people who have known me for over a year just recently found out that I had lost my leg."

—Kent

"I consider my prosthesis an addition to my body; but, I don't mind being without my leg at all."

—Mark

You may discover that you have two different body images of your self—one with your prosthesis and one without it. If you have two different styles of prostheses (or if you choose to use crutches or a wheelchair), you may find your self-image is altered depending upon which you use, and in what context you find yourself. For example, you may feel very comfortable at work wearing a hook, but more comfortable wearing a prosthetic hand when out socially with others. You may feel more comfortable meeting people for the first time wearing a prosthetic leg, rather that using crutches or a wheelchair.

Your attitude toward your prosthesis will change during different phases of your life, especially if you have grown up with apparent limb differences:

"When I was little, I didn't care if my friends or other people saw me without my artificial legs. Now, I'm ashamed to be seen without them; they are a part of me. When I was little, I hated my prostheses. I was always taking them off because I was more comfortable that way. Now, I'm more comfortable with them on; I don't want to be seen without them."

—Marie (15 years old)

Aside from these visual considerations, walking in a prosthetic limb at times may produce a number of odd noises. One potentially embarrassing sound occurs if air escapes from the top of the socket and sounds similar to flatulence. Also, there may be audible clicks or clunks in the knee or foot joints. The cosmetic cover may rub against the limb's interior, causing squeaks. A prosthetic elbow may produce noises when it locks into position. The good news is that there is an obvious solution to these "noisy" problems—visit your prosthetist, who will make adjustments in your prosthesis to get rid of the causes of these unwelcomed sounds.

RELATIONSHIP BETWEEN BODY IMAGE AND SELF-IMAGE

Your self-perception can make a big difference in your sense of well-being and in your enjoyment of life. A negative self-concept can lead to the loss of necessary motivation to proceed in your recovery.

For both the able-bodied and the disabled there is a significant relationship between body attitude and self-esteem. The way you respond to the physical changes in your body depends, in part, upon a variety of factors—your overall emotional balance, your life values, the priority you place on the lost limb, how well-prepared you were for the surgery, the responses you receive from family, friends, and colleagues, and whether or not you have met others with amputation who have successfully recovered and are enjoying their lives.

You may have difficulty accepting your body and assume that others do, too. You may project your own non-acceptance onto others, and needlessly alienate yourself from them. Compounding this alienation, after amputation you may suddenly find yourself lumped into the group that is considered physically handicapped, with all of the social stigma attached to it.

Some persons with amputation consider altered body image to be more of a handicap than their actual physical limitations. Some individuals, who have a poor self-image, will use their loss of limb as an excuse for not doing more with their lives. "You can't expect much from me. I'm not like you; I'm an amputee." Such self-pity and victim-like mentality are a way of defending oneself from failure and from reaching out into life. While this mentality may, in fact, shield one from risk, it does not promote a full, involved life.

Such attitudes contribute to poor self-esteem, depression, shame, and decreased-quality relationships with others. You probably know several "good-looking" people who do not feel great about themselves. Studies have shown it is not someone's actual appearance, but rather the body image that they hold that contributes most to feelings of self-worth. Therefore, someone who is deemed highly handsome or beautiful by others, may or may not feel good about himself or herself. On the other hand, someone who is not considered attractive according to social standards, may feel great about himself or herself. Body image and feelings of self-worth are highly influenced by each other. Have you ever had a good day, when you looked at yourself in the mirror and felt great? Conversely, have you ever had a day when you felt depressed, then looked in the mirror and hated what you saw? Self-confidence and self-acceptance can, therefore, be independent of actual appearance. In the following example, notice how the woman's husband and neighbor are more accepting of her limb loss than she is:

"There was a time when I was dating and thought it was important to have a set of prosthetic legs that was nice in appearance. When I met my second husband, I was wearing a long dress, so until I needed to walk, he didn't even know I had a disability. After we were married, I kept the lights off when we were in bed because I didn't want him to see my scars and my residual limbs. But he seemed comfortable, and, gradually, I became more comfortable, too.

I still try to cover up most of my body so I don't have to explain to anyone why this scar is there, or answer any other questions about my limbs. Most of the time I wear sweatpants because they cover my legs and are comfortable, but they are warm in the summer. I asked both my husband and my neighbor if they would feel uncomfortable if they saw me walking around the yard in shorts. They both said that it wouldn't bother them, but I am still not ready to do that."

—Molly

When a limb or limbs are amputated, it is natural to become self-conscious about your appearance. If you have lost an upper limb, there may be no way to disguise the loss. If you have lost a lower-limb, your gait may announce that there is something "different" about you. If you are self-conscious, you will be anxious about how others view and judge you. Being self-conscious is actually a state of great self-involvement, since you feel that all eyes are focused on you. When you are comfortable with yourself, you relax. You are relatively unconcerned by the evaluations and judgments of others.

It may take months or even years to integrate your altered body into your self-concept. As with other aspects of emotional rehabilitation, there is no set timetable for recovery. Each individual moves at his or her own pace—you will, too.

Beauty is in the Eye of the Beholder

It is said that "beauty is in the eye of the beholder." Whether you look at yourself in the mirror on the wall or the mirror of your mind, you are both the beholder and the beheld. How you *feel* about the way you look is of more importance to your self-esteem than your actual appearance. Therefore, it is helpful to alter thoughts and feelings about your appearance that do not enhance your sense of well-being. The benefits of cultivating a positive body image include the following:

• Feeling at ease with your body and accepting of it (even with amputation).

• Feeling less preoccupied with body image.

• Enjoying movement and your physicality.

• Enjoying your sexuality.

- Getting out of the trap of using societal standards to judge yourself.
- Improving what you can about yourself and accepting yourself as you are to achieve inner peace.

In short, the overall result of cultivating a positive body image is acceptance and enjoyment of who you are, with the body you now have.

It has been said the only material thing we truly possess is our body. We are born with it and relinquish it only when we die. In between, it is the one thing that can never be taken from us. It is the foundation of our physical existence; it provides the housing for our emotional, mental, and spiritual experiences. We must respect and care for it, and listen to its messages. Learning to view ourselves with compassion and a loving eye can truly improve the quality of our lives.

Accepting the Body You Have

"Except that my leg is gone, the amputation hasn't affected my body image at all. Occasionally, seeing that my leg is missing is a bit strange. I'll think, 'I've lost it, and I'll have to live without it.' I don't feel that the artificial leg is a part of my body, but it is a good feeling to have it there, taking the place of my real leg."

—*John*

Your body image influences your life choices and basic sense of well-being. According to Rita Freedman, Ph.D., in her book *Bodylove: Learning to Like Our Looks—and Ourselves* (New York: Harper and Row, 1988), one-half of all women diet most of their lives, and two out of three are depressed or have mixed feelings when they see their nude bodies in the mirror.

When you are preoccupied and unsatisfied with your appearance, you may tend to feel shame, guilt, and self-hatred. There is nothing wrong with wanting to look your best; appearance is a source of self-confidence and social power in our society. But when appearance becomes an obsession, your thoughts become self-destructive rather than life-enhancing.

Dr. Freedman talks about the concept of "bodylove" as a way of accepting one's appearance:

Bodylove is a mixture of emotions, attitudes and actions that allows you to enjoy the way your body looks and the way it feels. Bodylove enhances self-confidence and heightens physical pleasure. Like other loving relationships, bodylove includes caring and concern. There is joy in personal contact as well as tolerance of flaws. There is a unity that overcomes the separateness between mind and body. We all have the potential to love our bodies. Like any loving relationship, it takes work to realize that potential.

When you are able to accept your body just the way it is, you can enjoy its appearance, abilities, and sensations. When you can accept what is, and stop longing for what isn't, it is possible for you to live happily in an imperfect body. Remember, this is the only body you will ever have, so why not make peace with it?

All of us must learn to adjust to bodies that change as we age. Men often face problems such as balding, middle-age spread, and loss of muscle tone, while women cope with the changing texture of their skin, greying hair, and sagging breasts, among other changes. The sooner you develop an attitude of compassion for and acceptance of your body, the sooner you will be able to relax and enjoy your life, irrespective of your external appearance.

WAYS TO IMPROVE YOUR BODY IMAGE

Since your body image is internally generated, the power to change it lies within you. The following suggestions will assist you in making peace with your body and in improving how you perceive yourself.

1. *Appreciate the multitude of ways in which your body still serves you.* Set aside some time when you can have privacy. Sit comfortably and close your eyes. Take a few deep, slow breaths. With each breath allow more and more tension to flow out of your body. Feel yourself becoming more and more relaxed. In your mind, review all the ways in which your body serves you:

• Your heart constantly pumps blood through your body so that all of your cells receive the necessary food and oxygen.

• Your lungs work hard to remove carbon dioxide from your bloodstream, and replace it with fresh oxygen.

• Your amazing brain and nervous system synthesize an incredible amount of information from your entire body, and allow you to communicate what is happening both internally and externally.

• Your senses make you aware of the exterior world; they provide you with information that is both vital and pleasurable to your survival. . . .

Continue to use your imagination and run through the various organs and systems of your body. Allow yourself to feel wonder, appreciation, and gratitude for all that your body does for you—day in and day out. Inwardly thank your body for serving you well for so many years.

Next, turn your attention to your residual limb. Give thanks to your original limb for all it did for you. Feel a sense of appreciation and gratitude for all of the ways in which it served you so well, even though it was probably taken for granted. Feel a sense of compassion for your residual limb, for all that it has been through and all that it has suffered. Thank your residual limb for the ways in which it still serves you. Whether you use crutches, or a wheelchair, or a prosthesis, your residual limb is still working to help move you around in the world.

Now, view your entire body as a whole again. Consider how, even with all that it has gone through, your body continues to make your life possible. Consider the joys and wonders that would not be yours if you did not have your body. Consider the sensory and aesthetic pleasures you experience through your body. Consider the many benefits you may tend to take for granted—the joy of friendship, the beauty of nature, the pleasure of listening to music, the fascination of a good book, the enjoyment of a good meal—all of which would be totally impossible without your body. Sincerely thank your body for making all of these wonderful experiences possible.

After you have finished this exercise and move through your day, try to retain this sense of appreciation for all that your body does for you. Remember the question about whether the glass is half-full or half-empty; when you focus on what you have rather than on what you lack, you may very well find that the glass is not only half-full, but actually overflowing.

2. *Learn to view yourself more objectively.* If you look at yourself objectively in the mirror and describe what you see, you will find that the description in itself contains no value judgements. (For example, you may see a woman with brown eyes and dark brown hair. She has freckles and a dimple on one side of her mouth.) The assignment of relative value is something that you do in your mind.

Take time to leaf through the pages of a travel magazine. When you note the variety of shapes of human bodies, and the ways that persons of different cultures choose to adorn their bodies, it will become readily apparent that each culture has its own standards of beauty. If you tie your sense of well-being to external appearances and allow yourself to be a slave to the vagaries of fashion, you do yourself a great disservice.

3. *Respect your body. Listen to the messages it gives you, and take care of your physical needs.* Get adequate rest to refresh yourself. Follow a well-balanced diet, which will nourish you and provide you with the energy needed to keep up your vitality. Get adequate exercise to stay in optimal physical condition. Pay attention to the messages your body gives you, be they messages of pain or pleasure. When you respect your body by taking good care of it, self-acceptance is easier to achieve.

4. *Learn to accept your flaws and limitations.* They are only a small part of what makes you you.

5. *Consciously shift your body image into one that supports your well-being.* You can compare the process of defining your body image with the process of taking and developing a photograph. In the same way that many aspects of the photographic process are in the photographer's control, many aspects of your body image are within your control.

If you want to develop an image, you need to make a number of decisions. Will you shoot the image in the soft, natural light that is found outdoors, or in the harsh, artificial light of the studio? Will you shoot an extreme close-up of the object, which reveals its most minute details, or will you shoot it from a distance to produce an impression of the object as a whole? Will you shoot the object all alone against a blank backdrop, or surrounded by people and objects with which it bears a relationship?

Just as the discriminating photographer must make many decisions based upon the effect he desires, you must build your self-image based upon the effect you want to create in your life. Pay attention to the internal monologue that runs in your mind. Catch yourself when you are being self-critical and replace those messages with ones that are positive and enhance your sense of self. When you project yourself as comfortable and at ease with who you are, others will tend to be more at ease when they are around you.

IN CONCLUSION

It is my hope you use the information in this chapter to view yourself in the best possible light, surrounded by friends and family who love and appreciate you as you are, in an environment that brings you peace and contentment. When you look at yourself through the eyes of compassion and love, you will improve your self-concept. As you learn to accept yourself as you are, regardless of the size and shape of your body, or the number of limbs you have, you will find that you are comfortable with yourself. When you have the courage to embrace your uniqueness as a human being, you'll discover that the differences that make you "you" can be a source of strength and satisfaction.

15

MAKING MEANING
OF YOUR AMPUTATION

I almost entitled this "The Most Important Chapter in the Book." If I were told that an individual with limb loss could read only one chapter, this is the one I would recommend. In my opinion, the *meaning* you attribute to your amputation, and your *attitude*—the point of view and the life orientation through which you filter your experiences—are the key factors in your healing and recovery following limb loss.

This chapter presents a framework for creating positive meaning and a healthy attitude following your amputation. It builds on concepts discussed in previous chapters. Some of the topics include putting your life into perspective, the power of language, the healing potential of compassion and forgiveness, and the role of your spiritual life in your recovery. This information is offered with the hope that you will consciously use your amputation experience as a springboard for enriching your life.

THE POWER OF YOUR MIND

You experience what your mind thinks. This profound and very wise teaching, which has been handed down through the millenia, can qualitatively change the experiences of your life, including living with amputation. If you contemplate this concept, you will discover that you actually react to your thoughts and feelings about an event, rather than to the event itself. That which you believe becomes "truth" for you, because you act "as if" your beliefs are actual, objective reality. For example, if I believe that because I have lost a limb my life is ruined, or I am somehow less worthwhile than others, or I will never be happy, then I will make decisions and actions based upon those beliefs. I may not seek a satisfying career or a spouse who is my equal; I may not strive to attain other goals that I had previously held dear.

Therefore, your mind has great power to influence your state of well-being. Marie and Clint both intuitively understand this:

"If you think you are whole, you will feel whole. It's all in the mind. If I want to do something, I just go out and do it."

—Marie

"There I was in a hospital room feeling very alone. I realized what had happened and knew there was nothing I could do about it. My arm wasn't going to grow back. Right then, I realized it was the time to change the way I thought about things.

The hardest part was that I had been an auto mechanic. I liked to build things and work with my hands. Even before the accident, I had often thought, 'What would I do if I ever lost my hand?' Now I'm going to find out. I knew I had to make a decision, so I decided to do whatever I had to do to adjust to living without my hand. Half of it is in your mind anyway—half is in your body. I believed that no matter what happened, I'd be all right."

—Clint

As Marie and Clint wisely have realized, while it is true you cannot always control events in the outer world, you *can* control your responses to them. You may not be able to change events, but *you do have the power to change your thoughts about what has occurred.* You can correct distorted thinking and alter limiting or destructive self-talk.

Consciousness—Your Primary Tool

You already possess the tool you need to transform the quality of your life—your consciousness. What distinguishes man from all other creatures is his capacity for self-awareness. (The term "awareness" is used synonymously in this chapter with the term "consciousness.") Through awareness, you can recognize the places where you are stuck in self-imposed limitations. Without awareness, you will probably tell yourself that "this is the way life is"; in other words, you will believe in your own limitations. By acting as if these *self-imposed* limitations are real, you create self-fulfilling prophecies in your life. The following are examples of such self-imposed limiting beliefs:

Since I am someone who has had a limb amputated:

• I'm not worth as much as other human beings.

• No one will be attracted to me or want me, so I will always be alone.

• I might as well give up any aspirations of having a happy life, great relationships, a fulfilling career, an active recreational life, etc.

Repeatedly saying or even thinking these types of thoughts will create negative results. You will use them as a filter to interpret your experiences, and your limiting beliefs will become self-fulfilling prophecies. You will be less likely to make appropriate efforts where you should, and you will be prone to ignore real opportunities when they present themselves. You may not even recognize certain opportunities because you have been telling yourself that such chances are impossible for you.

Truly, the most remarkable individuals I interviewed when gathering information for this book are enjoying their lives to the fullest. It is not simply their accomplishments that are amazing, rather it is the *attitude* with which they approach life. It is their attitude that allows them the internal freedom to pursue their dreams. They have chosen to lift the cap off their limitations and go for the gusto. I'd like to mention just a few of these amazing individuals.

Margaret is a world-class skier who teaches disabled children how to ski. She has also starred in a television series, in which she played the role of a scuba diving instructor. She recently completed a twenty-two day trek in Nepal, hiking on one leg while using crutches.

Leslie is a physician who completed her medical training after triple amputation. She works full-time, is happily married, and is raising two children. She describes herself as a happy individual who enjoys the same satisfactions in life as everyone else.

Clint lost a hand in a fireworks accident. Within a very short time, he returned to his chosen career working as a car mechanic. He still enjoys a wide variety of recreational activities. Clint believes that adjusting to limb loss is as much mental as it is physical.

Question Who You Really Are

Another ancient teaching that still holds true today concerns the nature and cause of suffering. It states, *the pain individuals experience is, in part, caused by false identification with things external to themselves.* For instance, if you identify yourself with your career and equate your self-worth with your work—if you think of yourself as only a lawyer, nurse, engineer, car mechanic, etc.—the loss of your job is apt to devastate you.

Losing a limb forces you to question who you really are. When I came out of a coma and first looked into a mirror, because of the severe trauma I had undergone, I did not recognize the smashed-up face I saw looking back at me. I had to look into my eyes, the "windows of my soul," before I was able to recognize myself. Only then did I know that "I" was, indeed, in there. When I looked down and found an empty space on the bed where my leg should have been, you can bet I had to re-examine who I thought myself to be. If you believe you are *only* your physical body, then amputation will be devastating for you. On the other hand, if you believe the that totality of who you are is more than just your physical body, your adjustment will be significantly easier.

Ask yourself, "Who is reading the words on this page?" You might answer,

"I am." Well, how do you know that? It is your awareness that permits you to know your experience. This understanding is the first step in recognizing what has been called "witness consciousness." When you recognize your internal "witness," you recognize the basic awareness that underlies your experience. You can then choose to identify yourself with your awareness, rather than with anything else external. In other words, you can realize that although you may be strongly influenced and affected by what happens to you physically, the totality of who "you" are is far greater than your physical body. Your body may be missing part of a limb, but "you" are still intact. "You" are still uniquely you. "You" can still enjoy your life.

"Being disabled doesn't change you as a person unless you let it. You still have a heart with which you can love. You have a great gift in that you can empathize with others who have lost something because you yourself have had something taken away. It gives you strength from within."

—Molly

Witness consciousness can also be applied to your emotions and your mind. It is important for you to understand that you are not your feelings and thoughts. Although you experience feelings and thoughts, they are different and separate from you; inevitably, they will pass, but you will still be here. Discovering your witness consciousness can be a liberating and joyful experience.

Discover New Depths of Being

The more unyielding and confining your thoughts, feelings, and behavior, the more limited and constricted you will be in terms of internal freedom. When you can fully respond to the demands of the moment with an openness that is unconditioned by limiting beliefs, you will be more creative and free.

Since it is your mind that "creates" your subjective reality, you must learn to master it, rather than let it master you. Belief structures and patterns of thought tend to become crystallized, robotic, and habitual. The smaller your scope of life, the less choices will be available to you.

Sometimes it takes a shock—a jolt to everyday complacency—to snap us out of rigid thought patterns and to crack open our awareness to new possibilities:

"It sucks having to go through chemotherapy; but if I want to live, I have to go through it. Going through the cancer treatment process is a character builder. Being in the hospital really opens up your mind. There you are exposed to some of the hardships of life; you even see a few people die. It starts some gears spinning and gives you a better outlook, which carries over into other areas of life."

—Mark

"I know how to read people a lot better since my amputation. I know how to pick my friends. I look at things differently. Before I lost my leg I used to drink and party a lot. I don't abuse alcohol or drugs anymore; now I think it's a waste of time. There are other things to do that are so more stimulating! Things that I had just blown off before are more beautiful to me now. I can't say amputation has been all bad; I've benefitted from it in many ways."

—Bob

Loss of a limb is, of course, tragic. However, this does not mean that it cannot be useful in enriching your life and opening it up to new depths of being. When I underwent amputation, and subsequently experienced all that is involved in rehabilitation and emotional adjustment, my previous values and life priorities underwent a major shake-up and reordering.

Love, friendship, compassion, and kindness moved to the foreground of importance, while other aspects of my life such as work and material pleasures (which had once dominated more of my world), receded in importance. The shallowness of the world of appearances became obvious. Society's hypnotic pull toward valuing the superficial became apparent. The spark of Divinity within me and everyone else—that essential self that blazes with love and inner beauty—became clearly evident.

I share this with you because, in spite of my amputation and all I've been through, these realizations have made all I have undergone worthwhile. They have deepened my self-awareness and internal maturity.

THE CLASSROOM OF LIFE

Historically, the world can be likened to a classroom in which we are all students and our life experiences are lessons. This analogy can be useful in your recovery process. You can learn to convert your life experiences into wisdom by understanding their meaning and by learning their inherent lessons.

You can recognize the places in your daily life in which you get stuck in self-limiting beliefs, attitudes, and thoughts that produce undesirable re-actions. As you focus on these places and work to change them, you transmute your life experiences into wisdom. This wisdom can free you from destructive thought patterns and behaviors, and open the way for greater levels of internal freedom, love, and self-acceptance. These positive experiences add to the joy of living and contribute to your expanding realization of consciousness. Some have called this type of recognition about the purpose in living, "the only dance there is."

Think of the situations in which you find yourself reacting negatively. Try to free yourself from these reactions and heal any residual wounds from the past. If you don't learn the "lessons" inherent in the moment, don't worry—your life will provide you with other opportunities by repeating the lesson! For as long as your destructive beliefs, thoughts, and attitudes are still in place, you will continue to suffer their consequences until your consciousness is clarified in those areas. To put it another way, your mind sets up a structural grid through which you filter your experiences, in much the same way as the topography determines the course of a river. Change the structure of the topography, and the river will change course. If you want to change the course of your life, you need only change those destructive thoughts, negative attitudes, and limiting beliefs.

Learn Lessons from Others with Amputation

Those who have learned to cope successfully with limb loss have valuable insights to share. They can help you accept reality, cope with painful emotions, and develop a positive attitude. In this section, some of these individuals share the wisdom of their experience.

Some say it helps to put their amputation in perspective by considering it in relative terms. This is done by comparing their misfortunes to those of others, or by placing themselves in a hypothetical situation that is worse than theirs:

"Acceptance is the key to the whole thing. Life goes on no matter what. Anytime I start to feel down or sorry for myself, I can always find somebody who is in worse shape than I am, and that makes me feel fortunate."

—Kent

To promote acceptance, many suggest pursuing positive goals and keeping active in daily life:

"In the beginning, you have no place to go but up. It's just a matter of learning how to do things differently. Instead of bemoaning what you can't do, go out and create something to fill that void—develop new interests. Do whatever it takes; set little goals to get a sense of accomplishment—so that you are succeeding, rather than failing when you try to do something differently."

—Leslie

Some recommend surrendering to a greater wisdom and power than themselves ("Not my will, but Thine be done"). They stress how going through the amputation experience has given them strength in themselves and in their faith in a greater plan:

"I am very positive about my future, because I feel myself healing inside. Going through all this has given me a lot of inner strength and a lot of faith in that inner strength. I believe that everything that happens to a person in his life is supposed to happen. If you want to learn from it, you will."

—Judith

Most people recognize it is their attitude towards themselves that is of key importance in healing and recovery. A positive outlook directly affects the quality of living:

"Be positive! There are so many things you can still do; dwell on those, not on the things you can't. Right now, you might think, 'My God, the world's over. I'm not going to be able to do this or that.' But over time, you'll find yourself able to do more things than you believed possible. You might have to do them a little slower or differently, but you'll still be able to do them. Focus on what you want to do and work toward that goal. When you've accomplished one thing, it will be easier to accomplish the next, and soon you'll find yourself on a roll. It really does work that way."

—Margaret

Some say the experience has opened them up to a new appreciation of life and has given them a better overall perspective:

"Recognize the fact that you are still on earth. You are a living human being, and there are others who can't get around as well as you can. Learn to live with yourself. You are still here with your family and friends, which is so important. I look forward to the little things my wife and I do together. It is wonderful for me to see my children growing up, and to have grandchildren. I greatly appreciate that I am alive. I am here on earth. I still have my body."

—John

"A lot of times you take what you have for granted. I lost a leg, and I miss it now; I appreciate this artificial limb more than I did my real leg. I had never realized how much my wife loves me and how much she cares. Now I tell her so often how much I love her, it might sound a little corny to her."

—Fred

Many individuals stress that your state of well-being following amputation is ultimately up to you:

"If I were not a happy person, I would not want to talk about my amputation. But I feel it is important for people to know that they can still be happy in spite of losing a limb. If you are a happy person to start with, I really think you are going to be a happy person from here on in."

—Leslie

"You have to make it okay with yourself. You can deal with it, live a normal life, and be happy—just as happy as anyone else—but it is up to you. It is your responsibility to take care of yourself and to take charge of your life."

—Marcy

No one can say why some of us are given what may seem like overwhelming challenges in life. Just as steel is forged through fire, inner strength and maturity are tempered by how we meet adversity:

"I don't think of myself particularly as an amputee. After my amputation, I discovered that I had a lot of strength inside that I never knew I had. And that is something my husband and I both admire. I look at life with more of an even keel now. It's easier to look at the 'bad' things that happen, and know that I'll get through them."

—Leslie

"I'm very positive about my future. I don't spend much time thinking about myself as an amputee. In some ways, I am a more together person than others who may never have had to test their inner resources. I have been at rock bottom and dealt with a lot. Life should not have to be so tough, but sometimes it is. It's made me stronger; I'm a survivor."

—Marcy

Keep a Positive Attitude

As the song says:

> You've got to accentuate the positive,
> Eliminate the negative,
> Latch on to the affirmative,
> Don't mess with Mr. In-between.

Many individuals have the misconception that attitude is something you are born with, like hair or eye color. They believe that some people are stuck with bad attitudes while others are blessed with positive ones. If you are one of these people, know that attitude is something you have the power to control. Adopting a positive attitude can have a profound influence on the quality of your life.

In spite of their amputation, the following people have found happiness and fulfillment in their lives by choosing to maintain a positive attitude:

"Your limb has nothing to do with your mental attitude, or the way you interact with people. You can still do anything you want to do—anything. It's all in your head, not your hand or leg. Even though I am missing an arm, I can still ride my off-road vehicle, go camping, work on cars, and go fishing.

After I catch a fish, all I can think about is that fish flopping around on the deck—not that I caught it one-handed! So, hang in there. After you relearn how to do something, it becomes normal again. You're still going to make yourself happy. Your body, no matter how limited, is still the vehicle for that. Take advantage and use it as much as you can. You can do anything you want to do—anything!"

—Clint

"Your mind has control over your body. Learn to accept your amputation, and make the best of it—you are still capable of doing a lot. Concentrate on the positive aspects; if you dwell on the negative, you are just going to upset yourself. It will give you a feeling of inferiority, which makes it harder to pull yourself out. So start off with a positive outlook; accept the fact that life goes on. Your attitude plays the biggest part. Life is full of ups and downs, and you have to roll with the punches; get back up and make the best of it."

—Kent

In the field of aeronautics, "attitude" refers to the orientation of the airplane relative to three different axes of movement (forward/backward, side to side, and up/down). A pilot who doesn't control the attitude of his plane is likely to stall, lose power, and make unwanted contact with the face of a mountain or fall into a downward spiral until the ground intervenes. On the other hand, a pilot who controls the attitude of his plane will likely arrive at his chosen destination.

It would be wise to take a lesson from the experienced pilot. First take stock of your attitude. Are you headed up or down? Veering to the right or left? Spinning in one direction or another? Once you determine your current attitude, and you have explored your past to see the circumstances and beliefs that created that attitude, you can take firm hold of the controls and put your vehicle back on course. Having a destination clearly in mind, and checking your orientation periodically will make it easier for you to detect a shift in attitude and make the necessary adjustments for a pleasant and successful flight.

You are More Than "An Amputee"

Remember, your amputation is only one aspect of your life. As I integrated my amputation into my life and healed my emotional wounds, as well as my physical ones, I became "a person with an amputation," rather than "an amputee" who was struggling to live.

In the beginning, when you are struggling with adjustments to your amputation, it is hard to come to peace with your new realities. Over time, though, know that things will get easier. Most people who experience amputation go on to lead rich, rewarding lives.

The shock of amputation can serve to deepen your spirituality, opening your heart to greater love, which brings a deep inner peace. When you realize the power and mastery you can have over your own mind, and become confident of your self-worth, you will feel internally secure. This security will help you develop a sense of humor about life and about yourself; it will help you to be playful and lighthearted. Eventually, you will attain great peace and equanimity, and your inner love and compassion will grow.

THE POWER OF LANGUAGE

A friend of mine who is quadriplegic once pointed out that there is a fine line between those who are considered disabled and the non-disabled. In fact, she refers to the non-disabled as "TABs"—temporarily abled bodies. She is referring to the fact that, as medical technology continues to advance and we naturally age, many of us will live longer and develop some sort of disability that we must learn to assimilate into our everyday lives.

When you undergo amputation, you may suddenly find yourself being labeled. It's important to realize *you are not a label; you are not your physical condition.* You are not crippled, disabled, handicapped, or even physically challenged. Rather, you are an individual human being who happens to live with physical differences.

What's in a Name?

Our parents were wrong when they taught us the adage, "Sticks and stones may break your bones, but names can never hurt you." Words *can* hurt. Although they can lift our hearts, words can also drive us into despair. Throughout history, words have both unified people and incited rebellions. Labels have been used to segregate and divide people, often implying that those who are unlike us are somehow dangerous or inferior. Words have been used to make unfounded distinctions based on race, religion, sex, physical differences, and physical and mental ability. Oftentimes our use of language is based on fear, ignorance, and distorted information.

As a person with limb differences, you should describe yourself by emphasizing your humanness first. Rather than considering yourself "an amputee," refer to yourself as "a person with amputation." Rather than believing you are "disabled," think of yourself as "a person with a disability."

You may have heard of people referred to as "victims" of a disease or a physical condition—almost as if they are victims of a crime. Sometimes, people are said to be "afflicted" with a disease or condition, which implies that the disease is a form of punishment that has been delivered by a malevolent outside force. Instead of calling someone the "victim" of an amputation (or cancer, or diabetes), rather say, "He is a person who has lost a limb due to . . ." And never think of yourself as an "invalid." This literally implies that you are "not valid." Is this what you really mean to express?

Also, you are not just "a patient." Once again, this label puts you in a category in which your state of health is stressed as the most prominent part of who you are. In fact, many people with amputations are not ill and have no disease.

Some individuals are offended when they hear themselves described as "confined" to a wheelchair or "wheelchair bound." Wheelchairs are not confining, rather they are liberating in that they provide an individual with the ability to travel from one place to another. Although currently there is some controversy, even among "experts," concerning the terminology applied to those with physical differences, the World Health Organization makes a distinction among the following terms in ways that include physical, psychological, and social perspectives:

• **Impairment** refers to the loss or abnormality of a physiological, psychological, or anatomical structure or function. An example of physical impairment is the loss of a limb.

• **Disability** refers to a restriction in an ability to perform an activity that is considered normal for others. Not being able to run due to an above-knee amputation is an example of a disability.

• **Handicap** refers to a social disadvantage when interacting with others, or when trying to adjust to an environment. For example, I would have a handicap if I had to go up a flight of stairs and was using a wheelchair at the time.

From this discussion, you should realize how important it is to become conscious of the language you use, both in thinking about yourself and when speaking with others. Using appropriate terminology may seem of little importance, yet it can have both subtle and profound impacts upon your sense of self-worth, competency, and self-respect. Using accurate, positive language is an important part of recognizing that we are all essentially the same, despite any physical differences. We all deserve respect based upon our actions, not our physical conditions.

The Language of Suggestion

Through studying communication theory and the language of hypnosis, I became sensitized to the fact that we give ourselves many "suggestions" throughout the course of a day. These suggestions can actually function as a form of self-hypnosis. Understanding this concept can aid you in your recovery.

Beware of destructive suggestions. They can erode your sense of well-being and chip away at your self-esteem. You may give yourself suggestions through such practices as the unquestionned use of inappropriate terminology (as just discussed), and through negative self-talk (discussed in Chapter 13, "Self-Esteem").

It is important to always make statements in the positive rather than the negative. For example, think of what happens when you hear the command, "Whatever you do, don't think of a pink elephant." When given this negative command, you must first picture a pink elephant *before* you can internally compute that you were asked *not* to think of one. Now, imagine what happens when you tell yourself, "Don't worry." Of course, you will worry! It is far better to say to yourself, "Stay relaxed. You can be calm about this." By stating what you want in positive terms, you are more likely to improve your outcome.

Notice the difference in how you feel when you tell yourself, "I'll never learn to control my prosthesis," versus "I haven't learned to control my prosthesis *yet*." The first statement implies defeat; the second provides encouragement.

When you give yourself negative commands or negative suggestions, you do yourself a disservice. So, to enhance your well-being, pay attention to your suggestions to yourself, and keep those suggestions positive.

DEFINING YOUR SENSE OF PURPOSE

"One morning, about a year after my amputation, I realized that I was making breakfast, going to work, coming home in the evening, and even going away on vacation. It was what everyone else did in life, so why shouldn't I? I am able to do what they do. I make a living, I have a wonderful family, and I enjoy my life. What more can I ask for?"

—Leslie

Following amputation, you can either give in to despair, or convert your painful experience into one that embraces and enriches your life. There are two factors that can make a big difference in your recovery and well-being—the meaning you attribute to your limb loss, and your sense of life purpose. Meaning and purpose are intertwined; you make your own meaning and define your own sense of purpose.

You can do everything right in your rehabilitation (go to physical therapy, eat nutritious foods, exercise, have good relationships, enjoy a satisfying career, etc.), and still feel like something is missing in your life. Although you may appear to have it all, you may still feel an emptiness inside, a vacuum. You may feel that your life lacks a sense of purpose, direction, and value because of your limb loss.

Your sense of purpose, your priorities, your goals, your moral choices, your philosophy of life, and your spiritual orientation all contribute to the *meaning* you make of the events in your life. Meaning greatly contributes to your sense of life satisfaction. When you undergo amputation, the meaning you assign to your amputation makes a huge difference in how well you adjust to limb loss and its multidimensional effects.

Determining Meaning—A Personal Matter

The ways you come to determine meaning of your amputation are highly personal. They are influenced by your upbringing and values, and tempered by your life experiences. Your belief system and the filters you place on reality will all influence the meaning you ascribe to your limb loss.

Individuals respond to their loss of limb in a variety of ways. Some feel "crippled" for life, or believe that their value and worth as a human being is diminished; they then give up their hopes and dreams, and engage in self-destructive behaviors. On the other hand, some view their loss of limb as a challenge that calls upon them to bring forth the best in themselves, and they may even exceed previous dreams and goals as they tap into their strengths. Some may turn away from their spirituality and say things like, "How could this have happened to me (or my child)? There is no just God." Yet, others consider their limb loss a stimulus to deepen their religious convictions, and look deep within themselves for peace and wisdom.

You cannot change the fact that a limb has been amputated, but you *can* change the meaning you make of the experience. You can choose to become embittered; you can wallow in self-pity or despair; you can believe that your life might as well be over; and you can rant and rail at the heavens, "Why Me?" Or you can choose to find meaning in the experience. You can ask yourself, "What can I learn from this?" "How can I reassess my life priorities?" "What have I decided about life and living?" "Where is there love in my life?" "How can I turn this amputation into a life-affirming experience?"

In *Man's Search for Meaning* (Boston: Beacon Press, 1962), psychiatrist Victor Frankel describes how he and others survived a Nazi concentration camp by summoning up meaning in life, and a sense of purpose in the face of the utter horror of their experience. He states that the search for meaning is significant for us all, and that with a sense of purpose, we can survive and transcend even the most difficult of circumstances.

See how the following individuals found they could use their life experiences to enhance their sense of purpose and be of service to others:

"My pastor and I have discussed my purpose. I can minister to those who are hurting. I can share with them the strength that has come to me from my religious beliefs, from my church family, and from knowing God.

My spirituality has grown in a way that maybe it wouldn't have if I hadn't lost my legs. I took my legs for granted until I didn't have them anymore. I took life for granted until I faced the threat of losing mine. I began to see things differently. I realized my situation was forcing me to stop and take a look at what I was doing, and where I was going!"

—Molly

"I am a physician, and find that the experience of my amputation has helped me to interact positively with my patients. I can deal with a person who is going through something very difficult—trauma, cancer, or some terminal illness—and

I am able to share my experience with them, which is incredibly valuable. I tell them, 'I am missing both of my legs and an arm, but I'm working, I'm happy, and my life goes on.' I don't have to say a whole lot. I use my experience selectively to make people feel better, or to help them realize that things aren't as hopeless as they may seem."

—Leslie

Your sense of purpose and the meaning you ascribe to internal and external circumstances directly impacts the choices you make and the actions you take in your everyday life. When you have a clear sense of your values, you have guidelines with which to align your choices and behavior. Without this clarity, it is easy to flounder and allow yourself to be passively buffeted around by circumstances.

What is important to you? What do you value? What gives meaning and purpose to your life? Only you can answer these questions. For some, it's material success. For others, it's physical beauty. Service to others, work, love of friends and family, wisdom, and time for play and travel are common areas in which people find meaning in their lives. Still other individuals find meaning in good health, relationships, creative outlets, or personal and spiritual growth. The list goes on and on.

Ultimately, you are the only one who has the power to make meaning of your life and define your sense of purpose. No one else can do that for you. Others may share their point of view, or even try to impose their beliefs upon you, but only you can decide whether or not to rely on your own inner truth.

Take Time For Reflection

Set aside time for inner reflection, meditation, and contemplation. If you are spiritually oriented, turn to your faith and receive support from those in your religious community. Discuss your values with trusted family and friends. Read books or enroll in a class on values.

Make time to consciously evaluate your spiritual orientation, values, goals, and dreams. This will permit you to set priorities that are in alignment with your true desires and highest good; your actions will then be congruent with who you are, and you will be more self-accepting, self-affirming, and empowered in the course of daily living.

I invite you to take a few moments of your time to use your imagination and visualize yourself living in alignment with your purpose. How does your life look? How do you feel on the inside? What do you tell yourself about who you are and your life choices? What are you doing? How are you interacting with others? What is your typical day like? Adjust your vision of life until your inner voice says, "Yes!" then adjust your actions until you bring your vision into reality.

Keeping a journal is helpful. It helps you keep track of your personal goals. As the vision of what you want for yourself becomes clearer, you can modify your goals to reflect your new-found clarity. It is helpful to read what you've written once a day. In this way you will gradually manifest your vision by making decisions and taking actions that are in alignment with your goals.

Throughout each day, week, month, and year, you will have countless opportunities to make choices—some small and some large. Along the way, as you find your values becoming more and more clear, you can adjust your actions and beliefs to align with your goals. You will find yourself actualizing your vision, and rendering satisfying meaning to your life.

YOUR SPIRITUAL LIFE

It has been said that people who have strong faith manage to endure life even if their worst fears become realities. These people also believe that any pain that comes with life is worth enduring, because life itself has purpose.

In this brief discussion, I refer to the basic spirituality that underlies most religions, rather than to any one specific doctrine or path. The world's great religions have been compared to beads on a single string; this section refers to the string, rather than the individual beads.

For many people, spirituality provides a deep connection with that which is transcendental, that which adds depth and profound meaning to life. If you are one of these individuals, your experience of amputation may take on a new perspective in the framework of your religious or spiritual beliefs. It does not necessarily have to be a formal, organized religion that speaks to the spiritual part of you. Rather, it might be through your connection and commitment to others, to nature, or to work that gives you a sense of spiritual growth and fulfillment.

Your spirituality may serve as a steady home base in which you find repose from the ups and downs of daily living. Through it you may find meaning, strength, inspiration, and replenishment. Spirituality can provide you with guidelines for living and clarifying your values. It can encourage you to be hopeful and optimistic, which fuels your will to persevere during tough times. It can lead you to a community of others who are like-minded, and therefore help reinforce your faith. Further, spirituality can help you make sense of your life—the hardships and the suffering, as well as the joys. It can serve as a vehicle to help you transmute your everyday experiences into personal growth and wisdom.

By following your inner voice, you may discover you have profound wisdom from which to draw. This should give you a quiet satisfaction and a sense of being connected to something greater than your everyday concerns; it should keep you from feeling alone in a cold, uncaring universe.

You may recognize your unique place in the fabric of the cosmos, and realize you are a precious human being like no other. You may also find your heart opening to others with increased compassion and forgiveness. You may find yourself drawn to be of service to others. You may begin to experience a greater and greater sense that everything is going to be all right, no matter what happens in the exterior world. You know that there is more depth to life than simple outer appearances. Your inner peace is not dependent upon being in perfect physical health or having all four limbs intact.

As you connect more and more deeply with your inner self (some believe this to be synonymous with God, or that which is Divine), you will begin to recognize the love you have within and without, and be able to manifest that love more fully. Your experience of love will become more pervasive and unconditional.

Compassion

After your amputation, you may have feelings of self-pity, which are *not* the same as having compassion for yourself. Let's take a moment to examine the difference.

Self-pity implies that you consider yourself "less" than everyone else; you feel unworthy, incapable, and undeserving. Although this attitude is understandable, considering your altered-life circumstances, wallowing in it will impede your healing and recovery.

On the other hand, compassion heals; it strengthens self-esteem. As someone with amputation, having compassion helps you accept reality. This includes recognizing the challenges that you must face and realizing that your situation is indeed difficult. Compassion makes it easy for you to accept yourself as you are with your strengths and limitations. It opens your heart and allows you to demonstrate kindness, respect, understanding, forgiveness, and nonjudgmental acceptance. It is an interesting phenomenon that many people find it easier to have compassion for others than for themselves.

In their book *Self-Esteem: The ultimate program for self-help* (Oakland, CA: New Harbinger Publications, 1987), Dr. Matthew McKay and Patrick Fanning discuss three aspects of compassion that can be learned: understanding, acceptance, and forgiveness.

Understanding yourself in a given situation, means you have taken the time to objectively comprehend why you have reacted to inner or outer events the way you have. Nonjudgmentally, you have figured out how you operate. You don't necessarily have to come up with solutions to your problems. When you *accept* yourself, you acknowledge reality without making value judgements. *Forgiveness*, which is a natural outcome of understanding and acceptance, allows you to "wipe the slate clean" and move on. These three aspects of compassion do not imply that you approve of your actions or reactions; you simply acknowledge them without self-criticism.

The Power of Forgiveness

Forgiveness is a gentle refusal to defend ourselves against love any longer.

Gerald G. Jampolsky, M.D.
Teach Only Love

To forgive means to let go. Why is the topic of forgiveness included in a guide to living with amputation? If you haven't fully forgiven yourself or others for the causes, circumstances, results, or responses to your amputation—your own healing and recovery will be impeded.

When you condemn others, wishing revenge or punishment on them, you deny yourself peace of mind. But when you forgive, you release the past and let go of the idea that whoever caused you harm must be punished. The result of forgiveness is paradoxical—when you release the other, you also release yourself. When you forgive those who have "wronged" you, and wish them peace and the best possible life, you free yourself from being stuck in the past and harboring negative emotions.

The person who is most important to forgive is you! For you cannot have self-love without self-forgiveness. When you refuse to forgive yourself for your thoughts, emotions, or actions, you hold onto the past and cannot fully enjoy the present. Instead you are plagued by self-blame, guilt, and self-recrimination.

Some people are afraid if they "forgive," they must also "forget." This is simply not true! Forgiving does not mean that you repress your negative feelings and pretend they no longer exist. Acknowledging your pain is part of the process of forgiveness. It is also important that you remember what it was that triggered your sense of being "wronged," so you can learn from it and prevent your past from repeating itself in your future.

To forgive (either yourself or another person) requires a sincere willingness to let go of grievances and the desire to seek revenge. To practice forgiveness, use your awareness to catch yourself when you are thinking about revenge and punishment, or feeling guilt or resentment. Then consciously allow yourself to release these negative feelings, and send the person (or yourself) waves of forgiveness, compassion, and love. Say to yourself, "I completely forgive you, and release you from all of my negative associations with the event. I wish you the best in your life."

One way to assess whether or not you've really released your negative feelings is to vividly recall the event that provoked your anger, resentment, or guilt in the first place. If those feelings are no longer present, forgiveness has been achieved. Even when you intellectually recognize the benefits of letting go of the past, true forgiveness might still be difficult to achieve. Your own personal make-up will influence how easily you are able to forgive yourself and others. The degree to which you have been wronged might also influence your willingness to release the past.

DISCOVER WAYS TO NOURISH YOUR SPIRIT

Explore ways to nourish your living spirit (that part within you that connects you with Divinity). This can be done in a number of ways—participating in traditional religion; serving your family and others; advancing social, environmental, or artistic causes; or enjoying quiet, contemplative times or vigorous physical activity. The possibilities are limitless.

I have offered some ways to enhance that spiritual part of you. I hope you find the information useful. I also hope it inspires you to investigate further spiritual practices.

• Prayer, meditation, contemplation, or any activity that helps quiet the incessant chatter in your mind can serve to connect you with something other than your "little self" and its personal drama. Such contemplative activities allow you to touch something transcendental and bring you peace and contentment.

For some, there is nothing quite as awe-inspiring as making contact with nature—taking a walk along the beach, strolling through a beautiful park, or gazing upwards into the shimmering expanse of the midnight sky. Recognizing the handiwork of the Supreme Artist may nourish your spirit.

• A wide variety of inspirational books and audiotapes on the subject of spiritual practices is available at libraries and bookstores. Let your intuition guide you to that which will speak to you and expand your world view. There is also a great variety of metaphysical and spiritual groups in most metropolitan areas. If you enjoy personal instruction, or the support of like-minded individuals, check out the advertisements of such groups in local newspapers and bookstores. There may be a fellowship group at your church or synogogue that you have heard about but never investigated. Go ahead. Take the first step!

• There is great value to be gained from practicing any discipline regularly, whether it is meditation, prayer, or a physical discipline such as yoga. With regular repetition, your experience deepens and, like an interest-earning bank account, benefits will accrue on a daily basis.

Whatever form your spiritual nourishment takes, make it a regular part of your daily routine. How many days would you be willing to go without food or water? How many days would you be willing to go without human contact or stimulating entertainment? Once you get into the habit of feeding your spirit, you may find it as essential as other forms of nourishment.

IN CONCLUSION

When you undergo a personal crisis such as amputation, you are profoundly challenged on every plane of your being—physical, emotional, mental, and spiritual. The indisputable fact is that your limb is permanently gone. How you respond to that reality will determine whether or not you give in to despair, or use the experience to deepen your fullness of being. Undergoing amputation and recovery can prompt you to deepen your appreciation of being alive, and cause you to reorder your life priorities. This experience can open your heart to greater depths of compassion and love for yourself and others, and inspire a greater manifestation of consciousness in your life.

It's up to you! A life lived with amputation is not qualitatively any better or worse than any other life. In a process called alchemy, the ancients attempted to turn base metals into gold. In the same way, you can choose to embrace your experiences and transform them into wisdom. The meaning of living your life with amputation is whatever you choose to make it.

16

SEEKING PROFESSIONAL COUNSELING

No two individuals react the same way to loss of limb. Some people take it in stride, considering their loss only a minor inconvenience, while others struggle for years or even their remaining lifetime with the consequences of their amputation. The results of amputation can be stressful, confusing and, at least temporarily, can impact well-being. When confronting the internal and external changes wrought by losing a limb, life may seem inside-out and topsy-turvy.

The process of recovering emotionally from the multifaceted impact of amputation is, at the very least, extraordinarily challenging. There will be times when your emotional recovery progresses smoothly; yet, there may also be those periods when you find yourself stuck in the middle of painful feelings and limiting beliefs, or engaged in destructive actions that are harmful to your well-being. During these rough times, you can turn to family and friends, your spiritual beliefs, and support groups. Those close to you will love and support you to the best of their ability. At times, however, the process can be overwhelming, and it may be helpful to call in a professional.

This chapter presents information on when to seek the services of a professional psychotherapist and describes the types of issues that can be addressed through counseling. It dispels common myths about counseling and offers the following guidelines—how to choose a therapist; how to choose the best counseling approach for your special needs; how to establish treatment goals; and how to know when to terminate treatment.

WHY PROFESSIONAL COUNSELING?

I believe we all try to do the very best for ourselves that we can; yet sometimes we need additional input in order to discover new ways of thinking, feeling, and behaving. Working with a professional counselor, who is detached from your personal life and outside your immediate sphere of family and friends, can be a wonderful way to accelerate your healing process.

Psychiatrists, psychologists, marriage/family counselors, and other mental-health professionals can provide valuable assistance in helping you cope with the dramatic changes in your new life. A skilled professional can assist you in a number of ways. He or she can serve as a sounding board for your complaints, help facilitate the normal grieving process that follows limb loss, teach you skills to help cope with painful or confusing emotions, and guide you to reformulate a positive self-concept. A professional can also help you address issues such as changes in your family dynamics, concerns about your relationships and vocation, and fears about your future.

Working with a professional counselor also prevents you from overburdening your spouse, family, or close friends with your emotional concerns. More than likely, the people who love and support you are not trained to help you handle all of the intense issues that are provoked by amputation.

A counselor may serve as a bridge between you and other members of your rehabilitation team, and help remove any roadblocks that may be interfering with your rehabilitation. Some individuals with amputation—often the elderly—may also need help with finances, social activity, employment, and access to community services.

WHEN TO SEEK PROFESSIONAL COUNSELING

When is it a good idea to seek professional help in recovering emotionally from amputation? The answer is different for different people. Some may feel the need to work with a counselor immediately after their amputation, while others may not seek assistance until they find themselves stuck in emotional pain. Often it will be readily apparent to the people closest to you, the ones who love you most, when you are having difficulty coping and could use professional help.

If you find yourself experiencing any of the following—the inability to cope with everyday life, chronic or severe depression, or thoughts of suicide—it is especially important for you to seek professional assistance.

The Inability to Cope with Everyday Life

When you undergo the trauma of losing a limb, your ordinary lifestyle is interrupted. You must make a careful assessment, and attend to the far-reaching impact of limb loss on the many areas of your life. This may be an extremely stressful process.

If you realize you are having trouble getting through each day; if you are struggling with relationships, your job, the emotional adjustment to your limb loss, or caring for your health, seek help from a professional counselor. A well-trained professional will assist you in learning new coping skills and strategies; he or she can be an excellent sounding board for expressing your thoughts and feelings, and can provide an objective perspective to help you maintain inner balance.

Severe or Chronic Depression

It is natural to experience some level of depression after a traumatic event such as losing a limb. Generally, however, these feelings pass as you progress through your grieving and recovery. If you feel you are hopelessly stuck in depression, and that your healing process has stalled, professional assistance can provide a boost to facilitate your recovery.

If your symptoms are severe, you may benefit from a pharmacological intervention, such as an antidepressant medication. Psychiatrists are medical doctors and the only licensed professionals who can prescribe medication. If you're feeling so lousy that you can't even consider participating in therapy, because you think it is beyond your capability and energy level, proper medication may help you. It can raise your state of well-being and enable you to be more receptive to the idea of therapy.

In my opinion, antidepressants alone are not a good solution; they do not address the underlying problems that are at the core of your difficulties. However, antidepressants can be especially useful when taken in conjunction with professional counseling. You can gradually taper off using the medication as your sense of well-being and coping skills improve.

Thoughts of Suicide

Suicide has been called a "permanent solution to a temporary problem." After amputation, it is natural to question the value of your life and your ability to cope with your new challenges. If you find yourself feeling so hopeless and distressed that you are seriously considering "ending it all," *get professional help immediately!* Suicide is *not* the answer! A well-trained counselor can help you learn to feel good again.

COMMON ISSUES ADDRESSED THROUGH COUNSELING

In addition to addressing the primary issues that led you to counseling in the first place, you might choose to work on other areas of your emotional well-being. A counselor can be a wonderful guide to help you focus on areas that may improve the overall quality of your life. It is generally much easier to get where you want to go if you have the guidance of one who knows the territory and has the know-how to make the journey.

A well-qualified professional counselor can help you by:

• Reshaping your attitude toward yourself and your lost limb.

- Developing a base for your emotional support.
- Teaching you coping strategies.
- Getting you through stages in which you may be emotionally "stuck," such as grief, depression, anger, etc.
- Correcting your distorted thinking and limiting belief systems.
- Showing you how to make meaning of your amputation.
- Providing you with objective feedback to help you reassess what actually has and hasn't been lost in your life after your amputation.
- Easing any relationship and life-transition difficulties between you and family members, friends, colleagues, or others.
- Teaching you assertiveness skills.
- Improving your self-esteem, body image, and self-concept.
- Teaching you stress-reduction techniques.

Addressing these areas will help you transform your limb loss from a potentially destructive experience into a life-embracing one.

COMMON MYTHS ABOUT COUNSELING

There is a wide variety of myths that prevents many people from seeking professional assistance with their mental and emotional concerns. The most common ones are presented here.

"But, I'm not crazy!"

Some people still cling to the antiquated notion that you have to be certifiably "nuts" to seek professional assistance. It's time to put this tired old misconception to rest once and for all! Consider the following truth—it is a sign of sanity to be willing to deal directly with the issues that bother you.

"I should be able to work things out myself."

While self-reliance is to be applauded, if you believe it is a sign of weakness to ask for help in solving your internal dilemmas, you are depriving yourself of assistance that might be very beneficial. We all do the best we can for ourselves, given our own personal resources. The very point of going to a professional is to learn *new* ways of thinking, and to acquire *new* tools to help you work through those places in which you are stuck.

If you were going to start a new business, you would be considered wise if you consulted an expert in that area. Since counselors are experts in dealing with the kinds of coping issues you now face, you would be smart to avail yourself of their expertise. An objective, experienced professional can be an excellent resource for you, and a valuable part of your support network.

"I'm not into 'touchy-feely, airy-fairy, let's-share-our-feelings' stuff."

Many people (especially men) are repelled by the idea of having to talk about (gulp!) feelings. However, learning to cope with painful or puzzling emotions can greatly facilitate your recovery process following the trauma of amputation. (Chapter 7, "Coping with Your Emotions" presents this concept in detail.)

If you think that feelings are the only things one talks about in counseling sessions, you are mistaken. You can also focus on achieving your goals. This process can include clarifying just what your specific goals are, as well as designing strategies to achieve them. You can work on resolving whatever issues are creating limitations in your life. Thus, the aims of therapy can be very practical and down-to-earth.

"Underneath it all, it's really scary and painful in here."

Some people fear the counseling process will somehow open a Pandora's box of emotional turmoil. They are afraid that getting into certain issues will be unbearably painful.

Allow me to suggest that the emotional discomfort and pain you may be experiencing in your daily life is, in part, due to unresolved issues. Whatever events have happened in the past to cause you pain are over; by working on their emotional residue, you can free yourself from their effects. If you have underlying negative patterns of behavior, thinking, or feeling, and you do not break these patterns, they will continue to interfere with your well-being. Act positively to reduce inner limitations and empower yourself. "What we resist, persists." Amputation (and any underlying physical condition) is bound to stir up emotional chaos. By facing your uncomfortable feelings and fears, instead of ignoring or denying them, you can lessen their impact and help yourself transmute the pain into wisdom.

"Therapy is a lot of hooey! It doesn't help."

It is understandable that some people are cynical about the benefits of counseling, especially if they have never had any experience with it. It does involve an investment of time, money, and most of all, emotional commitment to your own growth. Just as in any other profession, there are effective counselors and ineffective ones; however, if you follow the guidelines that are presented in the following section, you will know how to choose a therapist who is right for you.

CHOOSING A COUNSELOR

Selecting the counselor who best suits your needs is critical. Just as it is wise to be a careful consumer when choosing a surgeon and a prosthetist, it is just as important to choose your counselor with care. Gather referrals from your family, friends, physician, or other health-care professionals. Local social service agencies, as well as members of your spiritual community and local support group are also good source referrals. If you interview a counselor who doesn't seem to meet your specific needs, feel free to ask him or her to refer you to another counselor who might better serve you. Most counselors will be happy to help you in this way.

Depending on your special needs, there are many counselors from which to choose—psychologists, psychiatrists, marriage/family counselors, rehabilitation specialists, counselors who work with children, and pastoral or other spiritual counselors. The important thing is to establish a good working relationship with your counselor. You should feel comfort and safety with your therapist. Both of you should be in alignment with your treatment goals and the methods used to achieve them. You should begin to experience positive results within a short period of time.

I suggest you choose a therapist who offers solution-oriented "brief-term" therapy. (Admittedly, this is my bias.) In this therapy, the counselor works quickly and practically to help you deal with your immediate concerns. In my opinion, a counselor who teaches you coping strategies is more effective than one who simply serves as a sounding board.

Important Considerations When Choosing a Counselor

There is, of course, no guarantee the counselor you choose will be the perfect match for you, or that your experience will be a successful one. However, there are steps you can take to make an educated, informed decision concerning your choice. Consider the following points:

• **Professional background.** What is the therapist's professional background? Is he short-term therapy oriented? Has he had experience working with individuals who have undergone life trauma that is, at least in some ways, similar to yours? It may be hard to find a therapist who specializes in working with persons who have undergone amputation, but relatively easy to find one who has worked with people who have experienced some type of loss, or a health problem that has greatly impacted their lives.

• **Financial considerations.** Find out the counselor's charges and discuss any financial matters with him. Many therapists adjust their fees on a sliding scale based upon your ability to pay. *Before* starting any therapy sessions, be sure to check with your insurance company to determine the type of coverage you have for counseling services. Some policies will pay

---

for one or two types of counselors but not others; some will limit the number of sessions within a calendar year; some will cover only severe cases in which a person is hospitalized. Many insurance companies pay a fixed price per session. Some will pay a percentage of the cost, generally between 50 and 90 percent. Be aware that most communities offer counseling assistance through social service agencies, which may operate on a sliding scale.

• **First-visit policy.** When researching and trying to learn about a therapist, it is often possible to call him and have your questions answered over the phone. Some therapists will allow you to come in for a brief preliminary session to answer your questions (there may or may not be a charge for this visit). This interview with the therapist will help you determine whether or not you may work well together.

• **Office location and hours.** It is wise to choose a therapist whose office is conveniently located and whose hours can easily fit into your personal schedule.

• **Length and frequency of sessions.** Most sessions run anywhere from forty-five minutes to an hour. Most people work with their therapist once, or perhaps twice a week during the beginning of treatment, depending on the severity of their symptoms. As you achieve your treatment goals, the sessions will gradually taper off. If a crisis arises months down the line, you may call your therapist for additional assistance and support. The length of your treatment time will be very individual; it is influenced by the nature and severity of your issues, your counselor's approach to therapy, and your commitment.

Careful consideration of these points will help you to make an informed choice when selecting a therapist. And remember, once you begin your sessions, if you feel you are not making any progress, or you feel a lack of rapport with the therapist, begin looking for someone new. It's your right.

THE BEST COUNSELING APPROACH FOR YOU

If you were a well-adjusted individual before your amputation, I recommend you seek a counselor who uses a brief-term, practical-oriented approach to therapy. Your amputation has, undoubtedly, given you immediate, practical issues to address. You must learn to cope with your emotional responses and make necessary adjustments in your everyday life.

I tell my clients I am interested only in their past history as it impacts their current life. If part of a person's past is significantly influencing current concerns, it is certainly important to deal with it. Although, admittedly, this is my personal approach, there are other, equally valid ways to work with your concerns.

Elements of Successful Counseling

One of the most important elements of successful counseling is good rapport with your counselor. Your counselor should create an environment in which you feel at ease and safe to explore your concerns and vulnerabilities. Your feelings should be validated, rather than discounted. You should be treated with respect and dignity, not told what to do. Together, you should work toward decreasing self-imposed limitations.

Recovering from loss of limb is an ongoing process. Patience and reassurance from others will reinforce your confidence. Your counselor should be steady, patient, nonjudgmental, and reassuring. He should acknowledge your very real physical and emotional pain. He should be upbeat, yet provide realistic expectations.

Being treated as a normal person, who just happens to have a limb missing, has been one of the most profound healing experiences for me. While friends and loved ones were going through their own adjustment to my loss of limb, my counselor took my amputation in stride. His acceptance of my physical disfigurement and emotional turmoil enabled me to accept my own body changes, and improve my shattered self-concept.

Knowing you are being accepted as a whole, complete person is a powerful tool for your healing. If you have recently experienced amputation, and this attitude is transmitted to you at this vulnerable time, it will aid in your recovery. When your counselor accepts you exactly as you are, by validating your current emotional state, you will feel understood and accepted. This, in itself, can be a powerful help in your recovery. In addition, it has been shown that counselors who demonstrate empathy, warmth, sincerity, respect, honesty, straightforwardness, and a willingness to share a little about themselves, achieve positive results with their clients.

SETTING TREATMENT GOALS

If you don't know your destination, you can't possibly expect to know when or if you have arrived there. One of your very first priorities when working with your counselor should be to define treatment goals for yourself. In addition to the goals themselves, you must also determine specific criteria for judging whether or not you have achieved these goals.

Setting your own goals will help you become an active participant in therapy. This allows *you* to make the optimal choices in your life. For example, you might set a goal to learn assertiveness skills. You would know that you were on your way to achieving this goal the first time you successfully dealt with an obnoxious person who treated you without respect. Or, you might set a goal to improve your general attitude. You would know you were achieving this goal when you became adept at catching yourself in the act of undeserved self-criticism or negative thinking.

Generally, a good therapist will not tell you what to do, or try to make your decisions for you. Rather, he will help you sort out your issues, teach you coping skills, and help you deal with troubling emotions.

EXPECT POSITIVE RESULTS

Before you can expect to see positive results from professional counseling, some groundwork must be established. First, you must have a good working relationship with your therapist in which you are comfortable enough to share your vulnerabilities and relevant personal history. Next, you must develop specific treatment goals. This process may take one or two sessions. (Sometimes this process in itself can begin to provide relief.) You should then expect progress with each session, which may range from small "aha's" to more major breakthroughs. You should take home coping tools, strategies, and concepts that can be practically applied to your daily life. In other words, your therapy should make a noticeable difference in your sense of well-being and ability to cope.

Naturally, some of your treatment goals will take longer to achieve than others; but, you should feel that you are making at least some demonstrable progress in achieving your goals. If not, discuss this with your counselor. If you are not satisfied with your progress, consider switching therapists. It may take more than one try to find a counselor who is right for you.

IN CONCLUSION

Counseling is an individual process. It is a blending of the counselor's skills and style with your individual needs and personal make-up. For best results, the two of you should be a "therapeutic match." Careful consideration of the guidelines presented in this chapter should help you achieve such a match.

Counseling can be a wonderful aid in your recovery process and in enhancing the quality of your life. You may even find yourself growing in ways that might never have occurred if you had not undergone amputation.

PART III

SOCIAL ASPECTS

17

DEVELOPING YOUR SUPPORT SYSTEM

Being social creatures we require interpersonal exchange to survive physically and to thrive emotionally. Caring relationships provide emotional nourishment, which enriches our lives. When you lose a limb, not only must you form a new relationship with yourself, you must also re-establish your relationships with others.

Society has a long history of prejudice and intolerance towards anyone who is "different." This includes those with physical differences. Your amputation may be perceived as threatening to others, including family members or friends, who project their fears about their own health or mortality onto you. They may try to keep you at arm's length, so they do not have to confront their own fears and insecurities.

The affection, acceptance, respect, and status you receive from family, friends, and colleagues contribute greatly to your sense of satisfaction with yourself and your life. When these relationships are impacted, your sense of well-being may be shaken. It is, therefore, beneficial for you to build a network of relationships that supports you emotionally. This chapter provides information to assist you in developing such a support system.

THE IMPORTANCE OF AN EMOTIONAL SUPPORT NETWORK

Since we are social beings, we tend to turn to each other in times of need. The far-reaching emotional challenges that accompany limb loss can seem, at times, far too overwhelming to handle on your own. Knowing you are loved and cared for, and that you have professional sources of support from which you can draw, can lessen the feelings of isolation and the heaviness of your burden. Family, friends, members of amputee support groups, mental and physical health professionals, and spiritual counselors may all prove to be emotionally supportive.

You may ask yourself why the need for a number of people in your support system. Why not rely on just one person—a spouse or a best friend?

The answer is really quite simple. Placing all of your support needs on one person can be an overwhelming responsibility for that individual. It is simply not fair. Remember, your spouse, friends, and family members are going through their own adjustment process to your amputation. They may need time to work out their own issues.

Encourage all of those who support you, but especially your primary support persons, to be honest with you. They should feel comfortable in letting you know when they are feeling overwhelmed or overburdened. Make sure they realize it's okay if they need a break. You can be more relaxed and breathe a little easier, when you know those who support you are open with you, and are able to maintain balance in their own lives. Honesty and a willingness to share what you are both feeling will go a long way to promote healing for everyone.

WHY SOME PEOPLE DO NOT SEEK ADEQUATE SUPPORT

There are a few common misbeliefs that prevent many people from seeking adequate emotional support during times of turbulence in their lives. Dispelling these misconceptions allows you to feel free to establish the support you deserve during this challenging time.

"I should be able to handle my own problems, tough it out on my own."

Although it is certainly admirable to be self-reliant, it is also a sign of wisdom to recognize when assistance can be beneficial. It has been said that no man or woman is an island, no one stands alone. It is a sign of humanness, not weakness, to turn to others for support and nurturing.

After undergoing amputation, your plate will be more than full when it comes to dealing with recovery. Be wise enough to obtain the support you need to make it through trying times. It is a misplaced "macho" belief that seeking help is a sign of weakness.

The misconceptions that you are supposed to bear your burdens by yourself and suffer in silence are, frankly, quite stupid! If your friend was injured, you would help him seek medical care. If your car broke down, you would bring it to a qualified repairman. If you had a business project to complete and were lacking the expertise to do so, you would seek the assistance of someone with that expertise. Why deny yourself the relief that can come through the emotional support of others?

"I don't want to be a burden. Others have their own problems."

If you have respect for the integrity of the person you share your concerns with, you should be able to trust that person to be honest with you. He or she should feel comfortable in letting you know whether or not it is a good time to discuss your issues.

The first and probably the most important thing is to establish that foundation of honesty. Then you can feel free to ask, "Do you have twenty minutes or so to spend with me? Is this a good time?" Once you have that person's assurance, you can relax and feel comfortable in opening up.

"My problems are worse than anyone else's. I'm ashamed (or embarrassed or humiliated) to tell anyone else what I am feeling."

When I participated in my first consciousness-raising groups in the 1970s, and again during my professional training as a group therapist, I began to recognize a certain pattern among new members. Most feared that what they had to reveal about themselves was so bad, that the other members of the group would be appalled. These new members were often surprised and relieved when the group took their revelations in stride.

You can diffuse many of your shame-based emotions when you discover others still accept you, even with your fears and vulnerabilities. You may discover others share similar emotions, or can relate to yours quite easily. One needn't have undergone amputation to know what it's like to deal with loss, poor body image, low self-esteem, or strained relationships.

BENEFITS OF SHARING YOUR CONCERNS

When you find an empathetic ear, you reinforce the comforting knowledge that you have friends and family who care about you—you are not alone. Others are rooting for your recovery and lending their support.

It is not only the actual words between you and a support person that heal, it is just *being* with someone who cares and demonstrates, both verbally and nonverbally, that who you are as a person has not changed since you lost your limb. This acceptance reinforces that you are not "less than" you were before. You are a deserving person, inherently equal to everyone else; your worth has not diminished simply due to amputation.

One of the most supportive things a very close friend has done for me over the years, is to accompany me from time to time on my visits to the prosthetist. Since these visits are usually at least two hours long, with lots of waiting time while my prosthesis is being adjusted, we have lots of time to "hang out" with each other. Her casual acceptance of me and my amputation has been a form of healing for me. She watches while I am being fitted, sees my residual limb, and has a realistic idea of the challenges I face. She calmly accepts my situation as nothing out of the ordinary, just a facet of who I am.

Expressing your feeling and sharing your concerns about what is going on can be like a safety valve on a pressure cooker. When you vent what is troubling you, you often feel better just for having gotten it out in the open:

"Deal with the anger, the pain, and the frustration. You have to deal with it! If

you need to, seek professional help, or talk to the pastor of your church or a good friend. Find somebody who will just listen; they don't have to say a word. As long as you keep what's bothering you stored inside, you are not dealing with it and it will tear away at you. You need to verbalize it so you can face it."

—Molly

It is not necessary for the person you are sharing your problems or concerns with to solve them. In fact, a good active listener will take in what you say, let you know you have been understood, and ask you questions that serve to deepen your own self-understanding. This, in itself, can aid you in finding your own solutions. This person can also catch you when your beliefs are unrealistic, nonconstructive, or even self-destructive.

BUILD A SUPPORT SYSTEM THAT REALLY NURTURES YOU

By developing a network of support for yourself, you can do much to assist your own emotional recovery. Family, friends, coworkers, others with limb loss, those in amputee support groups, health-care professionals, and those with a similar spiritual faith can all provide invaluable resources. This is especially true early in your recovery.

None of us can really know how we'll respond to a particular crisis until we are "tested"; this applies both to you, as you adjust to your amputation, and to those friends and family members who care for you. You may discover that the people you turned to for emotional support before your limb loss, may or may not prove as supportive following your amputation.

You may notice that despite the best intentions of some people, you are left emotionally depleted or agitated following their well-intentioned attempts at comfort and support. In striking contrast, others will leave you feeling strengthened with a heightened sense of well-being.

It is, therefore, a good idea to consciously choose those who comprise your support system. The guidelines in this chapter will assist you in making good choices.

Help Others Support You

You need to let well-intentioned friends and family know exactly how they can lend their support. Don't leave it up to them to guess how they can be most helpful. Let them know your needs. Aside from listening to your concerns, perhaps they can run errands for you, help you cook dinner, or babysit for your children.

When asking for someone's support, be clear and firm with your request. Remember, they have asked to help you. Don't let them take actions that are not helpful because you feel that saying so would hurt their feelings. For example, when I had first come home from the hospital after my accident, I really needed rest. However, I had a stream of loving friends who wanted to visit and cheer me. Soon, I realized these well-intentioned visits were causing me to expend a lot of energy—energy I needed for my recovery. I had to change my visitation policy in order to get the rest I needed.

How Others Can Nurture You

"I still hang out with many of the same people I did before I lost my arm—my family and my close friends. After my amputation, they cared for me in so many ways. They took me to the doctor, helped me financially, made sure I had food on the table, and took care of my animals. My family cared, my friends cared, my employer cared. This made a big difference to me.

Realize who your friends are—who is actually close to you and who really cares. You do need support, there's no doubt about that; everybody has a bad day. Good friends can make a big difference.

Even though you may have hung out with a person forever, he may not care enough to understand your new situation. You have to realize who your true friends are—the ones at the core of your life, the ones you want to spend time with and who want to spend time with you. I spend more time with my parents now than I ever did. They take me at face value."

—Clint

When you have people who care for you unconditionally, who accept you with all of your moods, with all of your strengths and weaknesses, through good times and bad, you feel affirmed in who you are. As a result, you become more self-accepting and self-loving. Having someone who cares about your internal state and roots you on during life's more difficult times is invaluable.

A good friend provides a reality check, and is willing to be honest and give you feedback; he is someone in whom you can confide your insecurities and innermost thoughts, someone who trusts you and in whom you trust. You may share an interest with a friend that you do not share with family members or even your spouse. Friends and loved ones provide an intimacy that is deeply nourishing emotionally and promotes a buoyancy to your spirit. Through intimate friendships you will feel a deep connection with others; they will help draw you out of your own concerns as your heart opens.

EXAMINE YOUR SUPPORT CHOICES

You may notice that being with some people strengthens your sense of well-being, while being with others leaves you feeling drained, anxious, or even angry. A friend of mine used to refer to certain people as "energy vampires"; after spending time with them, you feel as if your very life force has been sucked out.

It is a good idea to consciously examine those you choose for emotional support. Those you assumed would be supportive, may prove not to be, while others may come through for you in ways you never would have imagined.

Unwise Choices

Some people are not good choices for your emotional support system; without meaning to, they can actually impede your recovery.

When considering members for your support team, be aware of:

• The person who has a great deal of trouble accepting your physical handicap.

• The person who is so caught up in his own reaction to your amputation, that he cannot transcend himself to support you. As a result, you may find yourself having to care for him.

• The person who causes you to bring your coping tactics into play in order to remain centered around him.

These points are exemplified in the following account:

"My mother went into a state of self-pity. She thought God was punishing her. She wasn't helpful, and never expressed that she felt bad about what I was going through. Everything centered around her!

I'll never forget how my mother would not look at my leg. I came out of the shower once with just a towel around me, and she was horrified. It made me feel like a real freak! In order to protect her, I ran and put a long robe on, and said, 'Now, now. Don't get upset.' At the same time, I was pushing all my emotions down while thinking, 'Hey, I'm the one going through this. Not you!'"

—Judith

Another unwise choice for your support network is:

• The person who is too helpful, or exhibits an attitude of pity.

When others are overly helpful, or react with pity, you may be left feeling disempowered, helpless, and awkwardly uncomfortable. You can take others off the hook by letting them know your physical limits and capacities. Reminding them that you are still the same person you were before the limb loss will speed their adjustment to you. In doing so, you will regain your sense of mastery and self-respect.

In order to make others feel more comfortable around you, you might say something like, "I appreciate your attempts to help out, but I can do that myself. I'm still learning my own limits, and want to be as independent as possible. Please trust that I'll let you know when I need assistance." You might also say, "You seem a bit uncomfortable around me. That's understandable. Please relax. I'm still me, even without my limb. In time, you'll get used to me the way I am."

For your support team, also avoid:

• The person who does not know how to be a good listener.

• The person who denies the validity of your feelings, or who has unrealistic expectations for your recovery.

• The person who is repeatedly callous and insensitive.

"I was having so much trouble adjusting to the intense trauma I had experienced, I was placed on the psychiatric side of the hospital while I was learning to walk again. I would call home and tell my mom how upset and troubled and frustrated I was feeling. She would react by telling me I shouldn't feel that way. Her reaction really bothered me and got me even more upset and frustrated. I would also get angry at my pastor because he expected more progress from me than was realistically possible."

—Molly

When someone tells you to deny your experience, he is advising that you deny your truth. This is "crazy making," and does nothing to support your recovery; rather, it slows you down or holds you back. No one has the right to deny the validity of your feelings! You feel what you feel, whether or not those feelings are what others consider to be proper.

The timetable for physical and emotional recovery is unique for each individual. If you are like most persons, you are honestly doing the best you can to progress through your recovery; no one else has the right to impose their arbitrary schedule on you.

More unwise support choices include:

• The person who is a constant problem solver or advice giver.

• The person who imposes his own philosophy or religious beliefs on you in an attempt to make things better.

• The person who assumes too much of your care, preventing you from regaining your autonomy as rapidly and fully as possible.

Some people think they have all the answers to your problems—that they can "fix you" or make you better—and they try to take over your care. Although well-intentioned, these people deny you the right to work out your own solutions. They imply that you cannot do things without their help. They do not demonstrate respect for your coping abilities.

You need the freedom to explore and learn your limits, meet your own challenges, and gradually resume independent self-care. You must establish limits and assert your own independence. Over time, your needs may change.

If you have grown children, they may display a sense of duty and obligation toward you that interferes with your normal relationship. They may try to take over making decisions in your life—"Why don't you move in with us . . . move closer to us . . . let me handle your finances . . ." Caretaking that becomes excessive can rob you of your sense of control.

Losing a limb does not impair your ability to reason and make decisions. Help your children separate that which is their responsibility from that which is yours. Explore resources such as visiting nurses and homemakers; they will help you become as independent as possible. Your children can still contribute to your care, but it is important to strike an appropriate balance. This will relieve both you and your children.

Finally, do not choose the following types as members of your support network:

•The person who withdraws from you entirely due to your limb loss.

• The person who denies that anything at all is different since the amputation.

"When my condition was diagnosed, my brother was there. He is really a good guy, but he wasn't really supportive because he didn't know how to handle it. He acted as if nothing had happened. He expected me to do the things I used to do. When I brought up my cancer or my amputation, he'd feel uncomfortable.

Through the grapevine, the news of my amputation traveled to the place I used to work. I knew a lot of people there and they suddenly stopped calling me. This was hard for me to accept, but I figured it was because they were scared and didn't know how to react. I suppose it's the same with my brother. I guess they were just afraid of saying something wrong."

—Bob

Wise Choices

In developing your support system following amputation, you will have the opportunity to re-examine your relationships. When you honestly review your relationships, you will realize that certain individuals have rarely supported you in past crises and will probably be unable to now. Others may surprise you and prove to be wise choices for support.

The following types are likely to be invaluable members of your support system:

• The person who offers unconditional love, support, and care.

• The person knows how to be a good listener.

"My mother has been my main support during the hard times. When my cancer was diagnosed, she was there; when I had my amputation and all of my chemotherapy treatments, she was there. She was a constant source of support for me."
—Mark

Another smart choice for your support team is:

• The person who can accept your physical disability and altered lifestyle.

• The person who recognizes that who you are as a person has not been altered because of your amputation.

"My cousin never changed the way he treated me. If I needed to be lifted, he would lift me up. If I needed to be held, he would hold me.

Those people who didn't change their attitude toward me really helped me adjust. Had they treated me differently, I probably would have given up and checked into a convalescent home somewhere—but they never did. Just being there was the main thing. If it weren't for them, I really don't think I would have this positive attitude."
—Louise

Other wise support choices include:

• The person who supports that which is best and strongest in you.

• The person who encourages your healing and independence without being pushy.

"My family gave me a lot of support. They would say, 'Come on, let's go out and do this or that.' They never cut me any slack, and that was good. All my friends from high school were good, too. Nobody pitied me. I didn't know how many great friends I had until I had my amputation."
—Greg

Others who will serve to support you well include:

• The person who offers realistic feedback about your situation and experiences.

• The person who offers medical or psychological expertise in a caring manner and with a positive attitude.

"My prosthetist has been wonderful. She has always been open, and I know I can call her anytime. She always gets back to me if she's not there when I call. She also helps me simply by acknowledging what I've been through, and by telling me that I will be able to walk again and get along without a cane. I think that's really helpful."
—John

Most people are well-intentioned; they are as loving, caring, and supportive as possible. Yet some individuals may prove to be wonderfully supportive in some areas, and woefully lacking in others. Therefore, it is up to you to learn to accurately assess your relationships with others. Ask yourself, "What are this person's strengths and what are his weaknesses when it comes to aiding me in my recovery?"

Perhaps you have a few special friends with whom you can share your deepest fears and greatest successes, and know they will be there for you, no matter what. It may well be that another friend is helpful in accompanying you to medical appointments in order to help you sort out complicated information or simply to provide moral support. You may know someone who will simply be with you and allow you to feel his or her love—a person who provides you with the psychological "space" to be yourself, including all of your emotional ups and downs, without making you feel you have to put on a socially acceptable mask. This is a precious gift.

FAMILY AND FRIENDS

There is nothing that can take the place of the emotional support of those who love and care for you. When your healing process seems too overwhelming for you to bear alone, knowing that others love you and wish the very best for you in your recovery, can shore up your flagging spirits and be a soothing balm for your battered sensibilities.

The following stories illustrate the invaluable role of support from family and friends:

"My sister has been very helpful to me since my amputation. She pushes me to try to achieve reasonable goals. She is totally supportive. Everything that comes out of her mouth is positive, no matter what. I can remember one time when I was real sick, she constantly encouraged me by saying things like, 'When you get better, we'll go here or there.' Her words got me through it."

—Bob

"My husband is my main support. He refuses to let my physical condition get in the way of anything he wants to do with me, whether it is taking me camping in the mountains, carrying me up six flights of stairs to the top of a lighthouse, putting me on a horse, or taking me to the beach. He is willing to put in all the physical work if I am willing to go with him.

He is also very verbal. It's nothing for him to tell me four or five times a day that he loves me and how much I mean to him. When he gets in bed at night, he says things like, 'I just don't think you understand how much you mean to me, and how much I think of you during the day when I am at work.'

It was the tiny steps that made my recovery possible. I still have a notebook filled with ideas and topics my husband felt were necessary to address. Together we discussed his notes, which included such questions as: *What do you think we need to do to make things easier for you at home? How are you going to get yourself integrated back into your career and personal life? How can you continue to participate in your favorite hobbies?*

At times, I can remember not wanting to think about, let alone discuss, such issues, but he urged me. It was partly therapy for him, too. He couldn't do anything except provide support for me, which he was very good at."

—Leslie

"I couldn't have made it without my wife. The first thing she said to me every morning when I was in the hospital was, 'I love you.' It is important to know that somebody cares. Once I was home and started my rehabilitation, I would ask her to do things for me, and she would say, 'No, you aren't crippled; you can do it yourself.' She would make me do things on my own, so I wouldn't be so dependent. She was always there; if I cried, she was there; if I was happy, she was there; and when I seemed to be going out of my mind, she was there. She is always so positive."

—Fred

"Following my amputation, my mother was there nonstop for me. She would help wrap my legs, feed me, and do whatever else needed to be done. She gave me a lot of TLC, which I really needed at that point in my recovery. She was a great help to me.

My daughter was eleven months old at the time of my accident. While I was in the hospital, my sister constantly showed her pictures of me, talked about me, and brought her to visit, so my daughter would not forget her mother. Although it was especially difficult for her, my sister has come to accept that I have a physical disability. The last time she visited me, we played together in a sports tournament in which she, too, used a wheelchair."

—Molly

SPIRITUAL SUPPORT

Loss is a part of each and every life. Whether you have strong spiritual beliefs or not, when you experience a major loss such as amputation, it will hurt. At first, you may find yourself feeling dazed, bewildered, and confused. It is likely you will search for hope, purpose, and meaning. In this search, it is important to recognize that while your life will never be quite the same, it can still be good and fulfilling. If you believe in a Higher Power that guides human beings and cares about the outcome of your life, it may be easier to accept your new situation and your new challenges, secure in the faith that everything will somehow work out for the best.

For those who are spiritually inclined, turning to one's religious or spiritual path can provide great solace and meaning to a life experience

that may be difficult to understand. Some individuals turn to the traditional religion in which they were raised; others turn inward and draw
strength from deep within themselves:

*"I am not very religious; yet, I have found a source of inner strength within myself.
For a long time, when I was dealing with so much depression, I did focus on that
inner source of strength. It was helpful."*

—Molly

Your religious faith can be a base for the conviction that everything has
a purpose, and that you will be all right. Your amputation can be used to
propel you more deeply into your faith.

In times of grief, you can experience an overwhelming sense of loneliness.
While you may feel separated from others by your grief, it can be easier to bear
if you believe that God is near, understands your feelings, and cares about
your well-being. It may be that the spiritual teachings of your church or
synagogue, as well as the support of its members, can help you overcome a
sense of loneliness or hopelessness. An active prayer life or other inner
discipline may help you do the same. It is important to recognize that even
with the most profound faith, you will still need to work through the various
stages of grieving in your own way, at your own pace.

The religious community, itself, can be helpful in providing emotional
support and comfort. Responses from congregation members will likely
run the gamut from being very insensitive to very helpful, depending upon
the level of spiritual and emotional maturity of the individual:

*"I spent a lot of time talking with the chaplain at the hospital. I tried to figure
out why all of this had happened to me. Was I being punished? Was God
unhappy with me? We determined it had been an 'act of nature' that caused
the accident. It was an 'act of God' that my life had been spared. I had an
eleven-month-old daughter waiting at home for me. Here was a new need for
me just beginning.*

*My strength was going to be there through God, through my friends, and
through my pastor. I would be able to face daily tasks. I had to have lots of blood
transfusions, and my church family formed a blood bank and donated blood for me.
They sang at fund-raising events to make money for my hospital bills. I wrote to
each person who had donated blood, and I formed special personal bonds with them
by thanking each one."*

—Molly

Your religious beliefs can be extraordinarily supportive, or they can be
cause for further pain, depending upon what they are and how you apply
them to your situation:

"I grew up in a very religious family—with very fundamentalist Christian beliefs.

I had rejected many of these fundamental beliefs by the time of accident. A lot of family members and friends didn't know what to say. My very intelligent grandmother was praying that my legs would grow back. One of my family's favorite phrases was, 'Well, the Lord knew that you would be a great inspiration to everyone, and that you could bear this.' This attitude made me and my husband angry. We believed it was stupid—that warped concept of God—that He would injure people so that other people could be helped."

—Leslie

Individuals who have been relatively detached from their religion may suddenly find themselves praying to God for assistance, or blaming God, or railing out and asking an anguished, "Why?" I once spoke with a man who was a confirmed agnostic, yet following his child's trauma, was suddenly setting forth conditions to God—"If you don't bring my daughter through this, I'll never set foot in the synagogue again."

There a number of things that may be said by well-meaning friends in their attempts to support you in your recovery. Sometimes these well-intentioned comments can actually impede your recovery process, as just illustrated by Leslie. Minister and grief expert Bob Deits further explains in his book *Life After Loss: A Personal Guide Dealing with Death, Divorce, Job Change, and Relocation* (Tucson, AZ: Fisher Books, 1983), how certain beliefs can impede rehabilitation:

You did not suffer loss because you are bad or because God wanted to test or punish you. Another of the least helpful things you will hear is, "It's God's will.". . . In the long haul of grief recovery, such words hinder the journey back to wholeness rather than help it.

If you believe God has chosen to *take* your spouse or child or parent [or limb], you are going to have trouble grieving openly. . . . you will not allow important feelings like anger and bitterness to surface. To keep important feelings like these bottled up inside is to court long-term emotional and physical problems.

Turning It Over to a Higher Power

When certain situations seem impossible to cope with, some people take their pain and "turn it over to a Higher Power;" that is, they acknowledge that they require a power greater than themselves to surmount the challenges they face. So they ask for God's support and assistance in dealing with this pain. This allows them to be more at ease and to accept what has happened as part of a greater plan, and know that all will work out for the best.

This is exemplified in the following accounts:

"After my doctor told me I had cancer, I went out to my car and prayed, 'Dear Lord, give me peace and strength.' Suddenly, this feeling of strength just went

clear through me. I could feel it, and I was okay. That strength had been there all the time, but suddenly I could feel it running through me from my head to my toes; I had never felt that before."

—Judith

"My faith in God helped me get through the amputation and the chemotherapy. It was easy for me to say, 'Okay, God, apparently you have some plan that is going to work all this out—the chemotherapy and the amputation. I'll just put it in your hands, and you can take care of it for me.' Believing in a greater plan helped me relax a little bit more about my situation."

—Mark

MUTUAL SUPPORT GROUPS

"When I talk with someone who recently lost a limb, just my presence as someone who is successfully living with the amputation of both legs and an arm is impactful in itself. For a person who has had, let's say, a leg removed, simply being told that he or she will be able to walk again someday is not necessarily convincing. It does, however, make a big impact on that person to see someone who is wearing a prosthetic leg walk into the room. When I talk to someone who has just lost a limb, I talk to them about living their everyday life—just that."

—Leslie

There is absolutely nothing that can take the place of sharing your experiences with someone who has "been there." That person understands and truly empathizes with your pains, fears, and frustrations. Seeing is believing! When you see others doing really well and enjoying their lives, you know there is hope for you.

Although mutual support organizations are indeed available in much of this country, many persons with amputation choose to avoid them for a variety of reasons. Some of these reasons are practical, such as lack of proximity to a group or lack of transportation. Some individuals do not want to be reminded of their "status" as a person with amputation, and avoid association with others with limb loss. Others just do not realize the varied benefits a mutual support group may provide.

Of course, the choice of whether or not to participate in support organizations is up to you. If you are a person who does not wish to spend time socializing with others, just because you have amputation in common, I still encourage you to discover other areas of interest in which these groups might serve you. For example, you might have an interest in keeping abreast of current prosthetic advances, or you might want to become involved in influencing legislative matters that affect your health care. Perhaps you'd like information about specialized recreation programs and sports associations.

Both national and local support organizations for those with amputation meet a wide variety of needs and offer help on a number of levels. Among other things, these include mutual support organizations for those with amputation, as well as for families with children who have limb differences; information centers to help keep one abreast of the latest health-care consumer information; and groups that provide social and recreational programs for those with limb loss.

National Organizations

It is beyond the scope of this book to provide a complete directory of the many, varied resources available to you following your amputation. The two national organizations listed here each offer a wealth of resources for those with amputation, their families, and other interested individuals. I encourage you to explore these organizations to become aware of the resources they offer to improve the quality of your life.

The **Amputee Coalition of America (ACA)** is a national network of individuals, support groups, and health-care professionals who strive to improve the lives of those with amputation. The ACA provides assistance and support through education, consumer empowerment, and outreach. It offers:

• A wealth of information related to amputation and prosthetics, as well as word of upcoming meetings and conferences.

• Referrals to help put you in touch with local support groups, recreational and sports programs, and consumer assistance programs.

• Technical assistance to help set up and maintain support groups.

• A strong consumer and educational voice to the prosthetics industry, the insurance industry, the government, medical professionals, and the general public.

You can contact the Amputee Coalition of America by calling (800) 355–8772.

The **American Amputee Foundation (AAF)** is an information and referral source for those with amputation and their families. Supportive services also include peer counseling and some financial aid. Its National Resource Directory provides lists of amputee support groups and related support organizations in the United States (and a few in Canada), as well as a host of other useful resources including relevant publications, prosthetic and orthotic providers, and sports and recreation associations. To contact the AAF, write to P.O. Box 250218, Little Rock, AR 72225; or call (501) 666–2523.

Local Support Groups and Peer Support

One man with limb loss relates the following experience:

"I had a friend with amputation who had a very negative attitude. He would never leave his house. He stayed in a wheelchair and never wore his prosthesis. He was dependent on everyone. Whenever I saw him he asked me to run errands for him. He always acted like, 'Oh, feel sorry for me.'

Finally, one day he caught me at the wrong time and I said, 'You know, I don't feel a bit sorry for you. Life goes on and you can't sit here locked up in the house in a wheelchair. You have a perfectly good leg sitting there in the corner collecting dust. You want everybody that comes around you to feel sorry for you, and you are going to pull everyone down to your level.' He got really mad and said, 'I thought you were my friend. Get the hell out of my house!'

A few months later I ran into him. And guess what. He was wearing his prosthesis and walking! He thanked me for getting on his case; no one else ever had the courage to do that."

—Kent

In my mind, *nothing* can take the place of interacting with others who live with limb loss. Personally speaking, meeting other women and men with my level of amputation (or even more severe levels), who were living full, satisfying lives, was invaluable, especially during the early days of my rehabilitation. These people gave me the opportunity to comfortably seek information, ask delicate questions, watch them use their prostheses, and observe their loving spouses and well-adjusted children. I learned of their productive careers and fulfilling hobbies. I was encouraged to discover that, rather than being embittered, they were strengthened by their life experience. I had the opportunity to ask them, *"How do you do it?"*

Local self-help groups, composed of others with limb loss, can facilitate your recovery by providing mutual aid and social interaction. Some groups offer peer counseling. Members serve as role models for each other; it can be a tremendous boost to see how well others are thriving. Through this type of interaction you will discover that you are not alone. This can be an antidote to feeling isolated and believing that no one else understands what you're going through.

You can address issues and needs in ways that cannot be done elsewhere. Those experienced at living with amputation can help you develop realistic expectations. Medical professionals affiliated with support groups can answer physical or technical concerns. Interaction with others can also serve to make you aware of other concerns that you can clear with a counselor's assistance. You may want to discuss the effects of living life with amputation on you and your family. You can exchange information and receive practical tips about adjustments to daily living. You can learn about prosthetic advances, and become informed about related consumer health issues. If present, a skilled counselor can facilitate discussion and assist you in working on your emotional adjustment.

Local amputation support groups are found within or near most communities. They are invaluable resources. Get referrals through your prosthetist, physician, rehabilitation center, or national support groups, such as the Amputee Coalition of America or the American Amputee Foundation. Often, members of a support group provide peer visits to those who have recently undergone amputation surgery, or for those who are about to. Often the peer visitor is the first individual with limb loss a person with recent amputation has ever met. The peer visitor fulfills many functions, perhaps the most important of which is to provide an example of someone who has survived an amputation and is living successfully. This person can serve as an empathetic sounding board and can answer practical questions about day-to-day living, as well as discuss how he or she has coped emotionally with the challenges of life. Those with recent amputations report that peer visits are extremely beneficial:

"Meeting another amputee my age was helpful. I felt good seeing him, because I knew someday I would be able to do what he does. His leg was amputated about eight inches above the knee, way up there, and he does everything—runs, rides a bike, water-skis, and jet-skis. He is really active; his amputation hasn't stopped him. I can't wait until I get to that point!"

—Bob

"My prosthetist's wife had an above-the-knee amputation when she was a child, and she does so many things. It was great meeting someone like her and seeing that she was able to do so much."

—Leslie

All of these facets of peer support groups have been found to be beneficial and may facilitate your physical and emotional recovery. When you see for yourself individuals with amputation who are doing well—leading full, satisfying lives—you may draw the conclusion that you can, too.

IN CONCLUSION

Ultimately, it is you alone who must learn to live with the realities and consequences of your limb loss; others cannot do it for you, no matter how much they care. Yet, by developing a strong network comprised of those who really care about you, as well as those with professional expertise to improve your emotional and physical health, you can greatly lighten your load, increase your comfort, and ease your sense of isolation. I encourage you to consciously evaluate your current system of support. Is it all that it can be? If not, reach out and build yourself a support system that assists you in leading a full, rich life.

18

SEXUALITY

Sexuality is one our deepest avenues of human expression. When a limb is amputated, your sexuality may be profoundly impacted by your need to reconstruct your body image and self-concept. Like other persons who have undergone amputation, you may find it difficult to separate your sexuality from the emotional trauma that accompanies loss of limb. You must also learn to readapt interpersonally, as must those in a relationship with you. It is crucial that even without your limb, you feel "whole" and desirable to your partner.

This chapter presents an overview of the effects of loss of limb on sexuality. Practical suggestions are given for easing the adaptation process.

WHAT IS SEXUALITY?

Sexuality is more than reproductive organs and the act of sexual intercourse. Sexuality includes giving and receiving pleasure, sharing intimacy and affection, and communicating deep feelings. Through your sexuality, many aspects of both you and your partner come into play. These include how you relate with others; your feelings of self-worth and self-confidence; your values, inhibitions, and taboos; your communication style; and your personal history.

A person's sexual attitudes are shaped by a host of factors—gender, family background, society, culture, and religion; personal preferences and values; age; and life experience. Our attitudes may be complex since they are shaped by intellectual, emotional, conscious, and subconscious components. These attitudes can contribute to negative feelings about sexuality, such as guilt and anxiety. They can also contribute to positive feelings, such as love, deep caring, and affection, so you can experience pleasure, intimacy, and relaxation with your partner.

A person's concept of his masculinity or her femininity permeates everyday experiences in more arenas than the bedroom. For example, can a male with limb loss, whose work once included hard physical labor, accept a desk job and feel just as masculine? Can he feel just as manly if he can no longer participate in rough-and-tumble sports in the manner he used to? Can a woman who interacts with the public feel feminine if she is missing an arm? Can she feel womanly and attractive if her residual limb or prosthesis is readily visible to her mate or to others?

Does Loss of Limb Equal Loss of Sexuality?

Sexuality is a primary drive like hunger or thirst; this is not altered when you become physically challenged. Amputation of a limb in itself doesn't affect your sexual drive in any way, unless there is some underlying medical disorder. As mentioned, your sexuality is greatly influenced by who you are, your attitudes, and how you functioned sexually before the amputation. Both you and your partner are affected by the physical and emotional changes, so you must both adjust.

Oddly, many people automatically assume sexual interest and ability are somehow altered when a person loses a limb. You may suddenly find yourself treated as if you were asexual! This misconception can cause you and your partner undue anxiety and frustration. Note the following reaction from a male physician who had undergone recent amputation surgery:

"A good friend of mine is a urologist. After my surgery, I can remember asking him, 'Is this amputation going to affect me sexually?' From my medical training, I knew that it wouldn't, but my state of mind was such that I had to have it verified."

—Vincent

Most individuals with limb loss can engage in sexual intercourse. If, due to an underlying medical disorder, you are unable to have intercourse, know that there are still many avenues of sexual expression available. Your sexuality is still a way to deepen your relationship with another individual. You can continue to enjoy giving and receiving pleasure, along with releasing physical tension. Success in this area can greatly boost your self-esteem. It allows you to continue to express love, affection, caring, and intimacy.

After amputation, some individuals require a period of time to readjust to their sexuality both emotionally and physically:

"To me it was like walking, I had to learn how to do it again. At first, I didn't do it as well as I had before, but I was determined to find a way. Now, I have no qualms about my ability as a lover. I've always been able to satisfy women quite well. It was just a matter of finding a way to do it. It took a lot of practice."

—Henry

A Hush, Hush Topic

Individuals often keep sexual issues to themselves, since they consider their sexuality an area of utmost privacy. Thus, due to embarrassment and shame, problems may not be brought to the attention of professionals. Some people with amputation feel that their sexuality is an area of minor importance when compared with their orthopedic disability, so they do not focus on it.

The time of life when limb loss occurs may greatly affect its impact on sexuality. Obviously, a child or adolescent will have different considerations than a single adult, a married adult, or a senior citizen.

In many families, sexual issues may not be openly discussed, so it is even more difficult to do so if a physical difference is present; this is especially true for those at both ends of the age spectrum. Many parents already have an awkward enough time discussing sexuality with their child or adolescent. And older family members are sometimes treated as if their sexuality belonged to a previous stage of life. This is clearly not true for most senior citizens who enjoy vital, active sex lives!

It is important for you to know that sex-related issues are valid. Addressing sexual concerns helps you re-establish your self-worth. Returning to "normal" sexuality is a part of your rehabilitation process. So speak up! Speak with your partner. If warranted, speak with your physician, counselor, or sex therapist. Vital sexual expression is too important a part of life for you to passively allow it to disintegrate due to fears or embarrassment.

Self-Confidence and Attractiveness

As you might well imagine, the effects of loss of limb on sexuality, dating, and marriage can be far-reaching. Some women and men tend to have lowered self-esteem due to their altered physical appearance and their fears of not being able to compete with other members of their sex for mates. Often the single greatest fear of a female with an amputation is that she will not marry. In the teenage years, insecurities in these areas are especially heightened by dating situations.

Some who have recently undergone amputation fear that they will be rejected by able-bodied members of the opposite sex, and wonder if they will find acceptance only from others with limb loss. In general, though, most people who are missing a limb do not seek the exclusive company of other individuals with amputation.

As in other areas of social interaction, your own level of self-acceptance and self-confidence will often influence how you are received by others. If you are at ease with yourself, members of the opposite sex will find it easier to accept you.

Of course, there is a wide range of reactions by those who consider dating or marrying someone with limb loss. It is important for some individuals to have a mate that is able to participate fully in certain sports or other recreational activities. Others may not be able to get past their negative reaction toward the residual limb and prosthesis:

"My wife didn't like to have sex with me after my amputation. She was too freaked out by my leg. She'd lie next to me in bed, and if my leg touched her, she would get turned off. I was ashamed of her and the fact that she couldn't deal with it better. It was frustrating!"

—*Merlin*

Yet for the majority, the totality of who a person is holds far greater importance than does his or her loss of limb. Many persons with amputation state that the people they date (and often subsequently marry) have great depth of character, as evidenced by their willingness to accept the loss of limb. Other couples discuss how sharing the life crisis of amputation has served to deepen and strengthen their love and commitment to each other.

Amputation of a limb after marriage, especially an upper limb, can be a factor contributing to divorce; however, many marriages in which a partner has an amputation thrive and are stable. For information about the effects of amputation upon marriage in areas other than sexuality, refer to Chapter 19, "Your Family."

Effects of Amputation on One's Sex Life

Loss of limb appears to have a number of different effects on the sex lives of both men and women. For some, there is a decrease in sexual intercourse; in fact, a small number of individuals do not resume intercourse at all after amputation. There may be spoken or unspoken reasons for not resuming sexual activity. Some individuals justify their abstinence out of fear of injury:

"I had been married about thirty years when I lost my leg. One change in our marriage was that he slept in one room and I slept in the other. He was so afraid of hurting me that he would not have sex with me. I just accepted it because my leg was so tender that I was a little worried. We never had sex again after I lost my leg."

—*Frances*

Contrast the attitude of Frances and her husband with that of the following couple:

"Thank goodness my amputation hasn't stopped us sexually! My wife figured it would, but it hasn't; it just made us put the brakes on temporarily. My wife was afraid it would hurt me to get up on my knee, and she didn't want me to have a setback. One night, about three months after my surgery, we started having sex again. I just had to change my method a little bit. Now our sexual activity is about the same as it was before the amputation."

—*Fred*

Some people who have lost a limb become insecure with their sexuality or are fearful of rejection by the opposite sex. The decrease in sexual activity reported by some is not attributed to the medical cause of the amputation, nor is it due to the difficulty of body positioning during sexual activity. This suggests that the psychological issues of lowered self-esteem and body image may have a greater effect on sexual activity than physical body changes.

Generally, the sexual activity of a single person with amputation is altered more radically than that of a married person. In an effort to prove their sexual attractiveness, some individuals who have undergone amputation may experience a period of increased promiscuity. Some men require confirmation of their sexual prowess and/or of their role as family protector and provider. Men commonly fall into the trap of believing their loss of limb somehow means their virility is also lost. Women often feel unattractive. However, many persons state there is no change in the frequency or quality of their sexual activity following amputation.

Sadly, the insecurities of some persons with limb loss may cause them to be exploited as sexual objects by certain opportunistic individuals. The novelty of having sex with a person who has physical differences seems to be attractive to some people. There are other individuals, mostly men, who have a sexual attraction to women with residual limbs, and actively seek out partners who have had amputations. There also exist able-bodied individuals who are emotionally insecure, and who feel stronger and more potent when they are with a partner who has a disability.

WHEN THERE IS AN UNDERLYING MEDICAL DISORDER

Certain underlying medical disorders that cause amputation may interfere with sexual functioning. The conditions that accompany diabetes and vascular disease are the most common physical causes for impotence. Neuropathy (abnormality of the nerves) may lead to difficulty in ejaculation, although normal orgasm and sexual desire are not necessarily impaired. In some instances, when diabetes is controlled by diet and/or insulin, the impotence is reversible. Thus, careful medical supervision by your physician is vital for optimal health, which includes sexual functioning.

For some individuals with diabetes or problems with glucose tolerance, there may exist a progressive, irreversible condition so that erectile dysfunction occurs. Some men also experience lowered sexual desire and changes in orgasm and ejaculation. Vascular disease can interfere with erection by impeding blood flow to the penis. These physical changes, combined with the effects of the normal aging process, can be the cause of emotional upset and anxiety for men. A man may interpret these physical changes as a "loss of his manhood." When a man fears that he is no longer an adequate or capable lover, he may withdraw emotionally from his partner, further stressing the relationship. He may feel shame, lowered self-esteem, and/or depression, and imagine that he is no longer attractive to his mate.

If you have an underlying disorder that might be affecting you sex life, it may prove *very* helpful for both you and your spouse to have a frank discussion with your physician to learn how your medical condition can affect sexual function. Also, if you fear that sexual intercourse will somehow adversely affect your health, I encourage you to discuss these fears with your physician. Be sure to inquire about the effects of any medication you might be taking on sexual response. Find out how physical exertion will affect your health. Understanding the effects of your underlying medical disorder can provide great relief to both you and your partner, so you can then rebuild your intimate relationship together.

Generally, urologists specialize in diagnostic evaluation and treatment for impotence. A variety of medical interventions are available to counter this condition. Speak with your physician for more information about your options.

It is also a good idea to obtain a psychological evaluation when impotence occurs. Impotence can affect feelings of self-worth and greatly increase stress levels due to fear, embarrassment, frustration, and guilt. This may adversely affect your relationship with your partner. Counseling may help reduce the stress and increase the communication between you and your partner. With a combined approach of counseling, education, diagnostic evaluation, and treatment, impotence can often be successfully addressed.

ACHIEVING SATISFACTION

Even without intercourse, sexual expression can be mutually satisfying and pleasurable for both partners. Satisfaction does not necessarily imply orgasm. Sexual interaction is often used to express deep intimacy, caring, tenderness, and love. This expression does not require you to have a specific type of body, or to perform prescribed physical movements.

If intercourse is no longer possible, you can still share physical intimacy through caressing, kissing, and other forms of mutual pleasuring. You and your partner can choose to use sexual aids. Verbal and nonverbal communication, which includes language and touching outside the bedroom, contributes to sexual expression:

"After my amputation, I noticed that I wasn't able to function sexually. My doctor told me it was due to my diabetes, not the amputation. But you know what? In spite of this limitation, my wife and I feel much closer than we ever have. We talk more. I think I've kissed her more in the past three years than I have over our entire forty-five-year marriage. It's love, nothing else."

—John

WAYS TO MAINTAIN VITAL SEXUAL INTIMACY

Following your limb loss, there are a number of steps you can take and attitudes that you can adopt to help you and your partner foster sexual intimacy. The suggestions that follow are provided to assist you in creating a healthy, vital sex life.

Involve Your Partner Early in Your Recovery

It can be very helpful if your partner becomes accustomed to viewing and perhaps touching your residual limb early in your recovery. She or he might even massage your limb if you discover that this helps diminish phantom sensation or phantom pain. Your partner's involvement is also useful as a bridge to facilitate talking about your recovery and both of your expectations. If you begin this process while still in the hospital, you will have the additional resources of nurses, social workers, and physical therapists to assist in answering any questions you or your partner may have.

Notice the wonderful sense of healing and mutual support expressed in the following account:

"The first time she saw my leg was four days after the surgery. We sat there and took the bandages off together. When we looked at the limb, we noticed that the new scars and old ones created what looked like a 'face' on the end of my stump. At first, we laughed and started joking about it, but then I remember that we both cried, relieved that this sickness crap was finally over. We sat there holding each other, then we ended up making love, and it was no different from before. If anything, we felt even closer. It was very fulfilling, no trouble. Both of us reached orgasm, no problem at all."

—*Victor*

Experiment with Body Positioning

The mechanics of body positioning during sex might need to be altered to adjust for better balance and movement. Sometimes switching who is on top, or switching sides of the bed may be all that is necessary to ensure comfort. So, explore and experiment to discover what works for you and your partner. The exploration in itself may add new zest to your physical relationship.

Place Less Emphasis on Performance

Unfortunately, in our society, many people consider their sexual encounters performances that are judged and rated, rather than opportunities for mutual pleasure.

The quality of satisfaction you derive from sexual intimacy will be influenced by your individual preferences, your relationship with your partner, and your reproductive aims. Your physical capabilities must also be taken into account, without any comparison to some preconceived societal image. So, let go of worry, guilt, and shame about being physically different; it's a fact of your life now, like your height or your eye color. When you relax and accept yourself exactly as you are, you will find yourself appreciating your own unique gifts and personal style of interaction as a sexual being.

Sometimes it's easier for those who love you to accept the changes that have occurred, than it is for you to accept them yourself. Your partner's acceptance and unconditional love may ease the way for your own healing, as seen in the following case:

"At first, I was uncomfortable when it came to sex because of the way I looked. I was worried that my husband would catch me undressed with the lights on. Once, when we were going to make love, my husband started laughing. The hairpiece I wore to cover up my scalp burns was falling off and I guess it looked kind of funny. It took me a while to laugh, but finally I did. It helps a lot if your partner is comfortable with accepting the way you look."

—*Molly*

For some persons with an amputation, there is anxiety and fear of having to live up to someone else's expectations of the ideal lover. Some people are afraid to initiate physical intimacy. The best way to build up your self-confidence is by taking small steps, one at a time. You have to demonstrate to yourself and to your partner what is possible. As you are willing to be a bit vulnerable and take small risks, you will feel more secure within yourself and relaxed with your partner.

Realize That Sexuality is More Than Intercourse

Likewise, any effect that your limb loss has on your sexuality should not be a cause for guilt. Whatever is mutually satisfactory between you and your partner is okay.

Sexual expression includes much more than intercourse. There are many ways to give and receive pleasure, so give yourself permission to expand your definition of sexual expression. Whatever works for you and doesn't harm others is right. Be creative. Experiment within the context of your relationship.

Keep the Lines of Communication Open

Communication between partners is always of key importance, especially in so intimate an area as sex. The expectations of both partners and the reality of your physical capabilities need to be discussed. We often tend to make assumptions based on our own fears and insecurities, which may have nothing to do with what our partner is feeling. For example, many men worry about the size of their penis, while women are concerned with the size of their breasts. These areas of concern may not affect your partner's desire for you in the least. You may be sexy and desirable to your partner in ways you've never even considered.

It's important to do some reality testing. Most of us are not mind readers! Unless you ask your partner what he is thinking or feeling, you'll tend to make up answers. Your guesses can be way off the mark! This can lead to unnecessary anxiety and heartache. So, be sure to openly discuss your concerns as well as your partner's. This is good advice for all of us, able bodied or not. All good relationships include a willingness to be open with each other and to take risks, along with a delicate balance of give and take.

Initiate discussion. Your partner may be afraid of offending or hurting you in some way by bringing up sexual issues. Frankness and a willingness to be open and honest will promote trust and intimacy. It may be that both of you need to deal with pre-existing inhibitions and attitudes that have nothing to do with the loss of limb.

It is crucial that you address common concerns, such as the fear that sex will further injure you. Pain, discomfort, limits of mobility, and the process of an underlying disease do sometimes interfere with normal functioning. So let your partner know your limits. Once your limits are understood, you and your partner can relax and enjoy each other.

If you notice that your partner begins to behave in a different manner sexually, perhaps by withdrawing emotionally or by seeming uninterested, you may find yourself feeling rejected for unknown reasons. Have you become less attractive to your mate? Is there another lover? Sometimes neither of you will connect the differences to the underlying illness or the changes wrought by amputation. Thus, it's extremely important for both of you to openly discuss any changes you notice in your intimate lives. By sharing fears, insecurities, anxieties, and the sense of loss, painful misunderstandings may be averted.

Seek Counseling with a Professional Sex Therapist

Sexual counseling with a professional therapist is a good idea if one or both of you become stuck when working through sex-related issues. Counseling with a sex therapist may enable both of you to learn about alternative ways to enhance physical intimacy and achieve sexual gratification; it may help you both rid yourselves of limiting, inhibiting beliefs, and lessen the emotional turmoil that accompanies the physical changes brought about by the amputation. Sex therapy is often experience-oriented; the therapist will assign homework that may include performing exercises to reduce anxiety, or trying out new sensual or sexual techniques and communication methods.

EFFECTS OF AMPUTATION ON DATING

If a person is married when amputation occurs, he or she already has an established relationship, unlike the case of someone who is single. Let's face it, the prospect of entering the world of dating can be daunting enough for anyone, even without the added factor of amputation. Normal anxiety accompanies the risk involved in opening oneself up to someone new. So when the stress of having physical differences is added to this situation, dating can be very scary indeed:

"Dating after the accident was terrifying. I had been home from the hospital about three months when I went out with this guy I used to work with. I could tell he was terribly uncomfortable. I felt uncomfortable, too, because I had to have his help to walk."

—Molly

When you "put yourself out there" by entering the world of dating, you are taking risks and exposing vulnerabilities. It's true that you are exposing yourself to possible rejection, but the rewards of a satisfying relationship are well worth those risks. When you learn to disentangle your sense of self-worth from the possible rejection inherent in dating situations, you will feel much better about yourself. Your own level of comfort and ease will be noticed by the person you are with. A sense of confidence and good humor certainly helps:

"I used to think, 'Who would want to go out with me? I have only one leg.' I was surprised to find that it really didn't make a difference at all! Girls see that I have one leg and I rarely pick up negative attitudes from them. People are curious about my limb loss, but most don't really care—it's more your personality and the way you treat other people that is important. If you are going to be a butt hole, no one will want to go out with you whether you have one leg or two legs or four!"

—Mark

"During the time that immediately followed my amputation, I felt anxiety in the belief that I would never be able to get a guy. But once I was in a good place inside myself, I noticed that many men were attracted to me. The last time I was in a grocery store, a guy asked me out!

If you are taking care of yourself and the rest of your life is in order, dating is not going to be a problem. The guy I date now is a hunk—gorgeous, really built. I don't feel I have to choose a lesser man because I am an amputee. I don't feel I have to compromise because of my body."

—Marcy

The people you meet will naturally have different attitudes about your amputation that are based upon their personal history, priorities in a mate, and their strength of character. Contrast the difference between the responses of the following two girlfriends:

"I had a girlfriend for two years before I was diagnosed with cancer. When I lost my hair from the chemotherapy it hit her between the eyes that something was really wrong with me, so she left. It was easier for her to get out of the relationship than to deal with it. It was hard for me at first, but not anymore. Since she left, I've met girls of better quality."

—Bob

"At the time of my accident, my girlfriend was great. She stuck right by my side through the whole thing. She was my pillar of hope, my go-getter girl. She never cut me any slack. She never gave me any pity, and that was really good."

—Grant

Marie is fifteen years old. Due to a congenital problem, she underwent amputation of both legs as a young child. For her, dating has been, at times, a bitter and painful experience. Yet, recently she has met with some sweetness:

"Not having normal legs has affected my dating a lot. Initially, most boys like me for my personality and looks; but, when they find out about my legs, they drop me. It used to make me cry a lot. For a while, I decided not to tell any new boys I met about my legs. I would let them think I had a limp from a sprained ankle or something. But eventually they would find out. Now I don't care who knows about my legs, although it's still hard to deal with the negative reactions. I'm still in high school.

Right now there is a guy I like who doesn't care about my legs. I told him my story and he accepts me for what I am. He said that he doesn't go for girls just because they look good on the outside, but because of how they are on the inside. He is the first guy I have come across who is like that."

—Marie

If you have recently undergone amputation, you may be so enveloped in the cocoon of your immediate physical and emotional concerns, that you cannot yet imagine a future that includes dating, marriage, and children. Others with limb loss who have successful marriages and families can be inspirational models for you:

"When I was thirteen, a year after I lost my leg, I met a lady who was missing a leg. She wore a prosthesis, but she still had a normal life. She was married and had three beautiful daughters. Her husband seemed wonderful, and I remember thinking, 'Gosh, she has a great man!' It was important for me to see that someone could be attracted to a person who was missing a limb."

—Marcy

Many persons who have undergone amputation find themselves in relationships with people who have the ability to see beyond surface appearances:

"I think the amputation has helped my relationships with girls. I like to think that they look at me more for who I am personally, than how I look physically. So I weed out those girls that are shallow and get to know the girls that are really nice and like me for what I am.

I've asked the women I've dated since my amputation if it bothers them that I'm missing an arm. The answer is 'no' almost every time. It makes no difference to them. If the women I want to be with are not concerned by my arm, why should I be? It's awfully superficial. You find out who is worthy and who is not."

—Clint

It is important to recognize that many individuals with limb loss have met and married their spouses *after* the amputation. As the following story makes it clear, an important aspect of any successful marriage is talking things out well beforehand, so that each partner knows just where the other one stands and what to expect from the relationship:

"My husband says my amputation was never an issue with him; it never bothered him. The fact that he is very athletic was my main concern—if we got married, would he be off doing all the things he enjoys doing without me? Would we ever do things together? I felt very strongly about it and I wanted him to really think it out before he made a commitment.

As it turns out, we do most things together anyway. He still does the back country activities with other people, and that's fine. He tries to plan these trips when I am involved with a project at work. So we've worked it out. It isn't a problem."

—Margaret

IN CONCLUSION

Amputation poses a set of unique challenges to your self-concept that may impact your sexuality and pose additional challenges to dating and marriage. These can be met with a brave heart, a clear mind, a good sense of humor, and a firm resolve to weather the storm during rough times.

After limb loss, your sexuality can continue to be an expression of love and caring, as well as a source of intimacy and physical pleasure. Keep in mind that the relationships that thrive despite the difficulties brought on by limb loss, are often stronger, deeper, and longer-lasting than those that have never been tested.

19

YOUR FAMILY

In your individual life, you establish your own equilibrium, creating a balance between work and play, risk taking and comfort. In turn, you and your family members build a web of interaction that has a dynamic balance between personal and interpersonal concerns. The family can be thought of as a system—when one member undergoes a crisis, all are affected. Thus, even though you are the one who has lost a limb, your family members will undoubtedly experience emotional upset in coming to grips with your loss and the many changes it entails.

IMPACT OF THE TIMING OF YOUR AMPUTATION ON YOUR FAMILY

Depending upon where you are in your relationship and your stage in life, your amputation will have a differing impact upon your family. Are you a newlywed or someone in the early years of a marriage? Are you single or divorced? If so, an amputation may be particularly hard to accept. As with the person who loses a limb to sudden trauma, you will likely experience shock and bewilderment. How could this have happened to me, to my family? Suddenly your dreams may seem to crumble before your eyes—your future may appear to be slipping through your fingers.

If you had considered having children, amputation may cause you to question your ability to bear them or care for them. You may find yourself mourning the dreams of "how it might have been." If you have young children or grandchildren, you may find yourself bemoaning the physical limitations of your ability to play with them or take part in certain activities with them.

If you and your partner are older, and you have undergone amputation during your retirement, you may wonder why this had to happen during the time for which you worked so hard to prepare—a time when you and your spouse imagined yourselves relaxing and enjoying a care-free life together. You may have the added worry that your medical bills will drain the financial resources you had saved for your retirement.

If you are a widow or widower, you may find yourself feeling particularly isolated and alone. The task of caring for yourself without the benefit of a spouse can seem daunting.

There is a tendency for some who have lost limbs to withdraw and isolate themselves, feeling useless, unworthy, and depressed. This state of mind negates the reality of all that you are and all that you can still do and experience.

In addition to adjusting to amputation, it can be particularly disheartening if you must deal with the complications of a progressive disease as well. This is especially true if you, as a couple, finally feel adjusted to one challenge when some new complication arises. In this case, professional counseling may be helpful to teach you coping skills for handling life's ongoing stresses and decreasing your sense of isolation. Support groups in which others have similar challenges can also be helpful.

No matter what point in your life you undergo limb loss, you will likely have fears about its effects on your relationship with your spouse and other family members. It is crucial that you set aside time to talk with and listen to your spouse. Together, each of you should discuss your feelings and fears. Address your hopes. Talk about practical matters such as household chores, finances, and child-care responsibilities. If you feel the need, enlist the help of professionals to help you with financial planning, to teach you coping skills, or to put you in touch with community agencies that can help you. If one spouse feels overburdened, consider hiring outside help such as a homemaker or companion.

THE BURDEN OF GUILT

As discussed in Part II, if you require amputation, you may find yourself feeling responsible for having needed it. No matter what, the fact is you have indeed lost your limb and must come to grips with this painful reality.

In addition to self-blame, you may also feel guilty for the stress your amputation has placed on your family. Your guilt can stem from a number of factors including your new physical limitations, changed roles within the family, changes in your vocation and income, the need to spend savings on medical bills, and the fear of not being accepted by your spouse and other family members. You may also feel your spouse blames you for your limb loss and its ramifications on the well-being of your family.

Feeling responsible and harboring guilt and self-blame can promote anger, anxiety, and depression, which can interfere with your family relationships. You can best assist yourself and your family to return to a more normal balance by letting go of these harmful feelings and addressing the new challenges you face. When you recognize yourself getting caught in such destructive feelings, distance yourself from them and give yourself some compassion.

EFFECTS OF AMPUTATION ON MARRIAGE

In all healthy marriages, both partners must work to keep their relationship vital despite the ups and downs they face. Loss of limb can be a real blow to your self-image and self-esteem, which can result in feeling vulnerable in your most intimate relationship. You may fear your partner will reject you, find you physically unattractive, and lose desire for you. You may fear your relationship will deteriorate.

Marriage entails intimate physical and emotional closeness. When one partner loses a limb, both must deal with the physical disfigurement and normal emotional responses to the loss. There may be a shift in the balance of equality, since (at least temporarily) one partner is physically, and perhaps emotionally, more dependent. All of these changes may impact children and other family members, as everyone learns to cope with their loved one's new physical reality.

When one partner loses a limb, daily patterns of living and relating to each other are interrupted. The challenge of re-establishing intimacy and ease in the relationship should be of prime importance to both spouses. In order to meet this challenge, the emotional upheaval that accompanies the physical changes must be dealt with openly. In the arena of sexual intimacy, both partners must learn to feel comfortable with each other again. Working out this challenge together can be an awkward yet poignant experience that can serve to deepen your love and commitment to each other. It can ultimately strengthen the marriage.

For many, the totality of *who* a person is, holds far greater importance than any superficial loss. Amputation of a limb after marriage, especially an upper limb, can be a factor that contributes to divorce; however, in many of these broken marriages, there were significant problems before the new stress of amputation was added. On the other hand, many marriages in which one partner has an amputation, thrive and are stable:

"We had just gotten married when my cancer was discovered. I was twenty years old that June, and I lost my leg in August. Going through all this has made our marriage stronger. My husband has always been very proud of me—what I've done, how far I've come, and how I've accepted the amputation. He has been very supportive. It created a special bond between us. I have always been sure that my leg wouldn't affect our relationship, that it would never divide us."

—*Judith*

"Whenever I would get depressed, my wife reminded me that the world hadn't come to an end. She would say, 'I've got you and you have me, and I'm glad to have you here.' It was very touching and very loveable. Some people think of sex as the center of your life when you are married. I say, 'No way!' If you don't have that strong, supportive love between you, your marriage will never last. All this has definitely brought us closer together."

—*John*

"I think everybody who has had an amputation has also had thoughts in the back of their minds like, 'I'm not a whole person anymore.' 'She could do better.' 'She could go out and find somebody else.' That's when you get down to accepting a person for who he or she is, not for who you think they should be. They say 'love is blind.' Getting married just before my scheduled amputation reassured me that my wife really loved me for me. My amputation is just another part of my life. Like all married couples, we have our ups and downs and our spats. However, my amputation has never been the object of any of our arguments."

—Kent

"At first, I felt more uncomfortable about my amputation than my husband did. He had a way of making me feel at ease. He was interested in me, the person. He was more comfortable with my scars than I was. Both of us do miss certain things, like being able to walk side by side, since he usually pushes me in my wheelchair. Every once in a while he jokes that he pushes his wife around and he is the only one who can get away with it."

—Molly

EFFECTS OF YOUR AMPUTATION ON YOUR SPOUSE

Your mate must go through considerable adjustment to your amputation. He or she is bound to experience a host of feelings and responses that may be extremely challenging. With so much focus on you—your health and well-being—your spouse may feel a bit neglected. It is also natural for him or her to feel some anger and resentment about the blow that life has dealt and its effects on your relationship and dreams for the future. Your spouse may also feel a bit trapped by the circumstances that you both must face.

In my own case, I was severely injured when I was crushed in an automobile accident. My husband-to-be visited me daily in the hospital, and played host to my parents (who had moved into my home during my recovery). He also fielded innumerable phone calls and questions from friends and loved ones. Once I was home, he performed countless activities. He fed me, helped me bathe and dress, and changed my bedpan (Ah. True love). He cooked for me, took me for daily rides in my wheelchair, and drove me to various health-care appointments. He was phenomenally supportive.

One day, I can remember him being very upset. He told me that of all the people who called to see how I was, very few asked how *he* was doing, how *he* was holding up and adjusting to all the stressful changes *he* was experiencing. He was feeling discounted and underappreciated.

Your husband or wife will probably go through a turbulent period in which he or she has some difficulty in accepting the changes to your physical body and the reality of all that your limb loss entails. During this time, your spouse must learn to find a balance between helping to care for your needs and caring for his or her own. Mates may resent their altered roles and responsibilities. You may feel guilty for their burden. Both of you may feel selfish and self-centered for having the feelings you do.

In *Building a New Dream: A Family Guide to Coping with Chronic Illness and Disability* (Reading, MA: Addison-Wesley Publishing Company, 1989), Dr. J.R. Maurer and Dr. P.D. Strasberg further explain:

> Spouses can also feel guilty for feeling angry or disappointed. Anger and disappointment, though, are normal reactions to a life crisis. It is not helpful to discount these feelings . . . rather they should be recognized and acknowledged. The well spouse has lost things even if they have their health. They have lost a healthy husband/wife who contributed to the family income and care of the children and provided help around the house. They have to reorganize the way they live their daily lives. Sometimes a spouse considers leaving the marriage. This is also a common reaction and does not mean that one is evil or disloyal. For some marriages, a severe disability or illness does cause so much emotional disruption that divorce is inevitable. If the marriage was filled with conflict before the illness or disability, it may be too hard for the couple to overcome old resentments and find ways to overcome the new difficulties that illness brings in order to feel productive and happy together. However, it is not impossible.

You and your mate need uninterrupted discussion time during which you can express your fears, sorrows, and concerns. You'll need to restructure your responsibilities and grapple with the new challenges you now face. Communication is of critical importance during this stressful time. Too much estrangement can cause one or the other of you to withdraw emotionally from the relationship. Set aside time for yourselves to check in with each other. One of you can talk while the other actively listens, then you can switch roles. This type of interaction can clear the air and open the way to increased intimacy, empathy, and understanding. This is a critical time for the two of you to be open and share your fears and concerns. In this way, you can support each other and come up with creative approaches to the challenges you both face.

By sharing your crushed hopes and fantasies of "how it was supposed to be," you will grow closer together. By sharing your sadness, disappointment, and guilt, as well as your new hopes and dreams for your lives together, you can come up with creative solutions and new visions of a quality life. You can draw from each other's strengths. By sharing your true feelings, you will not cause your partner to feel worse than he does already. You can work out new goals for your future, discover those goals that have been unaffected by your amputation, solve problems, and make decisions together.

The Desire to be Desirable

"My wife and I were sexually intimate while I was still in the hospital. Even so, I went through a period of time thinking, 'Why would she want to be with me when she could be with a whole person? Are things ever going to be the same?'"

—Kent

Since your relationship with your husband or wife is one of the most important in your life, your partner's attitudes can deeply impact the reformulation of your self-concept, your sexual security, and your overall well-being. If your spouse still treats you as if you are desirable, it is much easier for you to come to terms with your altered body. The more comfortable your partner is with you, the more you can relax within yourself and enjoy your sexuality.

Consider the following story of this remarkable woman who has amputation of three limbs:

"My husband approached me sexually within the first week-and-a-half of my recovery. I was flabbergasted! I couldn't imagine somebody 'coming on' to me while I was swathed in bandages with nothing where my limbs used to be. I thought it was the most amazing thing that anyone could do.

My amputations have made it more difficult to be as spontaneous sexually as it would if I had all my limbs (I can't sneak up behind my husband and 'put the moves' on him). And that has been frustrating! It's been helpful to have an affectionate spouse who has made extreme efforts to really be physically and verbally supportive. My husband goes out of his way to convince me that I am still sexually attractive."

—Leslie

Some individuals with amputation fantasize about having an affair or will actually have one, in part, to prove to themselves that they are still desirable to the opposite sex. The spouse of the person with limb loss may also want others of the opposite sex to reinforce his or her sense of attractiveness, particularly if there has been prolonged illness and a period without usual sexual activity. Sometimes the spouse will feel guilt or shame for having these feelings. Fantasies are normal and can enrich your internal sexual life. Giving yourself permission to enjoy your fantasies does *not* mean you have to act them out externally.

Once again, it is crucial that you take stock of what is really going on inside each of you and honestly share these feelings with each other. By understanding each other's conflicting emotions, without blame or judgment, together you may come up with potential solutions and healing will occur. For more information on the effects of amputation on sexuality, refer to Chapter 18, "Sexuality."

When Your Partner Behaves Differently

If you notice that your partner begins to behave in a different manner sexually, perhaps by withdrawing emotionally or seeming uninterested, you may find yourself feeling rejected for imagined or unknown reasons. Has your amputation made you less attractive or even repulsive to your mate? Is there another lover? Because of all the changes you have both experienced due to your limb loss, it is extremely important for both of you to openly discuss any problems you notice in your intimate lives. By sharing fears, insecurities, anxieties, and the sense of loss, painful misunderstandings can be averted.

When There is a Progressive Medical Disorder

When you have undergone amputation due to an underlying disease process, it is often more challenging for you and your family to return to a state of equilibrium in your daily living. Rather than allowing you to settle into a new level of stability, an underlying disease may bring with it a series of setbacks. You may re-experience grief again as each setback brings a new loss to mourn. By recognizing that you and your family will be subject to recurring cycles of chaos and stability, you will expect this to happen and be better prepared to face these cycles with equanimity. In the case of an underlying disease process, professional counseling may be helpful in teaching you coping skills to better handle ongoing stresses.

Your spouse still needs to participate in activities that are pleasurable and revitalizing for him or her without feeling guilty or selfish because you may not be able to join in. You, in turn, need to relax, let go, and allow your spouse to continue participating in these activities without complaining and acting bitter about the way things are.

Be sure to plan some activities you can do together, and make dates to do so. Perhaps you can develop new interests in which you find satisfaction and fulfillment. You must both learn to balance caring for yourselves and each other.

ROLE CHANGES WITHIN THE FAMILY

Family members tend to take on certain roles—some that are traditionally defined by society, and some that are unique to our particular families. With today's economic realities and the loosening of stereotypic roles for both sexes, these roles are becoming somewhat more fluid. One parent may be responsible for the greater part of earned income; one may be responsible for managing the household. One may pay bills, serve as the accountant, and make major financial decisions. One may tend to oversee the family's social life or take a more active role in caring for the children.

Loss of limb may, at least temporarily, throw these family roles off track. Perhaps your spouse, who relied on your ability to bring in a certain amount of income, must now take on greater responsibility to compensate for this financial loss. If you are at home more, you may take on more responsibility for the children.

It can be a deep blow to have to give up one's position as chief homemaker or breadwinner. You may feel you have lost part of your identity if you are no longer able to carry out the roles you once used to define yourself within your family unit. You might feel guilty for not holding up your end of household responsibilities. You may feel impotent since there is nothing you can do to change the situation. All of this may lead to feelings of frustration, anger, bitterness, and resentment of the other family members.

The necessity to shift roles can upset the usual family equilibrium and provide stress for all family members. It is important for all members to feel good about themselves and believe they are worthy individuals. You may question your own worth when your roles change. On the other hand, this whole process can actually serve to strengthen the family and enhance the self-esteem of all, as each member offers creative solutions, and all pull together to meet challenges.

Accepting Changes in Your Independence

After living an independent life, it can be hard to accept becoming temporarily or permanently more dependent on a spouse. It can feel shameful or humiliating to rely on a spouse for simple aspects of self-care. Believe me, I was not thrilled to have my husband-to-be carry out my bedpan, or push me in a wheelchair when I was too weak too walk. Loss of self-sufficiency and control over the environment can be a bitter pill to swallow. It is, therefore, empowering to discover those things you can still do, and then do them. Perhaps you can adapt the chore or adapt yourself to be able to accomplish the same end.

Your spouse may become resentful and angry at the increased demands, and begin to feel as if she or he is a maid or servant rather than an equal partner. He or she may become physically or emotionally exhausted. Be aware of maintaining a balance. If need be, hire a personal attendant, visiting nurse, or a neighborhood teenager to prevent overloading your mate. An important part of maintaining a balance is making time for relaxation and fun. In addition, you each need private time to pursue your own interests.

Sometimes, by undergoing a crisis together, you and your spouse will learn to appreciate each other in new ways. You will recognize ways in which you are interdependent and your relationship will be strengthened, as seen in the following case:

"Having gone through this trauma when my husband and I were both young made

both of us realize that although life is here now, it could be gone very quickly. That first year after my amputation, we both talked a lot about how lucky we were, and we realized how important our time was with each other. It helped us to set our priorities at a younger age than a lot of people may do. We became very aware of our security, for our future and our kids.

When we'd get into an argument, suddenly one of us would say,'We shouldn't be doing this. We have had worse things happen to us. This isn't the end of the world.' My amputation caused us to work hard together to make our marriage work. It also made us realize that, although we had always thought of ourselves as independent, we really depended on each other. We were a team."

—Leslie

Too Much of a Good Thing

Your parent or spouse may become so focused on caring for you that he neglects other members of the family and his own needs. This person may be trying to "make up" for what has happened to you. He may feel guilty for his own good health, or feel that he had somehow contributed to the cause of your amputation. Neglecting the needs of others in the family causes imbalance of the family system and can provoke resentment and frustration.

Well-meaning relatives, such as parents, siblings, or your children, may also assume this type of over-involvement. It may be that, in caring for you, they now feel useful; caring for you gives enhanced meaning to their lives. When you are discouraged from assuming full independence and autonomy by these well-meaning family members, it's time to put your foot down and have a good discussion. Let them know you appreciate their efforts, but it's important that you regain control of your life and resume full activity as soon as possible.

THE DECISION TO HAVE CHILDREN

There are a number of factors every couple should consider before making the decision to have children. For a person with amputation, there are additional factors to be considered. What was the cause of your amputation—do you still face a potentially life-threatening disease such as cancer? In which stage of life are you? How well have you adjusted to your limb loss? How has your amputation impacted your life? Will you be able to devote the time and physical energy that is necessary for raising a child? If you have carefully weighed these factors, and there are no medical reasons to stop you from having children, then, by all means, do as your heart tells you.

Ultimately, you are no different from any prospective parent who must weigh factors such as financial stability, career demands, energy level, stage in life, and a willingness to spend at least eighteen years to help guide a child into responsible adulthood.

The following stories illustrate the variety of attitudes of those with limb loss and their decision on whether or not to have children:

"I do want to get married, but I don't want to have kids. It's not that I don't like kids, it's just that I would be afraid that they might be born with the same deformity I was born with. I would never want them to have to go through what I did."

—Marie

"My husband and I plan on having children. I don't consider my amputation a reason not to have them. And I don't think my limb loss will have any bearing on raising them. I'm going to be in better shape, because they're going to run me around. I know my husband will be great with kids; he's the type who will get involved with them."

—Margaret

"One of the first things I considered after my amputation was having a hysterectomy. My husband adamantly opposed the idea. He convinced me that someday we might want kids. And he was right!

During my first pregnancy, which wasn't planned, my biggest concern was for my child—how fair would it be for him or her to have a disabled mother? Jokingly, my husband and I decided that the kid would probably hate us when he or she was fifteen anyway—every teenager does.

My pregnancy was not complicated; it was, however, a little inconvenient. At the time I still used a wheelchair. I was also finishing my medical residency, and living by myself in a modified apartment. Ultimately, the pregnancy and birth of our daughter worked out well. Three years later, I gave birth to our second child, a son. Today, my daughter is seven and my son is four. They are wonderful!"

—Leslie

"I already had a child when my leg was amputated. The idea of having a second child caused us to consider a number of factors—with my physical limitations, could I go through a pregnancy and raise a child? After talking with my gynecologist, we decided to have another child. As the delivery time got closer, we went to the hospital and practiced the whole thing—the labor and the delivery. My doctor and I decided to leave my prosthesis on during the delivery so I was able to use the stirrups. As soon as the baby was born, they removed the prosthesis so I was able to rest and recuperate without it. The whole thing went really well."

—Molly

EFFECTS OF AMPUTATION ON PARENTING

When a person loses a limb, the normal expected patterns of the life cycle within a family may become disrupted. If you have lost a limb and you already have children, you may question your ability to raise them. As you recover, you may find yourself becoming fatigued easily. You may experience physical pain or discomfort. You are also in the process of coping with new experiences as you progress through your recovery—learning to use a prosthesis or wheelchair, adapting to changing family roles, and perhaps learning a new vocation. With all of these stresses and challenges, you may find yourself becoming short-tempered with your children. Small frustrations may bother you more than ever before.

While you are involved in such things as doctor's appointments, physical therapy sessions, and appointments with the prosthetist, your children may find themselves more and more in the company of babysitters and relatives. You may fear the effect your amputation will have on their development. Because of your time-consuming involvement in your recovery, you may feel your children are cheated out of spending time with you. You may yearn for the kinds of physical activities that other families take for granted.

It can be very difficult for you as a parent to place your own recovery needs ahead of the care of your child, even when, rationally, you know it is necessary. This is especially tough when interacting with young children, who are not yet mature enough to understand the nature of what you are undergoing. They may feel neglected or abandoned and may act up, displaying extreme behaviors to gain your attention. It can be emotionally difficult for you as a parent if you feel you are disappointing your children. You may be tempted to compensate by giving them material things, or by overextending yourself physically, which can tax your energy level.

All of us want to shield our children from the harsh realities of life. We want them to know only security, safety, and happiness. We want to shelter and protect them with our love. However, do not overlook the fact that even young children have very good survival instincts; they are very resourceful and resilient. Your children will soak in your love and support no matter what the condition of your physical body. A loving touch, kind words, and an empathetic ear do not depend upon the number of limbs you possess.

"Having kids as a person with a disability has not been a problem, so far. In fact, it has allowed my kids to grow up independently. I can't run to help them or prevent them from doing things. So my husband and I have always encouraged them to learn what is reasonable on their own. They are very protective. Whenever they see people in a crowd start jostling me, they try to keep them away."

—Leslie

Your love and support do not depend on your ability to be a super sportsperson, or to join them in every physical activity in which they are involved. Accept the fact that your amputation might limit your participation in some activities with your child and exclude you from others. As a parent, it can be painful to watch your child participate in activities that you had always assumed you would be a part of. In time, you will reconcile yourself and discover that there are still many activities you can enjoy together.

EFFECTS OF AMPUTATION ON YOUR CHILDREN

The effects of your amputation on your child will depend upon your child's developmental capacity for understanding. A very young child will have a different interpretation of what your amputation means than will an adolescent or fully grown child. The following sections discuss these differences and offer age-appropriate tips for parenting that will ease your child's adjustment to your limb loss.

Young Children

Young children have very imaginative minds. They may feel responsible for your amputation and somehow blame themselves. For instance, they may think you are being punished because of *their* misbehavior or bad thoughts. It is particularly important to find out what they believe has happened to you and why. Dispel any myths they might have—for instance, that you are going to grow another limb. Using concepts at a level they can understand, explain very simply why your limb was amputated and explain that it is permanently gone.

Because of your amputation, your young child may fear for the integrity of his own body. He may believe that losing a limb is contagious, or that a similar accident or disease will befall him. Assure your child that this is not the case. Just because you have lost a limb, your child should not believe that he will, too. While these misconceptions may seem foolish to an adult, they can be very real to a child. It is far better to take the small bit of time necessary to dispel these myths, than it is to allow your child to nurse morbid and unreasonable fears in silence. Don't be afraid to show your child your residual limb and your prosthesis. Your accepting attitude of your body will help your child accept it, too. Answer your child's questions simply at his or her level of understanding.

Let them know that you are still the same person—their mommy or daddy—and love them just as much as before. They still need you. This can be especially difficult if you are temporarily incapacitated. You need to do your best to assure your child that you will be there for him or her. Remember that losing a limb does not take away your ability to spend quality time with your children. There are still many activities you can enjoy together, even if you are in a wheelchair or use crutches. You may have to adapt your physical activity, but there is still much you can do. Your spouse should also spend special time with your child.

Young children may also harbor negative feelings toward you. Your amputation may cause them to be fearful, anxious, or worried. They may feel anger toward you since you can't play with them as before. On top of this, they might feel guilty for feeling angry or hostile. Allow your child to go through his own adjustment to your limb loss. Understand there may be emotional outbursts or withdrawal, as your child adjusts to the new realities in the family.

Young children can be like emotional sponges, absorbing your feelings, even when they are not verbalized. They may be very sensitive to your mood changes, and mirror your fears and anxieties back to you. Lying or covering up your true feelings will only confuse your children and cause them to question their own perceptions. Always be straightforward and honest. This will strengthen them and reinforce their confidence in their own perceptions. Let them know that together you will be able to handle whatever comes up. Try to keep in mind that while you are adjusting to your new realities, your children must adjust, too.

Once you understand that your children are undergoing their own adjustment to your amputation, you'll realize it is normal for them to react with confusion, distress, fear, and anger. Rather than telling them they shouldn't be feeling what they are, let them know you understand. Help them find outlets for these feelings, such as open discussions in which they can vent their emotions, or vigorous play to discharge pent-up energy.

Your children might harbor a number of concerns, including the fear that you will die and leave them. They often act out their feelings, rather than express them directly. Keep an eye out for behavioral changes at home, in school, and with their peers. Observe changes in appetite, sleep, or activity levels. Watch out for personality alteration. Is your quiet, well-behaved child suddenly prone to tantrums and misbehavior? Is your outgoing child suddenly withdrawn? These are tip-offs that your child is in a state of inner turmoil. Ask questions. Find out what your child is thinking or feeling. Allow your child to go through his or her own adjustment. Offer steady love and support. Continue to answer questions simply, and dispel any misconceptions. Let your child help with household tasks without turning him into a servant. Discuss familiar ways in which you can still interact, and discover new ways to play together as a family. A family or school counselor may prove helpful if your child has problems making adjustments to your limb loss.

Children have a great desire to fit in with their peers, and they are vulnerable to the opinions of their friends. Thus, your child may be embarrassed or even angry about the fact that you are physically different from his or her friends' parents. One mother approached this problem in a novel way:

"Kids in school were making fun of my nine-year-old daughter for having a mom who had no legs. My daughter was actually angry with me for being this way. She

wished I wouldn't come to school anymore. It was like having the rug pulled out from under me to hear that her friends were making her feel uncomfortable because of the way I looked.

I went to school and talked to the kids who were doing the teasing. I explained to them why I was in a wheelchair. It was a little unsettling. I asked one of the kids to get a basketball so together we could shoot some baskets. Meeting them on their own turf was more comfortable for me than just sitting in my chair and telling them about myself."

—Molly

On the other hand, some young children do not perceive a parent with amputation as unusual or different:

"Children of a parent with a disability such as mine perceive unusual things as normal, like having an elevator in the house. Once, when my children were very young, my sister came for a visit. They wanted to know where her wheelchair was and why she didn't use a cane. They thought every mom did.

I can remember one night when my six-year old came into my room crying. When I asked her what was wrong, she said, 'Oh, I am so ugly.' I assured her that she was not ugly, but rather a beautiful little girl. But she said, 'Mom, you're beautiful. I wish I was as pretty as you.' I was amazed to learn that my daughter hadn't looked at my amputation as a physical detraction."

—Leslie

As a parent, you may tend to isolate your young children from anyone who has undergone amputation. You may view this as a way to shelter them from reality and prevent them from developing any fears as a result. This is a big mistake! Children are naturally curious; they are generally honest and direct with their questions, and they deserve honest responses. Don't underestimate children; they have a tremendous capacity for resilience, and generally adjust quite well to change.

By isolating your children from a grandparent or another relative with amputation (or your own limb loss), you deprive both of the richness of interaction. Offer your children the chance to learn about the realities of life that befall loved ones. Give them the opportunity to provide age-appropriate comfort and support, and give the person with amputation the opportunity to share his or her life experience.

Older Children and Adolescents

One of the major developmental tasks for a teenager is to gradually emancipate himself from dependency on the family, so he can learn to live an independent life. When a parent or family member undergoes amputation, that teenager may be called upon to assume additional chores and responsibilities. It is perfectly appropriate for your teen to contribute in these ways; however, a balance must be struck so he or she is able to take care of responsibilities, and still have time for normal activities with peers. Your adolescent is not yet a mature adult and needs the time and space to develop independence and a sense of self-identity; this may be hard to do if he or she becomes a primary nurturer of a parent or grandparent. Your teen may feel conflicted—guilty and selfish for wanting to separate, and resentful for having to stay.

As you may well recall from your adolescent years, teens tend to be extremely self-conscious—aware of their own bodies and those of others. Extremely vulnerable to peer pressure during this age, your teenager may find it especially difficult to accept your altered body. I clearly remember dressing like my friends, talking like my friends, and wanting to fit in with my social circle. Your teen may be embarrassed to have a parent who is physically different.

As J.R Maurer, M.D. and P.D. Strasberg, Ed.D. explain in *Building a New Dream: A Family Guide to Coping with Chronic Illness and Disability* (Reading, MA: Addison-Wesley Publishing Co., 1989):

> Teenagers . . . may not want to invite friends to their home or have parents attend school functions. This may be difficult for the parents while it is going on, but, in time, teenagers do mature. It is important for the ill or disabled parent not to give up important once-in-a-lifetime events, such as graduations, concerts, sports events, etc., because of their teenager's insecurities. Firmly, let them know you plan to attend these things, but give them permission to spend time with their friends if they prefer.

You serve as a model of strength for your child when you demonstrate that life goes on even though misfortune has occurred. You model dignity and self-respect when you participate actively in life. When your teen learns about your amputation and all it entails, his world view becomes enlarged and enriched. Maturity is enhanced, and you may be helping to shape your child's values about what is really important in life, such as the value of looking beyond the exterior to someone's inner being.

During the period when you and your spouse are caught up in attending to your recovery needs, it is especially helpful to expand the sources of emotional support for your children. Friends, relatives, and church or community groups can help during this time. If you are a single parent, outside support systems can be extraordinarily useful.

Discipline

You and your spouse are still your children's parents, no matter what age they are. Losing a limb does not mean you have lost your role as a protector or advisor to your children. Discipline should continue just as it did before, even though it may be physically more difficult to keep up with your children. Children may be able to run away; yet, they must learn to face the consequences of their actions. Small children, in particular, must learn to obey, so they do not place themselves in physically precarious situations. The following parents talk of the importance of discipline:

"I haven't experienced any more difficulty than a normal mom regarding my toddler's discipline. I'm probably just firmer in some areas than some other mothers might be. For instance, I expect my child to obey me when I say, 'Come here!' Obeying could affect her safety because of my inability to chase her."

—Nancy

"My children are now nine and seventeen. When they were very young, disciplining them was very hard because of my physical limitations. At an early age, my kids learned all they had to do was get behind the couch to get away from me. I spent a lot of time chasing them, and it made me angry when they played this game with me. They acted victorious when they were able to make it behind the couch before I could catch them."

—Molly

Be on guard not to use your physical condition as grounds to manipulate your children. Don't use guilt as a motivator to get them to follow your wishes. It may be especially tempting to use such tactics if your energy is low, your emotions volatile, and your temper short. Nevertheless, this kind of manipulation breeds resentment and anger, and is definitely not worth it in the long run.

Your concept of how your children need to behave may undergo some modification. You may decide that some of the small chores you required of your child before your amputation may not seem as important now. For example, rather than insist your child clean up his room, you may tell him to close the door to his room instead. In other words, you may benefit from using more discrimination in deciding which issues are worth pursuing, and which could have more relaxed standards. Both you and your child will benefit, since you will be able to use your energy for more important issues, and your child will not feel constantly nagged.

You may find that your children are very protective of you. While this is touching, be sure they do not take on responsibility that oversteps the bounds of what is reasonable for a child. Their love and support can soothe your soul in ways that the affection of others cannot. There needs to be a balance; your children's own developmental needs must be met.

By coping successfully with your limb loss, you have the opportunity to enrich your child's experience of what it is to be human. You model integrity, strength, honesty, and the ability to deal effectively with challenges. You provide an opportunity for your child to take on age-appropriate responsibility. Through your example, you demonstrate the value of love, compassion, and support. The entire family can learn the benefits of teamwork, flexibility, and meeting life's challenges creatively.

Grown Children

"All this did not really affect my relationship with my children that much, except that my daughter makes more time now to see me, even though she has her own business. As a matter of fact, she dropped everything and took care of both my wife and me when I was hospitalized. She was there whenever my wife couldn't be, which made a big difference."

—John

Sometimes older children, or adult children, will come to the assistance of their parents who have undergone amputation and aid with household and financial responsibilities. Although this may be welcomed and appreciated, you may also feel that you are losing control over your well-being, and being replaced by the next generation; you may begin to feel resentful that you have become a burden. It is sobering to exchange the roles of nurturer and nurturee, after so many years in which you, as the parent, were the prime source of support. As we become more advanced in age, whether or not we have lost a limb, it is common for adult children to assume more of a nurturing role. This requires adjustment on the part of both parent and child.

As with other family members, it is very helpful to have open dialogue about the changes that have occurred and the resulting feelings. You are still a source of love and support for your adult children. You can still share the wisdom gained by your life experience. They are often happy to contribute to your care, but they must also tend to their own needs and the needs of their families.

KEEPING THE FAMILY STRONG

Without a doubt, your limb loss will individually affect each member of your family as well as your family unit as a whole. Read through the following suggestions, which are offered to assist you in supporting the health and integrity of your family.

Cultivate Outside Support

No matter how much family members love and support you, there are limits to how often they are receptive to hearing about your recovery process. They are going through their own personal adjustment to the changes your amputation has made. Therefore, it's a good idea to air your feelings occasionally with someone who is outside your family. In this way you will be "heard" by someone who is not "in the thick of it." This person might be a friend, counselor, member of the clergy, or a peer support group member. Through this person you can vent feelings and frustrations in order to gain a new perspective. You don't need advice or solutions, just someone who will listen with an open heart and mind, and validate your feelings without judgement.

Have Family Meetings

Try to hold family meetings, perhaps weekly, to air feelings, to answer questions, and to work on solutions together. You can discuss sharing of household chores, and plan activities in which you can all participate. Find out what each of your family members is thinking and feeling. You may be amazed to discover their feelings to be different from what you believed them to be. By bringing issues out in the open, your family will discover that you can handle their responses. They will see that their honesty will not launch you into despair; rather, it will bring you all closer together. Children of all ages like to feel as if they are helping out and making a contribution to the family. Assigning them appropriate tasks in this regard will promote their acceptance of changes in the family and enhance their self-esteem.

If your child begins to demonstrate differences in social behavior, eating habits, or sleeping patterns, it might be wise to address such matters during a family meeting. You might gently bring up the subject by saying something like, "It's understandable for you to be concerned about my health and have questions and thoughts that might be scary. Can we talk about these things?"

Realize Your Limitations

During the period following your amputation surgery, you may be more fatigued or tire more easily; you may have physical limitations and other health-care concerns. It may be hard to admit that you must lighten your load; but it's common sense to do so. No one will think any less of you. And be honest with yourself. After all, no one knows your capacity better than you! It may, however, take you a while to figure out just what that capacity is.

There are so many "firsts" after amputation—the first time you return to a familiar activity, or the first time you engage in a new one. By all means, test your limits. When you find out what these limits are, allow others to assist you when you need help. Let go of the "shoulds." It's not etched in stone anywhere that you, personally, need to fulfill every function that you did before your amputation. Allow others to help out. Delegate responsibility. Do whatever you can that will still permit you to have a healthy balance of activity and rest.

Continue Roles and Activities When Possible

Participate in household jobs and activities as much as you can. Find out from your prosthetist, your physical or occupational therapist, or others with a similar level of limb loss, how you can adapt yourself or the desired activity, so you can still perform it. For example, before my amputation, my husband and I often hosted parties that included dancing. During my recovery period, when I was still using a walker, the idea of a party with a lot of dancing was emotionally too painful for me. So, we adjusted by hosting dinner parties for a while instead. Sometimes we had parties during which only a short part of the evening was dedicated to dancing.

Remember, having undergone amputation does not change your ability to be supportive to your spouse and children. Your brain was not amputated! You can still help with homework, offer your advice and opinions, make financial decisions, etc. Dwelling on limitations does nothing to further your recovery, and is bound to launch you into despair. Concentrate on what you can still do—and that's a lot! Widen your interests and discover new activities that you can enjoy with your family.

Make Time for Play and Relaxation

Undergoing the crisis of amputation can make life seem so serious. You and your spouse may feel there is so much to do between normal household upkeep, child care, medically related appointments, and physical therapy that you neglect to make time for fun. This is a big mistake! You may think you can't afford the time to play, but the truth is you can't afford *not* to play. You each need time alone to refresh and renew yourselves, as well as time for dates with each other to keep your relationship kindled and balanced. Make time to relax and revitalize yourselves, whether this means having a romantic dinner, sitting together in a park, or going to a movie. All work and no play makes for a dull life.

You also need to make time to be with your children to relax and play together. Even when you are caught up in the many necessary tasks of recovery, it is wonderfully healing for everyone if you can maintain a normal balance of play and fun. So be sure to plan family outings and other activities that everyone can share together. The sooner you can establish a good balance of work and play, the sooner you will feel that your life has gotten "back to normal."

Peer Support Groups

Support groups composed of others with limb loss can be of invaluable assistance for you and your family. You can share your feelings, decrease your sense of aloneness, and discover how others have coped with the challenges you face. Family members can air frustrations and vent feelings.

You can learn of the creative solutions that others have come up with to address the changes in family roles and relationships. For more in-depth information about the advantages of peer support groups, please refer to Chapter 17, "Developing Your Support System."

SEEKING PROFESSIONAL ASSISTANCE

If the stress on you or your spouse becomes too great, or your children are having a hard time adjusting to the changes in the family equilibrium, it is important to seek professional assistance. Professional counseling can benefit the person experiencing adjustment difficulties, as well as other family members. Sometimes it is useful to have a few family sessions. Professional assistance can also help when either partner becomes angry, resentful, or severely depressed. A counselor can help your child express feelings, teach him coping skills, and assist him in learning to accept all that has occurred. For a more in-depth discussion on this subject, refer to Chapter 16, "Seeking Professional Counseling."

IN CONCLUSION

Human beings cannot exist in isolation. We lack the specialized physical attributes that other species rely on for survival. Our young are dependent upon adults for many more years than the young of other species. We need our families to provide a source of ongoing love, acceptance, and emotional renewal. For this very reason, your family unit can be a source of incredible strength.

It is my sincere hope that as you become alerted to the common sources of discomfort, friction, and stress that can affect a family unit when one member undergoes an amputation, you become determined to draw strength and courage from one another, and nourish each other with love and compassion.

20

DEALING WITH SOCIETY

> It can be congenital or it can happen at any age, to people of widely
> different social circumstances. The similarity of our condition is, how-
> ever, social, for no matter who we are or how we got into our unenviable
> condition, the able-bodied treat the physically handicapped in much the
> same way. Disability is defined by society and given meaning by culture;
> it is a social malady.
>
> Robert F. Murphy
> *The Body Silent*

If, like me, you have lost a limb due to trauma (or some other cause
requiring surgery with little warning) you know the feeling of having a
body that is intact one moment and "disabled" the next. No matter why
you have lost a limb, you will discover that some people will treat you
differently. You will find yourself suddenly lumped by society into a group
you had never considered would include you.

One has only to turn on a television or read a magazine to realize that
our society promotes everything youthful, beautiful, and healthy as good
and desirable. Those with a disability tend to lose status as a result of
society's lack of regard for anyone who is outside the norm. Due to negative
stereotypes, many individuals in our society presume that all people with
disabilities are similar to each other.

The ways people may interact with you as a result of your amputation
are presented in this chapter. Common misconceptions about those with a
disability are dispelled. Several individuals with limb loss discuss how
they have dealt with the responses of others. Suggestions are offered for
handling sticky social situations that may arise simply because you now
appear to be "different."

MYTHS AND STEREOTYPES

At one time or other, we are all faced with stereotypes, prejudices, and
myths that hinder our interactions with others. For those with physical
differences, the barriers to normal interactions with others often include

misbeliefs and negative attitudes that are based on ignorance and misunderstanding. Accurate information is the key to dispelling such harmful misconceptions.

Some common myths and misconceptions that surround people with disabilities are presented below. (Information adapted from Easter Seal Society pamphlet PR-42.)

Myth: The lives of people with disabilities are totally different from those of able-bodied individuals.

Fact: People with amputation and other disabilities go to school, get married, work, have families, do laundry, buy groceries, pay taxes, get angry, laugh, cry, have prejudices, vote, plan, and dream like everyone else.

Myth: People with disabilities are brave and courageous.

Fact: Adjusting to disability requires adapting to a new lifestyle. Just because you have lost a limb doesn't mean you have suddenly become a "super person." Individuals with amputation have the same range of degrees of bravery or courage found in the rest of society.

Myth: All persons who use wheelchairs are chronically ill or sickly.

Fact: A person may use a wheelchair for a variety of reasons, none of which may have anything to do with lingering illness. Many persons with amputation have no associated illness.

Myth: Wheelchair use is confining; users of wheelchairs are "wheelchair-bound."

Fact: A wheelchair, like a bicycle or an automobile, is a personal, assistive device that enables a person to get around faster or more easily.

Myth: Persons with disabilities are more comfortable with "their own kind."

Fact: Years of grouping persons with disabilities into separate schools and institutions have reinforced this misconception. In fact, most individuals who have lost limbs do not exclusively seek the company of others with amputation.

Myth: Non-disabled persons are obligated to care for those with disabilities.

Fact: Although some individuals may choose to offer their assistance, most persons with disabilities prefer to be responsible for themselves.

Myth: Curious children should not be allowed to ask individuals about their disabilities.

Fact: Children are naturally curious. Although you may be embarrassed by your children's questions, you imply there is something "bad" about being different when you scold them for asking. Most persons with disabilities don't mind the honest questions of children and will respond to them in their own ways. If they do mind, they will let you know.

Myth: There is nothing one person can do to help eliminate the barriers confronting those with disabilities.

Fact: Everyone can contribute to change. You can help remove barriers by doing the following:

• Understanding the need for accessible parking and leaving it available for those who need it.

• Encouraging participation of persons with disabilities in community activities by making sure the events are accessible.

• Advocating a barrier-free environment.

• Using proper words and terms when referring to those with disabilities (a person with a disability, *not* a disabled person); speaking up when negative words, phrases, or stereotypes are used by others in describing those with disabilities.

• Writing a note of support to producers and editors of books, movies, plays, and television shows when they portray people with disabilities as being just like anyone else.

• Accepting people with disabilities as individuals who have the same feelings and needs as you or anyone else.

• Hiring qualified persons with disabilities whenever possible.

Clearing up these myths allows those of us with disabilities to be judged by our own merits. It encourages others to treat us with the respect and dignity we all inherently deserve.

PREJUDICES AND THE RESPONSES OF OTHERS

Me prejudiced?

Like anyone else, you might have prejudices toward those you perceive as "different." I invite you to take some time to examine your own attitudes and beliefs about those with disabilities. How do you respond to others who have mental or physical differences? Do you shy away? Are you repulsed? Do you make gross generalizations about how life must be for them? Do you consider them to be essentially different from you?

Without even realizing it, you may have taken on society's beliefs, prejudices, and values; these attitudes may even be reflected in your attitude toward yourself. Notice the following prejudicial attitude on the part of a woman who lost her limb *despite* her training as a physician:

"I was dismayed to find myself in a wheelchair. I somehow assumed that being in a wheelchair meant that something was mentally wrong. I made a great effort to be animated enough so that people would know I was only physically disabled and not a mental case."

—Leslie

If you feel that you are somehow "less" than you were before you lost a limb—less worthy, less deserving, less entitled to a full rewarding life—you will tend to extend those harmful beliefs in your interactions with others. For example, you may isolate yourself by avoiding social gatherings or stop engaging in activities in which your limb loss may be apparent. You might feel you constantly have to prove your worth or "explain yourself" to others. *You are still the same person you were before the amputation. You are still equal to everyone else. You were born deserving and worthy; it is part of your birthright. This does not change just because you have undergone amputation.*

Your Vulnerability

Living with an amputation may render you highly susceptible to the responses of others, especially in the early days of your recovery. Negative responses can, at times, launch you into despair, since it is partly through the feedback of others that you formulate your new self-image. So the reactions of significant others, particularly spouses, physicians, and prosthetists, may take on special significance. It is, therefore, very useful for your emotional recovery to spend time with others with amputation who are doing well, feel good about themselves, and are enjoying their lives.

Individuals with limb loss react in varied ways to the responses of others. Some say that over-helpfulness, as well as expressions of pity and "understanding," are often humiliating and emotionally disturbing. Others appreciate these attempts at emotional outreach. The frank curiosity and open remarks of children are painful to some; but attempts by parents to stifle their children's natural curiosity can be even more upsetting to those with a disability. How you respond to others depends upon your unique makeup.

Most people with amputation claim they go through a period in which they are hypersensitive to the reaction of others. Some deny it. This stated indifference may be a cover-up for sensitivity, hurt, and anger. In time, the hypersensitivity may diminish. Occasionally, some persons will deflect their own discomfort by attempting to embarrass or shock others with their residual limb or prosthesis:

"The most ignorant ones are the adults. They stare at you but won't ask you questions. I don't like people to stare at my leg. Usually, when someone starts staring at me, I will look at them, stick my stump out, and say, 'Want a picture?'"

—Fred

"I say things to shock people occasionally. If someone is being a real jerk, I'll tell them I had my leg cut off, or that it was bitten off by a shark."

—Mark

The more apparent the physical abnormality, the greater the impact on how a person is viewed by society. Facial disfigurement or an upper-limb amputation is generally harder for most people to accept than a lower-limb amputation. Individuals are often ashamed to acknowledge their fear and revulsion at seeing those with physical differences, so they may conceal it by avoidance, pity, or over-helpfulness. Some able-bodied individuals actually expect the disabled to withdraw socially, and are resentful of those who lead full lives.

I clearly remember the range of strange reactions I received from others when I first lost my leg. The reactions suddenly began to make sense when it occurred to me I was like a movie screen onto which people projected their fears, prejudices, and beliefs about disability and mortality. It became increasingly clear to me that many of the responses I was receiving from others actually had *little or nothing to do with me personally.* As someone who has lost a limb, perhaps some of the following experiences I had may be familiar to you.

Several months after my accident, one friend confided that he could not bring himself to visit me in the intensive care unit. He realized that the graveness of my condition was stimulating *his* fears about death. Another friend who became very involved in my nursing care confessed that she realized part of her doing so was "selfish"—she viewed my convalescence as an opportunity to show others in our community of friends what a good person she was.

A strange phenomenon occurred in public places. Being in a wheelchair with one leg amputated seemed to be an invitation for complete strangers to approach and tell me their life stories, or stories of people they knew. I heard stories of heart attacks, strokes, and all kinds of physical disabilities. I was given all sorts of advice, philosophies, and expressions of sympathy from these total strangers.

It amazed me that when I used a wheelchair, many people reacted to me as if I were mentally retarded or incapable of speaking! They would ask my companion, "What happened to her?" and then proceed to make comments about me as if I were also deaf! In restaurants, some waitresses would ask, "What would she like to order?"

When you recognize other people are seeing you through the distorted lens of their own experience, it is truly freeing! You realize there is no need to take their remarks personally. What they say or how they react is often more of a statement about who they are than who you are.

At a time soon after amputation, when my own self-concept was shaky, and, like all of us, I was incorporating the responses of others in rebuilding my self-image, this realization was a big relief. It enabled me to step back mentally, and emotionally separate myself from the reactions of others. I became much more flexible in responding to the reactions of others. I learned to be more relaxed, and I developed an expanded sense of humor, as did the woman in the following case:

"You have to have a sense of humor—you just have to. Especially in the time immediately following your amputation, you are going to find yourself in new situations over which you have no control. For instance, air escaping from your prosthetic leg can sound like farting. I was really embarrassed about this, but it was something I had to live with. I learned to joke about it. A sense of humor is a survival tactic for sure."

—Margaret

While you cannot control the reactions of others, your own attitude is an important factor in influencing how others respond to you. When you are self-accepting and at ease, the more likely you will diffuse the anxiety of others, encouraging them to become more comfortable and accepting.

"When people had a hard time dealing with me, and they didn't know what to say or do, I maintained the attitude that it was their problem, not mine. Soon, people began to realize that I was coping with my amputation very well, so they should, too. When people discovered that I didn't mind talking about my cancer or my amputation, they usually began to feel comfortable around me."

—Margaret

We expect others to be normal. Our notion of what constitutes "normal" serves to help us make sense of our vast world. I find it fascinating to observe people's responses once they discover I have had an amputation. Often, they appear to be, at least momentarily, jarred by their discovery. I watch them go through shifts in their behavior while they attempt to integrate this new bit of information.

Here follows the experience of one individual:

"It's hard to tell that I am an amputee. I've worked with people for three years who still don't know. It's funny that people who don't know me treat me just like anybody else, but I see a change when they find out I have an amputation. They are nicer to me all of a sudden. It makes me feel like the man with a hundred million dollars—do they like me for me or my money?"

Reactions from Children

Children are generally more honest and natural in their responses to those who appear "different." They often exhibit a frank curiosity and ask very pointed questions about obvious limb loss. This directness can be a cause of chagrin to their parents who may be more concerned about being socially correct.

Those with limb loss have mixed responses to the directness of children. As the following examples illustrate, some find the honesty and curiosity of children refreshing; others find these same traits to be embarrassing or annoying:

"Kids are harder on me than anything. They don't know what they are doing. When I go to get my mail and I don't have my leg on, kids always gawk and stare. They make me very uncomfortable. I'd rather walk into a group of adults than children any day!"

—*Judith*

There is no doubt that the responses of parents and their children to the same circumstances can be wildly different. Seeing someone with an amputation is certainly no exception:

"Kids are so much more open about it. They'll say things to their parents like, 'That man has only one leg!' Their observance is often followed by the obvious question, 'Why?' Sometimes I try to explain what happened. Most of the time, they really don't understand; half the time their moms shut them up before they can say or ask anything else."

—*Mark*

Some individuals find the attempts by parents to suppress their children's natural curiosity more disquieting than the children's responses:

"Most little kids say, 'Look, he's got a broken leg!' Once, when I was swimming at a public pool, this little girl, who must have been four, watched me walk to the edge of the pool, take off my prosthesis, and dive into the pool. She kept going underwater to look at my leg because she was really fascinated. I didn't mind. Actually, I don't mind the reactions of kids at all. It's their parents that bother me. Sometimes they grab their kids as soon as they say something, or they tell them not to look at me."

—*Kent*

There are certain times when the innocent and unrepressed responses can be awkward for all of the adults involved:

"Kids are very curious. Often I'll hear them ask their mothers if I have a broken leg. They know something is different and they stare at me. They are definitely not shy. Usually, the parent tries to hush the child. I try to explain about my leg in simple terms. I remember one time in a grocery store a young child saw me and started screaming, 'Mommy, that lady's leg is cut in half!' I was dying of embarrassment. What could I do? I just sort of smiled and walked on."

—*Judith*

Offers of Assistance

Many people are happy to help when they see a person with amputation (or someone using crutches or a wheelchair) attempting a difficult task, such as opening a door while carrying groceries. Others seem to go into shock, apparently forgetting whatever social graces they were taught, and stare dumbfoundedly at the sight of someone who is obviously different physically.

There is also a wide range of reactions by those with amputation to offers of assistance. Notice the strong reaction of a young man who is very proud of his independence:

"It used to annoy me when people opened the door for me. It happened so often that I really resented it. It must have been a real shock for them when I got upset, but I felt that I could open doors myself."

—Mark

Compare Mark's response with that of Marcy, who overcame her initial discomfort with asking for help when she needed it:

"I used to be uncomfortable asking others for help, but I learned to deal with it. For example, I don't have any trouble moving my cart around at the grocery store. However, on days when I'm too tired to push the cart to my car, I'll ask for help. Also, as an art major, I often have a lot of stuff to carry at school. I've gotten really good at asking the guys in my class for a hand when I need it. They never seem to mind."

—Marcy

Sometimes, support from others is expressed as a sensitive refusal to cater to the person with limb loss. Such firmness encourages that person to do whatever he or she can whenever possible, thus fostering independence:

"I had a great girlfriend, great friends, and great support from everybody when my leg was amputated. My friends didn't cut me any slack, and that was good. Only my mom babied me, and that eventually got so bad that I had to say, 'Mom, stop, please.'"

—Grant

Some individuals appreciate assistance from time to time, yet want to spare others awkwardness or discomfort:

"I used to have trouble knowing how to ask for help when I needed it. Since I work in such a controlled environment at the hospital, there are some things I simply cannot do; so my colleagues will often bring me lunch or coffee, and pull chairs

around me to talk or eat. During those times when I don't want help, I go out of my way to say,'No, but thank you very much for asking.'"

—Leslie

DEALING WITH THE RESPONSES OF OTHERS

When you first learned of your impending amputation, or—as in the case of trauma—you discovered the harsh reality of your situation, no doubt it took you a period of time to adjust to the idea. This adjustment also holds true for those who first encounter a person who has lost a limb. Unless they have had some personal experience with amputation, they are likely to be shocked or confused. Many will need time, just as you did, to overcome their initial reaction.

"Initially, because they don't know how I feel about it, most people don't talk to me about my amputation until they have known me for a while."

—Mark

While adults will be, at the very least, curious when they detect your missing limb, most are sensitive enough to respect your privacy:

"People stare at me, but they have never been rude to me, nor have they ever laughed at me. Some people are curious and ask, 'What happened?' 'What does it feel like?' 'How does your artificial leg work?' Although it was difficult for me to talk about my amputation at first, eventually I became more confident, and now I am comfortable talking about it."

—Grant

Many individuals have preconceptions about people with amputation:

"Once, when I was all dressed up, this guy mentioned that I was really pretty, and that I held myself together really well. That made me mad—what am I supposed to look like?"

—Marie

"Most people who use handicapped parking spaces are older. When I pull into one of these spaces, people often stare at me because I am so young. They wait until they see me get out of the car and pull out my crutches before they walk away."

—Marcy

Your Responses to Others—A Personal Choice

It is important to remember that no matter how respectful others are of your privacy, or how outwardly inquisitive they may be, it is up to you to decide how you choose to respond. Explore and discover a level of disclosure with which you are comfortable. This may vary with how you are feeling at that particular moment—how playful, moody, or relaxed you are. Your responses are entirely up to you. There is no one right way to address the ignorance and curiosity of others:

"At first, I thought if people asked about my leg I would have to tell them what happened. Eventually, I realized that if I didn't feel like talking about it, I didn't have to. Sometimes I feel the need to protect myself. If I am having a bad day, or simply don't feel like discussing my amputation, I politely respond to the questions with, 'It's a long story,' which usually veers the discussion in another direction. You really have the right to be yourself. It gives you strength."

—Marcy

In the following example, notice the strategy Fred developed in helping both himself and others get used to his new condition:

"After my operation, as soon as I was able, I sat outside in front of the house in my wheelchair. Kids would pass by on their way to and from school. I would be out there on purpose to face the public and to get used to my amputation. I thought the hardest part would be facing the kids, but they are not so bad. My smallest grandchild was afraid of my leg at first, but I didn't push myself on him, and now he is comfortable coming over and sitting on my lap."

—Fred

As you become comfortable interacting with others, you may choose to assist others in feeling comfortable, as well:

"From the very beginning I felt that it was going to be up to me to make people feel comfortable with my amputation. It was up to me to educate them. It has been fifteen years now, and I still feel strongly about this. Rather than have people stare at me and whisper, I encourage them to ask questions."

—Margaret

In the process of dealing with others, many have found that humor can be a wonderful tool to make everyone feel more comfortable. Whether you use it to keep a buoyant attitude about yourself or to put others at ease, humor can provide a welcome relief from a potentially stressful situation:

"I find it easier to relate to people if I can joke with them or make light of my situation. This is the easiest way for me to deal with people. For example, early in my recovery I joked about taking up roller skating, since I didn't have many more bones to break."

—Leslie

Others will often take cues from you in how they should respond to you.

You will probably notice that when you are natural and at ease with others, they will be natural and at ease with you:

"Early on, when I was in a wheelchair, people often stared at me because I was so young (and young people are not supposed to have such things happen to them). Their first glance is trying to figure out what happened. They usually don't ask, they just stare a lot. I learned early on that I had to project myself as a normal person in order to be treated like one. I had to be talkative and friendly."

—Leslie

Ways to Deal with Others

Here are a few key points that may prove useful in dealing with others:

1. The reactions of others speak more about them than of you. You will never be able to control or change the reactions of others. What you can control are your own responses. People's reactions tell volumes about their upbringing, character, and level of maturity. It is, therefore, very useful for you to learn to separate your well-being from the reactions of others. Your responses to others do the same. If you make a firm internal commitment to treat others with dignity, respect, and compassion, you may find that they will treat you the same way.

2. The ways in which you relate to yourself and then project your self-concept can influence how you are perceived. If you consider yourself defective, crippled, "less than" others, or shamed, you will communicate those perceptions to those around you. If you appear depressed, defeated, or collapsed in self-pity, others will be likely to agree with you. On the other hand, if you present an air of being at peace with yourself, and are friendly, you will tend to elicit positive responses from others. Of course, this advice needs to be balanced with being authentic in your emotions. No one is telling you to deny your true feelings, just to be aware of the messages you are sending others.

3. You are the one who decides how much to tell others. You need only share as much of your personal history as you want. If you ever feel pressured by someone to divulge more than you wish, be honest and tell the person you are not comfortable talking about it. Most people will respect your response.

4. Keep a sense of humor. There are so many unforeseen events that life brings to our doorstep, so many unusual individuals with whom we must interact—a sense of humor is really essential to promote your equanimity. So, if someone is getting your goat, try to shift your perspective. Imagine that person standing there in Mickey Mouse underwear, or picture him as a small child whose mother is trying to make him eat his

broccoli. Do whatever you have to do to see the situation with different eyes. Remember that familiar line: *Someday I'll look back on all this and laugh.* Why wait? Laugh about it today.

There are a variety of ways to respond to any situation. Keep the following principle in mind. *Those with the most behavioral flexibility have the most freedom.* If you always respond to a certain person or situation in the same way, you are a slave to your own habits. You have limited your options and, therefore, possess limited outcomes to your actions. Break those habits. Try something different. Change your approach. Maybe allow yourself to do something outrageous (that doesn't cause harm) just to see how it feels.

IN CONCLUSION

There have been significant improvements in society's acceptance of disability in recent years. Buildings, public transportation vehicles, public facilities, and laws have been altered to be more "handicap friendly." More physically challenged children are being mainstreamed into regular classrooms. Schools as well as the media are educating people to be more accepting of those with differences. It has even become somewhat fashionable to include actors who have disabilities in movies and television programs. However, erasing social prejudices and negative attitudes that have been around for thousands of years is not a simple task. The reality is that following your amputation, you may find yourself having to deal with the ignorant responses of those with whom you come in contact.

Most people are well-intentioned and will treat you with respect. Realizing that you are still the same person you were before the amputation, and that you still have equal worth, will allow you to feel more secure and distance yourself from the social awkwardness and ignorance of others. I encourage you to try out a variety of responses in dealing with those you encounter. And keep your sense of humor while demonstrating love and compassion in your interactions.

21

VOCATION

Work and play are the two poles of a continuum that establish a dynamic balance of the activity in our lives. For all of us, these complementary aspects of our experience can greatly contribute to the satifaction of our lives. When you return to work following your amputation, you join the ranks of the 18 million Americans with physical or mental disabilities who are part of the work force in this country.

This chapter presents a discussion of some of the issues related to your vocation such as the challenges in returning to work, fears about the workplace, and issues related to your co-workers. It also provides an overview of vocational rehabilitation, as well as tips on finding new employment.

LOSING WORK—A PROFOUND LOSS

We all complain about work from time to time—having to get up early, punch a time clock, or deal with a difficult boss. Yet, when our ability to work becomes limited, we may find that we miss the activity. Our lives may seem out of balance because we no longer feel productive. (This point is illustrated by those lottery and sweepstakes winners who continue to work in the same job they had before they became financially independent.)

As the following story illustrates, some individuals who undergo amputation find the possibility of losing their chosen field of work even more difficult to accept than the loss of the limb itself:

"My heart is in working on cars. That's what I love to do. The first few weeks after my amputation were hard for me because I didn't know if I could continue working at a job I knew and loved. I also worried about how I was going to pay the thousands of dollars worth of medical bills that had accumulated. I wasn't as concerned about the loss of my hand as I was about the loss of my career."

—Clint

When you are not able to work, you may feel shame and embarrassment, as well as a blow to your self-esteem, sense of competency, dignity, and self-identity. You may find yourself mourning the loss of work in much the same way you grieved over your lost limb. In addition, you may feel you have lost the ability to be a financial provider. Believing you are no longer able to contribute in the same way to your family and community, you may fear loss of social status.

For many, work provides a source of self-worth. It may be emotionally difficult to give up work when you are used to being busy and productive. It may be hard to feel dependent upon others for income. Work also expands your world of social interaction. In fact, some individuals center their entire social life around their co-workers. The friends they see in their off-time are the same people with whom they work.

The ability to return to your former work will, of course, depend upon your prior occupation and whether you still have the physical ability to perform your job. It also depends upon whether or not your workplace or job tasks can be adapted so you can still fulfill your job-related responsibilities. Many occupations that are executive or professional in nature do not require a lot of physical labor; rather, they rely on thinking, speaking, and decision-making skills. If you happen to have this type of job, your loss of limb may not interfere with your ability to continue working in your chosen profession. However, if you have earned your living by using your physical body primarily for such tasks as lifting, carrying, or performing delicate hand operations, you may not be able to continue your former job. You may need job training in a new or related field.

Common Work-Related Fears

Losing your job may understandably provoke a number of anxieties and fears—the need to retrain and find new work, the possibility of having to deal with new stresses at home as family roles become altered, and concerns over financial matters. You may realistically fear loss of health insurance, pensions, and other benefits.

If you have "defined" yourself largely in terms of a job that you can no longer do, the result may be a personal identity crisis. You may have determined your sense of self-worth, in part, by being able to do your work and contribute to your family and society. No longer having a job may result in shame, embarrassment, feelings of inadequacy, and self-re-crimination.

You may try to perform your job at the same level of functioning you had before your surgery; but, you might find yourself physically and emotionally exhausted. You may be able to do your old job with modifications, yet find yourself frustrated with your new physical limitations and energy levels. If you use these types of criteria as measurements of personal success, you may deem yourself a failure and sink into depression and despair. And this will contribute to stress at home with your spouse and family.

Even if you are still able to do your work competently, you will inevitably face new challenges, as you and others adjust to your altered body and the social awkwardness of being perceived as "different." At work, as well as in other areas of your life, the more comfortable you are with yourself, the more at ease others will be, too. For some, it may take a bit of time and experience back on the job to regain full confidence.

Hear what Marcy has to say about the value of confidence on the job and the benefits of being willing to take risks:

"I designed advertising banners for businesses. My amputation never hindered me in my work, even though I had to deal with the public constantly. I felt very secure in my job and confident in myself, yet there came a time when I needed to move on to greater challenges.

Quitting my job to go back to school was a big step. It made me pretty nervous and scared at first, but I was determined to move on in my career. There's a lot of growth in store for me and I am going to risk going out there and finding a new job. My self-esteem has grown in that I have overcome my initial fears about taking risks. My core is becoming very strong."

—Marcy

Some individuals state they have actually gained self-confidence through the recovery process that followed their limb loss:

"Going through the amputation has changed the way I think about everything. I wouldn't be doing what I'm doing now—helping a lot of people through work in the prosthetic industry—if it hadn't been for my own amputation. I get a lot of self-satisfaction from working with others; it's just natural for me.

My amputation has helped me gain confidence in myself. I feel I can deal with almost any situation. I don't see myself as being different from anybody else."

—Grant

Be aware that there has been some exploitation of those with amputation in the workplace. Some employers may attempt to hire you at a lower salary level than so-called "able-bodied" workers. Additionally, promotions to higher positions and pay may be slow in coming. These types of exploitation are illegal. Some people have allowed themselves to be taken advantage of by charitable organizations to raise money; others have been used by medical personnel for publicity, or as models for teaching, without receiving financial compensation.

Financial Concerns

If you have to change your job, and your new income is lower than your previous one, this can be a blow to your self-esteem. You may feel shame, frustration, anger, and anxiety about meeting financial obligations. Although your family may be empathetic and supportive, they may also suffer resentment if they have to adapt their lifestyle to meet with new financial realities. Money that had been previously slated for college educations, vacations, clothing, cars, etc. may become depleted due to health-care costs and lost income. This might be especially hard on older children and young teens, who often lack a solid grasp of economic reality. If you and your spouse had been looking forward to a certain level of financial freedom in your retirement, you might have to adjust your dreams. If you are already retired, you may fear using up money saved for those "golden years."

It is very important that your entire family come together for frank discussions of the financial facts; share your emotional responses to what is happening. The family is a team in which all members must pull together to meet new challenges. Each member can think of new ways to contribute to the well-being of the family, or come up with novel solutions to deal with times of stress. Of course, the idea is not to burden your children, but to bring the issues into the open. Children are very perceptive and intuitive; they will sense when there is extra tension in the family. If your spouse or older children wish to find work in order to contribute to the family's financial stability, this may require adjustment on everyone's part. Meeting these challenges as a family unit can bring you together as you serve as mutual support for each other.

This may be a good time to set up a meeting with your accountant or a financial planner to help you figure out your assets and liabilities, and then come up with a workable plan with realistic goals. Set up a meeting with a social worker to discover if you are elegible for benefits from a disability program, local community services, Social Security, or Workman's Compensation (if the cause of your limb loss was work related).

VOCATIONAL REHABILITATION

"The most exhilarating experience I had since my amputation was working a full eight-hour shift while standing on my 'legs' for the first time. It reassured me that I could be independent. I knew I would be able to support myself."

—Carol

Your state's Department of Rehabilitation can assist you in your recovery process, whether you need help in obtaining work or keeping your present position. A rehabilitation counselor will explain your rights, and assist you in identifying and obtaining acceptable employment. Generally, a medical evaluation is required to determine your ability level, as well as your physical limitations. Treatments may be suggested to aid in your recovery. A vocational evaluation will help you decide the kinds of work you are able to do. These evaluations will also help determine if you are eligible for further rehabilitation services.

Vocational rehabilitation may be necessary if your former work requires physical strength or agility that is no longer possible. Once a rehabilitation counselor has helped you define your physical limits and your vocational aptitudes and interests, you may require assistance in adjusting your career goals. Together you can come up with a plan to achieve those goals. Your counselor can suggest interviewing strategies and show you ways to best present yourself as a job applicant.

Once you have found work that suits both your physical requirements and emotional temperament, your frustrations will often diminish in intensity. Returning to the workplace will also give you another focus in your life, making it easier for you to keep from dwelling on other problems.

Financial assistance may be available to you through local, state, or federal agencies. Other types of services offered by such agencies may include job training, help in learning job-seeking skills, provision of transportation to and from a job site or training center, and the supplying of necessary tools and equipment. Some agencies offer help in obtaining necessary licenses for your chosen work, or help in modifying and customizing equipment to meet your needs. Other services may include helping you with job placement, coaching you on your work site, and following up to be sure you and your employer are satisfied.

In the following case, the initial loss of work for Kent was difficult and anxiety-provoking. It turned out, however, that a training program provided him with the possibility to grow through a new career. He rose to meet new challenges and discovered new satisfactions:

"I had been in the Navy for many years. Four days after my amputation, I returned to work. Unable to perform my old job, I was given a good desk job as a watch coordinator. After a short time, I was given ten days notice on my job. Everything hit me at once. With a wife and newborn at home, I didn't know where to turn. My pension helped, but it wasn't even enough to pay the rent.

I discovered the Veterans' Administration has a number of excellent job-training programs for those with disabilities. I was accepted into a program for interior design. The program covered tuition, books, and shop fees for schooling up through a bachelor's degree. I now have a new career that I really enjoy."

—Kent

Interviewing Tips

Job interviews can be daunting for anyone. In addition to following the basic rules for a successful interview, the person with amputation has the added challenge of demonstrating how his disability is not a liability.

During an interview, it is important to appear relaxed about your amputation. Demonstrate how you take your limb loss in stride. For instance, if you have an upper-limb amputation and wish to shake hands with your remaining limb or prosthesis, feel free to do so. Most people will feel comfortable in following your lead.

Be sure to emphasize your abilities, achievements, education, and experience. And remember that a job interview is a two-way experience. Use the opportunity to learn as much about the position and the company as you can.

Be as open and honest about your amputation as you choose to be; but remember, you are not required to answer personal questions that have nothing to do with the position for which you are applying. You may find that you have to spend some time educating others, whether in an interview or on the job. The following incident illustrates just how unmindful people can be, even when they are trying to be sensitive and understanding:

"Once I was interviewed for a position with a graphic design shop. The shop consisted of two large rooms that were divided by a single step. Instead of being interested in my abilities, the first thing I was asked was if that step would be a problem for me. I told the interviewer that I lived on the second floor of an apartment house that had no elevator, and the step would not be a problem."

—*Marcy*

Returning to Your Former Job

Before returning to work, you need to be far enough on the road to physical and emotional recovery to assume job-related responsibilities. Since you have had to deal with the life-altering experience of losing a limb, you may find that your vocational priorities have shifted. Your old job may or may not hold the same importance for you that it once did. This is certainly an excellent time to reassess your priorities; finding meaningful new work or retiring may be a part of this process.

If you return to a former job, be prepared for some changes. Your employer will naturally be concerned about your ability to perform your job at full capacity. He or she may fear that you will need to take off a lot of time to attend to health-care concerns. Anxiety about how your care will affect health insurance costs is another likely employer reaction.

If you return to work shortly after your surgery, it is conceivable that you will, indeed, require a substantial amount of time for such things as prosthetic fittings, physical therapy, medical care, or possibly legal proceedings related to the cause of your limb loss. Enlisting the aid of your employer or immediate supervisor can ease this difficult transition period. Making him an ally in your rehabilitation will make him more likely to cheer you on and provide assistance when possible:

"Four weeks after I lost my hand, I went back to work at the garage where I had been a mechanic. My boss was great. At first, he asked me to run the office for him; but within two weeks he let me start working on cars again, a little at a time. And I was still in bandages! His support and confidence in me was a stabilizing factor."

—Clint

When you return to your job, it will likely be stressful at first. It is important to assess how well you can deal with work-related stresses as you adjust physically and emotionally to your limb loss. The level of your amputation and the resulting physical limitations, as well as the degree of visibility of your limb loss, will, of course, impact the ways you will have to adjust to life in the workplace. You must deal with how your amputation will affect your job performance. You will likely have to adapt yourself and/or your workstation, as well as deal with the reactions of colleagues to your limb loss. If your job includes interaction with the public, you must learn to handle those interactions as gracefully as possible.

What about inquiring colleagues? How should you handle their questions? This is really up to you. Your openness will likely depend upon your prior relationships with your co-workers and their comfort level with your amputation. Keep in mind that if you are at ease with your physical changes, you open the way for others to feel comfortable about them, too. And remember, you don't owe anyone any explanations. If you wish to share details of your limb loss, then do so; if you would rather not, then don't.

Spouses can be helpful by keeping your employer informed while you are still recuperating. As soon as you are able, be sure to talk with your employer about your current status and work-related expectations. It may well be that you don't know what you're capable of until you try it out. If you find you are not able to return to your former position, your employer may have another job in the company for you. However, if you are able to return to your former position, it is wise to start off with a light work load. Don't allow yourself to become overwhelmed by tasks that are beyond your abilities. As you regain strength and agility, your ability levels might change, and you can add more job responsibilities. As seen in the following story, you are the only one who can truly assess your own capabilities at work:

"I was fortunate that I had chosen a profession [physician] that I was able to go back to after my amputation. Of course, I wasn't able to do as much physical work as I used to. I found that I functioned best in a teaching program where I was able to share personal experiences and opinions. I like what I do, and I love working with residents and medical students."

—Leslie

Your health-care professionals may have valuable suggestions to assist you in adapting yourself or your work environment to best meet your needs. Speak with your physician about any underlying physical concerns related to your job. It may be very helpful to meet with a physical or occupational therapist, or even bring this person to your workplace to help you discover creative ways to approach certain tasks; he may show you the best ways to deal with your physical limitations, and how to avoid taxing your energy reserves. I did this when I first returned to my job in a clinic as a physician's assistant. Because I was in a wheelchair at the time, my physical therapist observed me at work, then showed me ways to adapt to my tasks.

Discuss your physical capabilities with your prosthetist. He might come up with prosthetic options to make it easier to accomplish physical tasks. Your workplace environment may be modified, if it is not already handicapped accessible. You might also speak with members of your local amputation support group to find out how others have dealt with the same kinds of challenges you now face. A vocational rehabilitation counselor might also provide helpful input.

Thus, with a bit of flexibility and a willingness to adapt (on the parts of both you and your employer), you may find it possible to return to your former job. Or perhaps you will be compelled to move on to a different type of work that may be more in line with your current priorities or physical realities. Working again can go a long way in restoring a sense of normalcy to your life. You'll discover that your willingness to take risks and master new skills will enhance your self-concept and sense of competency.

THE AMERICANS WITH DISABILITIES ACT

In 1990, the Americans with Disabilities Act (ADA) was signed by President George Bush to ensure that some 43 million American citizens with disabilities have the same civil rights that others enjoy. Considered the most important civil rights legislation enacted by Congress since the Civil Rights Act of 1964, the ADA legally prohibits discrimination against anyone based upon physical or mental disability in the areas of employment, public services, transportation, public accommodations, and telecommunications. This landmark bill thus opens the way for many physically challenged individuals to more fully participate and contribute to society.

The ADA states that job applicants must be evaluated solely on the basis of their actual abilities. As long as an individual is capable of performing his job, an employer cannot refuse to hire him because of his disability. This is true even if it means the individual requires reasonable accommodations—such as an easily accessible and usable restroom, or ramps, wide doorways, and clear paths for wheelchair access. If necessary, an employer is required to make these accommodations, unless they would create "undue hardship" for the employer, based upon factors such as the size of the company and the financial resources available. Furthermore, employers are not allowed to limit, segregate, or classify an individual because of his disability.

The ADA applies to employers of fifteen people or more. ADA regulations apply not only to individual employers, but also to employment agencies and labor organizations.

The Equal Employment Opportunity Commission (EEOC), and state and local civil rights agencies that work with the commission, enforce the ADA. This prohibits discrimination against disabled individuals in the private sector and state and local governments. The EEOC also receives and investigates discrimination charges.

Know Your Rights

As someone with a disability, it is important for you to be aware of your rights in the workplace, as well as your responsibilities and the responsibilities of your employer. Answers to the following questions should aid you in your awareness:

Does an employer have the right to ask me questions about my disability?
Absolutely not! An employer is permitted to inquire only whether or not you can perform necessary job tasks. Once the job has been offered to you, you can be asked to describe or demonstrate how, with or without reasonable accommodation, you will perform the job. It is now illegal for an employer who is interviewing you for a position to require you to state in your job application whether or not you have a disability. Even if you have an obvious disability, the employer cannot ask about the nature or severity of your condition.

Can an employer require me to have a medical examination?
An employer has no right to force you to take a medical examination before offering you a job. However, he may offer you the job on the condition that you pass a medical examination; but only if the same is true for *all* new employees. As long as you are capable of performing the responsibilities of the job (with or without an accommodation) he cannot refuse to hire you. In short, no employer can refuse to hire you solely because of your disability.

Once you have started work, your employer can require you to take a medical examination only if it is related to your job and necessary for the conduct of the business. The same applies to asking questions about your disability. If the company has an employee health program that conducts voluntary exams, he may provide medical information to the agency that oversees the state worker's compensation laws. In such cases, all results must be kept confidential.

If the employer has two job applicants who are equally qualified, and one is disabled, what is the employer's obligation?

A disability itself cannot be the basis for the final decision on which applicant to hire. The purpose of the ADA is to prohibit discrimination on the basis of disability; however, it does not mean that an employer must hire you over other qualified applicants just because you have a disability.

What happens if I become disabled while on the job?
Your employer is obligated to try to accommodate you in your same position if possible. If necessary, you may be transferred to another position for which you are better qualified.

What if my employer is excused from making job accommodations for me?
If your employer is exempt from making job accommodations, you can choose to pay for all or part of the accommodations yourself. However, your salary cannot be lowered to pay for the cost of the accommodations.

For further information regarding your rights in the workplace, contact your local branch of the Equal Employment Opportunity Commission, found in the phone directory under "U.S. Government Offices."

RETIREMENT

If you were just putting in hours until your retirement, you probably won't be heartbroken if you have to stop working. However, if you want to keep working, but cannot due to your physical limitations, you might have a harder time adjusting to retirement. There exists a danger that you may equate the fact of no longer working with no longer being a useful member of society. If this is the case, you may tend to withdraw socially and give up on life. This is tragic and unnecessary!

There are still many ways you can stay active and make a contribution to your family and the community. Being at home more, you may discover new levels of intimacy and interaction with your family. You may involve yourself more fully with your children or grandchildren. Retirement can provide you with a wonderful opportunity to engage in recreational activities for which you never had enough time.

There are a number of volunteer positions available that might allow you to serve others while continuing to use your skills. It might be natural for you to become a peer visitor, assisting others who have recently lost a limb. In doing this, you can make a unique, emotionally satisfying contribution. You may find that you finally have the time to work for groups or agencies in whose causes you always believed but never had time for—environmental protection groups, literacy programs, your local church, or a political candidate whome you support.

IN CONCLUSION

Work helps give meaning to our lives. It helps to define who we are and where we fit into society. Perhaps some of the happiest people alive are those who are fortunate enough to find an easy match between their natural interests and their vocation. Whether you are able to continue in your previous career, or whether you are forced (or choose) to find a new one, the important thing, aside from earning an adequate income, is that you are at peace with what you do for a living. Use this as an opportunity to re-evaluate your options.

What is it that you really want to do? The word vocation comes from the Latin *vocare*, which means "to call." What type of work calls forth your interests, talents, and abilities? What type of work calls forth the best in you while meeting your financial needs? One day you might look back at this time in your life and feel grateful that you were pushed forward into a new, satisfying direction.

22

RECREATION

No matter what your age or ability level, recreation can revitalize your body and spirit. Your limb loss need not interfere with your enjoyment of life. This chapter presents an overview of the psychosocial as well as the physical benefits of recreation; it also explores some common concerns about participating in such leisure activities. Several recreational opportunities are suggested, along with a sampling of ways to successfully adapt to them.

As you deal with your immediate health concerns following surgery, recreation may be the last thing on your mind; but as you go through rehabilitation and progress in your recovery, you're going to find yourself needing new outlets. After all, how much time can you spend as a "couch potato"? It's important for you to take charge and discover the many opportunities that are available to you. Your life is what you make it. Go out and get involved!

Recreation is very individual. What is recreation for you may be very different from what recreation is for me. One person might find a vigorous aerobic workout at a gym pleasurable, while another is exhausted at the very thought, and prefers instead to take a quiet walk in a park or along a beach. Another person may prefer the intensity of competitive sports, or the stimulation of travel, or the creativity of the fine arts.

If certain activities give you feelings of pleasure, accomplishment, and purpose, by all means, pursue them! These feelings need not be diminished once you have undergone amputation. There are so many opportunities available today, at so many levels of interest, your amputation need not stand in the way.

IMPORTANCE OF RECREATION

Involvement in hobbies, sports, or other recreational activities provides an excellent outlet for expression of your unique talents, interests, and personal style. In addition to the creative satisfaction and social interaction brought about by pastime activities, engagement in such activities can be enjoyed purely for the inherent pleasure they offer.

Physical and Psychological Benefits

The benefits of regular leisure activity—whether it is a vigorous physical workout or a less strenuous, more serene activity—are apparent. Recreational involvement serves as a diversion when you are going through rough times—the sheer pleasure of the activity adds enjoyment to living and provides a balance to the more serious aspects of life.

A program of regular physical exercise offers many physiological and psychological benefits, all of which contribute to a healthy lifestyle. Physically, exercise can help you regain past abilities; improve your strength, coordination, agility, endurance, and cardiovascular fitness; reduce musculo-skeletal tension, blood pressure, and overall stress; maintain your optimum weight; and increase your sense of well-being and vitality. When you are physically fit, you have more energy. This enables you to function better with a new prosthesis or wheelchair, and it helps you gain a greater sense of mastery and control over your body as you learn to adapt to physical limitations.

Following amputation, while you are adjusting to the realities of your loss, it's common to experience feelings of alienation from others. Involvement in recreational activities can help you feel less alone. Joining a sports program or other group activity, for instance, can provide a wonderful opportunity for healthy interaction and friendly competition with others. In the setting of relaxing play, you can take risks and explore your strengths and limitations. This allows you to perceive yourself in new ways that may enhance your self-esteem.

Through participation in special interest groups or sports clubs, you are bound to make new friends, extend your social interactions, and learn to become more accepting of your limb loss. Often the opportunity exists to meet others with amputation, share experiences, and find out how they have coped.

Common psychological benefits of recreation include enhanced feelings of well-being, increased self-esteem, improved sleep patterns, better concentration and alertness, less depression and anxiety, decreased stress, reduced dependence on mood-altering drugs, physical and emotional discharge of frustration and anger, and opportunities to interact with others.

Involvement in a recreational activity can enhance your sense of competency by shifting the focus from your disability to your abilities. Outside interests can provide you with a sense of purpose, and let you know you are still a viable part of society—that your life isn't over because you have lost a limb. There are so many things you can still do—and do successfully—if you just keep an open mind and are willing to explore your options.

Think of how good you feel when you're doing something you enjoy. Through new interests you may realize talents you never knew you had. For example, you may discover you work well on a computer, that you have a flair for flower arranging, or that you are a competent athlete in a wheelchair sport. Some individuals find success and satisfaction as peer counselors, helping others with amputation adjust to their new challenges.

The Age Factor

No matter what your age, you can benefit from play. If you are elderly, it is especially important that you keep physically active—participation in activities that keep you in good shape is beneficial for both body and mind. There are misconceptions concerning the desire and ability of elders to participate in recreational endeavors. The truth is, you are never too old to enjoy!

For children, participation in sports and other recreational group activities provides opportunities to promote physical and psychosocial development. Involvement promotes social interaction, enhances self-esteem and feelings of mastery, and allows a child to just be "one of the kids." It can lay the foundation for your child to develop a lifelong interest in maintaining optimal physical fitness through a variety of well-balanced activities. This helps a child integrate into his peer group and the larger community.

Common Fears

Your own motivation and the support you receive from others are key factors in your participation in a leisure activity. Some people, however, are hesitant to get involved due to any one of a number of reasons. Pain from prosthesis, prolonged recovery time, underlying medical conditions, phantom pain, and residual limb pain are a few of these reasons. Limiting factors such as the inability to run, lack of energy, and decreased endurance can also inhibit participation. Another common reason is a fear of embarrassment at not being able to perform the activity as well as others.

If your lack of participation is the result of pain or irritation from your artificial limb, realize that these problems can often be addressed by your prosthetist. Depending on the activity, you may opt not to wear the prosthesis at all. For example, many people who have lost a lower limb find it easier to ski and swim without their prosthesis.

Try not to let self-consciousness or embarrassment be your reason for not joining an activity. As a peer visitor for my local support group, I once visited a woman who had an above-knee amputation. She lived in a condo complex that had a community pool. A man lived in the complex who also had an amputation, and whom she observed swimming a few times a week. This woman, however, was so self-conscious about her own limb loss, she was not able to bring herself to swim in the pool—although she longed to do so. This was certainly her loss.

If you are hesitant to engage in an activity because you are self-conscious of being seen by others, I urge you to take some risks and do whatever it takes to participate in the activity. It has been my experience that, initially, most people are curious about others who are physically different. People may stare at first, and perhaps make a comment or ask a question or two, but, generally, they will ignore you after that. After all, most people are more concerned with themselves than they are with you.

Again, I encourage you to work through your self-consciousness. By letting it get in the way, you are imposing additional, unnecessary limitations upon yourself. The rewards for working through your self-consciousness are great. In addition to experiencing the joy of enhanced self-confidence and self-acceptance, there is also the inherent pleasure derived from the activity itself.

Before Participating in Vigorous Physical Activity

It is important for everyone—those with and without disabilities—to engage in an overall program of self-care that includes exercise, good nutrition, and stress reduction. Leisure activities can play an integral part in such a program.

Be aware, however, that many recreational activities involve some measure of physical risk. Before participating in a new sport or other vigorous activity, consult with the appropriate health-care professionals. Determine your physical limitations to prevent exacerbating any orthopedic problems or underlying medical conditions, and decide if you can help yourself get into shape before starting the activity. A physiatrist, or other type of informed physician, and/or a physical, occupational, or recreational therapist can be excellent consultants in helping you develop an overall program for fitness. They may help you discover creative ways of adapting to certain activities. Your prosthetist may modify your prosthesis or offer special assistive devices that better enable you to engage in the activity of your choice.

Whether or not you have a disability, it is best to start off any new physical activity slowly. By gradually increasing the demands you place on your body, you can safely build up strength, flexibility, and endurance. Use common sense. When you are fatigued or feel you may be over-stressing yourself, either stop the activity or rest a bit before continuing.

In summary, no matter your age, level of amputation, or number of remaining limbs, you can still participate in many recreational activities. You can do this by engaging in a professionally guided program of fitness to optimize your physical abilities, working with your prosthetist to adapt your prosthesis or other assistive devices, adapting or modifying the activity itself, joining sports organizations for those with physical disabilities, and working to adjust any limiting thoughts and beliefs that interfere with your ability to feel good about yourself and enjoy leisure activities.

POPULAR RECREATIONAL ACTIVITIES

"I love to hike and I love the outdoors. Last year, my husband and I took a twenty-two day trek in Nepal. I trained to get into good shape and keep from getting injured. I did the whole trek on one leg with crutches. It was great—so much fun!

I've always had the attitude that my amputation wasn't going to stop me from the activities I enjoy. My approach in performing the activities may not be conventional, but no matter what, I'm going to figure out a way to do them. I still play tennis, volleyball, and softball, and I enjoy cross-country skiing and golf. For these sports I wear my prosthesis. I also swim, river-raft, and kayak."

—Margaret

"I had a horse within a month after my amputation. It took me a while, but I finally built up enough strength to saddle him. Believe me, putting a saddle on a horse that was sixteen hands high was a pretty big deal! It was also important to me to be strong enough to lift myself onto that horse. It proved that I was independent."

—Marcie

"I have always been an avid fisherman. After losing my hand, I had to learn how to cast again and manipulate the equipment. I had to learn how to tie a knot in a piece of string that was only a hundredth of an inch thick—talk about difficult. The first few times I went fishing, I had some trouble, but I still caught fish. Each time it got a little easier. I gradually learned to adapt by manipulating things differently. Once I figured it out, fishing became as normal for me as it did when I had both hands."

—Clint

Your choice of leisure opportunities is limitless, and depends upon your interests, physical abilities, and motivation. The activities you choose may require very little energy or all-out physical effort; they may be performed alone, with a partner, or as part of a team.

The activities presented in this chapter are just a small sampling of all those possible. I encourage you to do some exploration on your own. Excellent sources for available opportunities are your local amputation support group, as well as your health-care providers. In addition, there are excellent local and national sports associations for those with disabilities, such as National Handicapped Sports and the National Amputee Golf Association. Most recreational activities can be adapted for wheelchair users. Examples of wheelchair sports include track and field, road racing, archery, skeet shooting, table tennis, weightlifting, and team sports such as basketball and quad rugby. Wheelchair Sports U.S.A. can provide you with information about such sports programs in your area. And the American Amputee Foundation and the Amputee Coalition of America can provide information about activities in which you are interested. (For further information on these and other sports organizations, see "Groups and Organizations" beginning on page 323.)

Although much can be gained from participation in physically challenging activities, great satisfaction and fulfillment can also be achieved through quiet, less-active types of entertainment. Playing an instrument, painting, sculpting, and taking photos can all be quite rewarding. Many who have lost an upper limb can perform these activities with one hand. If, however, you cannot, your prosthetist may come up with some clever adaptation that will enable you to enjoy the activity. Keep in mind that performing with an adaptation may include trial and error; but, with effort, you should be able to work out a viable solution. Your enjoyment is certainly worth the effort.

What follows are a few leisure activities reported to be most popular for those with amputation.

Swimming

Swimming is a wonderful and very popular leisure activity for those with amputation. From a physical standpoint, swimming is great for your cardiovascular system and muscular endurance. As an added bonus, it simply feels great. When I began swimming again after losing my leg, I can remember how I revelled in the freedom the water afforded me.

You may have to adapt your strokes to compensate for the effect of your limb loss on maintaining your balance in the water and performing the stroke itself. Generally, this can be readily accomplished. Although most individuals with lower-limb loss choose to swim without one, a special waterproof swimming prosthesis provides added propulsion and ease in getting in and out of the water. Wearing a prosthesis also reduces edema in the limb.

If you have only one remaining upper limb, you may still be able to swim well without using a prosthesis. Or you might choose to wear a waterproof prosthesis to increase the power of your stroke. (This can be especially helpful if you swim competitively.) Another way to enhance stroke power is to affix a training paddle, instead of a prosthesis, to your forearm. Your prosthetist can show you other available assistive devices and prosthetic options for swimming.

Golfing

"In golf, your handicap is nothing more than a number. It is not related to your physical well-being. Golf has provided me with an outlet to get outdoors, play a game I truly love, enjoy the camaraderie that exists within the game, and return to a more mainstream style of life."

—*Tony*

Golf is not only an extremely popular sport for those with disability, it is also one of the most adaptable. Although balance and the ability to swing the golf club are necessary functions for every golfer, this sport allows each individual to have his or her own unique style. A wide variety of prosthetic or orthotic devices are available to assist and enhance one's ability to play the game. Those in wheelchairs can also participate.

Depending upon the golfer's physical circumstances, each has the option to wear or not wear a prosthesis. Certain assistive devices may help certain individuals. For example, a rotator or torque absorber in the ankle of the prosthetic leg will ease lower-body turn during the swing. The removal of spikes from the golf shoe(s) may assist the foot to turn, especially in the lead leg.

Some with below-elbow amputation play one-handed. However, most opt for a prosthetic device that helps them gain bilateral assistance. The standard hook or myoelectric prosthesis can be used. To have a bilateral swing, however, a wrist device that can move multi-axially is a must. There are a number of prosthetic devices that have evolved to meet this need.

Speak with your prosthetist or contact the National Amputee Golf Association (NAGA) for information about available options. NAGA also conducts a program called First Swing . . . Golf for the Physically Challenged. A "Learn to Golf Clinic" is part of the program and is open to any individual with a disability who would like to learn, return to, or improve his or her golf game. For further information, call the National Amputee Golf Association at (800) 633–NAGA.

Snow Skiing

Many people with amputation find snow skiing a wonderful form of recreation. Those who enjoyed skiing before losing a limb, generally find that with the necessary adjustments and some helpful adaptations they are able to pick up this sport again with relative ease. Given the proper instructions and assistive equipment, even those who have never skied before can learn to do so, no matter what the type or level of limb loss.

In addition to the pleasures of skiing itself, some people say their success in this sport opened them up to the possibility of expanding other horizons in their lives:

"Attempting to ski so soon after my amputation was good for me. I had skied ever since I was young, so I was able to pick it up again pretty quickly. Being able to ski again proved to me that I could still do things that I was able to do before the surgery. It gave me the confidence to try other things."

—*Margaret*

"I had been a runner before I lost my leg at age twenty-three. The doctors told me I would never run again, nor would I be able to stand up for many hours. I moved to Wyoming where I taught myself to ski. I discovered that it was a great sport for those with amputation. Unlike many other sports, when you ski, you don't have to overcome gravity. Gravity works with you. After a while, I found myself skiing all day long. Being able to do that made me aware that I had the endurance to go back to work full time.'

—Carol

Although individuals with below-knee amputation can ski successfully both with or without their prosthesis, most choose to remove it. Many choose to use "outriggers," which are forearm crutches with ski tips attached to the bottom. When used in place of ski poles, outriggers help the skier maintain balance and improve maneuverability. Those with bilateral below-knee amputations often wear their prosthesis and use regular ski poles. Many people with above-knee bilateral amputation choose to ski with either their usual prosthesis (or a shorter one) with the aid of outriggers. And sleds and mono-skis are available for those with high levels of bilateral lower-limb loss.

If you have an upper-limb amputation, you may be able to ski very well without poles, or with the aid of a single pole. If, however, you wish to use a second pole, there are a variety of devices to help you. A pole strap can be tied to anchor a split hook to the ski pole. A special prosthetic "ski hand" is also available.

Whether you have upper- or lower-limb loss, there are many prosthetic adaptations and assistive devices available to increase your comfort and performance while skiing. Speak with your prosthetist or sports organization for more details. Most states offer classes in skiing through National Handicapped Sports (NHS), an organization that also arranges competitive events. Contact the NHS at (301) 217–0960 for further information.

Dancing

Beginning to dance again was symbolic for me. I felt that the joy of movement had indeed been restored to my life. For couples who have enjoyed dancing together, knowing they can still share in this fun and romantic activity may help restore the sense that things are all right. Dancing can also help enhance coordination, balance, and endurance.

If you have a lower-limb amputation, you can enjoy dancing in a wheelchair. With practice, you can master dance moves while wearing a prosthetic leg. If you are missing an upper limb, you may choose to participate one-handed, or while using a passive cosmetic hand or a padded hook. Speak with your prosthetist about what might best suit your needs.

Other Popular Activities

Know that most sports and other physically challenging leisure activities can still be enjoyed, especially if the proper adaptive equipment is used. Baseball, basketball, football, soccer, volleyball, and other ball sports are popular choices for many with amputation. Other popular activities include hunting, horseback riding, and even mountain climbing! Boating, fishing, water-skiing, and windsurfing are other sports that can be successfully performed by those with limb loss.

It's important for you to give the activity of your choice a fair chance. With the proper instructions, assistive devices, and practice, you can experience great enjoyment from any one of a number of activities. But it's up to you to get out there and do it!

Competitive Sports

Be it the satisfaction of surpassing a personal best performance or participating in intense competition between highly skilled athletes, for some individuals, nothing beats the invigoration of competitive sports. Many with amputation claim that their involvement with sports has been a pivotal factor in their physical and emotional recovery. Through mastering a sport, many individuals with amputation claim they have achieved enhanced physical skills, a boost in self-confidence, and the confidence that they can master other life challenges.

"After I lost my leg, I had to learn that it was not the end of my life. When I first showed up at the ski races, I was getting beat by everybody, so I set some goals for myself. I trained seriously and began to excel in racing. This personal achievement has given me the confidence to deal with any situation. I also get a lot of satisfaction showing other people what they are capable of.

Being in the Olympics was a great experience. The best feeling I had came when I walked out there after the races and 44,000 people were cheering! If I can maintain the attitude I developed from competitive sports—setting goals and not limiting anything I do—I will do great in all the areas of my life. I never say, 'I can't'"

—Greg Mannino
World-champion Alpine ski-racer

You don't have to be an Olympic-caliber athlete to enjoy competitive sports. There are opportunities available at every level.

WHEN TRAVELING

Many individuals with limb loss are avid travelers. Whether you travel for pleasure or for business, you will want to make taking your trips as easy and comfortable as possible. For instance, whenever I travel by plane, I call ahead to discover if the distance I have to cover in the terminal is great enough for me to request a wheelchair. Always trying to anticipate possible problems, I usually pack extra prosthetic supplies such as blister tape and scissors. I usually bring a collapsible shower seat with me, and, if I am going to be away for a long period of time, I pack my spare prosthesis.

In the United States, air travel has been made easier for those with disabilities by the passage of the Air Carrier Access Act (ACAA). The ACAA prohibits discrimination against persons with disabilities by monitoring the airline industry in three areas: aircraft and airport accessibility, service requirements, and administrative considerations. For example, airline personnel are trained to better assist passengers with disabilities; new airplanes are required to have a wheelchair-accessible lavatory and an onboard wheelchair; and ticket counters, baggage facilities, and gate areas must be wheelchair accessible.

If you do even a small amount of traveling, you will find, as I have, that being prepared for unforeseen circumstances will give you a sense of security.

IN CONCLUSION

Recreation is play and play is fun! It is great for you physically, emotionally, and socially. It revitalizes your spirit. No matter what your age or level of amputation, you can still participate in a wide variety of leisure activities. With proper instruction, prosthetic and adaptive devices, and practice, you can still enjoy almost any activity. As in other areas of your recovery, a positive attitude and motivation will make a difference.

"I believe anything is possible; but, first you've got to listen to your body. If you are still recovering from your surgery, you are going to be weak—at this point you can't expect to go gung-ho into a sport or other physical activity. Just be realistic and give yourself a little time. You are your own worst enemy if you believe that because you have lost a limb the recreational side of your life is over. You've got to get out there and try! If you really want to do something, you will find a way to do it. This is not the end of your life—it's just a new chapter."

—*Margaret*

What is it that will "re-create" freshness, vitality, enthusiasm, and joy in your life? Sports? Travel? Quality time by yourself or with friends and loved ones? Creative expression through the arts? Only you can answer this question. During recreation the focus is on your abilities rather than your disabilities. No matter the number or condition of your limbs, you can re-create an active, vital lifestyle. So enjoy.

IN CONCLUSION

When you undergo amputation, you are profoundly challenged on every level of your being—physical, emotional, mental, and spiritual. The indisputable fact is that your limb is permanently gone. How you respond to that reality will determine whether or not you give in to despair, or use your experience to deepen your inner maturity and heighten your appreciation of living. Although the challenges you must face may seem more readily apparent, the opportunities are equally dramatic.

In the beginning, when you are struggling with your physical and emotional adjustment, it is harder to come to peace with your new realities. Over time, know that you will forge your own path to healing. When you realize that the totality of who you are is far more than your physical body, your adjustment will be significantly easier. Your body may be missing a limb; but, "you" are still uniquely you. You can still enjoy your life. Who you are is so much more than "an amputee."

It's up to you! A life lived with amputation is not qualitatively any better or worse than any other. Enjoy your life now; don't tell yourself you must wait until you are through with your recovery. Consciously choose to embrace life; commit yourself to it. When you say "Yes!" to life, you meet reality head on, rather than resist it. You embrace "what is," including the frustrations and challenges, as well as the joys and triumphs. You use your reality as an impetus to achieve greater levels of knowledge, wisdom, and love.

Become your own best friend. Cherish yourself—be gentle, compassionate, accepting, and loving. Laugh freely. Live in the present, while preparing for tomorrow by visualizing a positive future for yourself and your loved ones. Then hold onto that vision. Align your head, heart, guts, and spirit, and then take action to bring your vision to fruition. Saying "Yes!" means being an active participant in your life, rather than someone to whom life happens.

The "shock" of amputation can serve to prompt you to reorder life priorities, deepen your spirituality, and open your heart to greater depths of compassion. No one can say why some of us are given what may seem like overwhelming challenges. Just as steel is forged through fire, inner strength and maturity are tempered by how we meet adversity.

It is my hope that the information presented in this book will not only answer factual and practical questions about limb loss, but that it will also inspire you to make positive meaning of your experience. By assimilating the concepts and trying out the suggestions, you will gain the confidence to know you can successfully cope with whatever comes your way. If you have comments about the usefulness of this book, or suggestions as to how it might be improved, please feel free to write to me in care of the publisher.

You already possess the primary tool necessary for transformation—your consciousness. As you increase your conscious awareness, you will be able to recognize the places in which you are stuck in self-imposed limitations of thought, belief, or behavior. You can then take action to free yourself. With awareness, you will be able to recognize that the totality of who you are is far greater than the number or shape of limbs you have, and you will render your life rich with meaning.

GLOSSARY

Abrasion. A scraped or worn area of the skin.

Above-elbow amputation (AEA). The removal of an arm at a level above (proximal to) the elbow. Also called above-the-elbow amputation.

Above-knee amputation (AKA). The removal of a leg at a level above (proximal to) the knee. Also called above-the-knee amputation.

Adapt. To modify for easier use or improved function.

Advocacy. Active support or assistance of a cause, idea, or policy.

Alignment. The relative positions of the prosthetic socket, knee, and foot.

Ambulate. To walk.

Amputation. The traumatic loss or surgical removal of all or part of a limb or organ.

Amputee. A person who has undergone removal of all or part of a limb (or limbs). *Please note:* The word "amputee" defines a person by his disability, rather than his humanness. It is more sensitive to refer to someone with amputation as "a person with limb loss" (not "an amputee").

Ankle disarticulation. An amputation in which the foot is removed, the shin bones are left naturally pointed, and the heel pad is sewn back in place.

Anterior. The front side.

Atrophy. The shrinkage of muscle tissue.

Below-elbow amputation (BEA). The removal of an arm at a level below (distal to) the elbow. Also called below-the-elbow amputation.

Below-knee amputation (BKA). The removal of a leg at a level below (distal to) the knee. Also called below-the-knee amputation.

Bilateral amputation. The removal of both arms or both legs.

Brace. A device used to support a part of the body.

CAD/CAM. Computer-aided design/computer-aided manufacturing, sometimes used in the making and alteration of prostheses.

Chronic pain. Pain that persists over a prolonged period of time.

Congenital limb deficiency. Refers to a limb that is either absent or developmentally abnormal at birth.

Contracture. The shortening of muscles, tendons, or ligaments, which causes a decrease in the range of motion of those tissues.

Cosmesis prosthesis. Refers to the aesthetic appearance of a prosthetic limb.

Disability. A restriction in the ability to perform activities that are considered normal for others.

Disarticulation. Amputation through a joint.

Distal. Anatomically, a position far from the origin or line of attachment, as a bone; opposite of "proximal."

Double amputation. The removal of one upper and one lower limb.

Edema. The swelling of tissue.

Endoskeletal prosthesis. Similar to the human body, this type of prosthesis has a soft outer shell with a stiff core to support weight and function.

Exoskeletal prosthesis. This type of prosthesis has a hard outer shell, which is generally more durable than the soft cover of an endoskeletal prosthesis.

Extremity. Refers to a limb. An upper extremity refers to an arm or upper limb; a lower extremity refers to a leg or lower limb.

Femur. The thigh bone.

Fibula. The smaller of the two bones of the lower leg, the fibula is located towards the outside (lateral) part of the leg.

Forequarter amputation. The removal of the entire arm, shoulder, and shoulder girdle.

Gait. A particular way or mode of walking.

Gangrene. Death and decay of body tissue, often in a limb, due to injury, disease, or lack of blood supply.

Geneticist. A physician with specialized training in genetics. Genetic counselors, who may be nurses or paramedical specialists, can discuss the ramifications of diagnosed hereditary disorders.

Handicap. A social disadvantage one might have when interacting with others, or when trying to adjust to an environment.

Hemicorpectomy. *See* Translumbar amputation.

Hemipelvectomy. *See* Transpelvic amputation.

Hip disarticulation. Amputation in which the entire thigh bone (femur) is removed.

Hypertrophy. An increase in the size of muscle tissue due to use.

Impairment. A loss or abnormality of a physiological, psychological, or anatomical structure or function.

Insert. A cup-shaped device that can be made of one of several materials that fits inside a below-knee prosthesis for improved fit and comfort.

Ischium. The lowest of three major bones comprising each half of the pelvis. Also called the "sit bone."

Lateral. Anatomically, a position toward the side or the outside of the body. The opposite of "medial."

Liner. *See* Insert.

Marriage, Family, and Child Counselor (MFCC). A counselor who specializes in working with family systems.

Medial. Anatomically, a position toward the center or middle of the body. The opposite of "lateral."

Microprocessors. These small electronic circuits, which are used in personal computers, are a component of "smart knees." They help adjust the knee for increased stability, flex control, and speed and swing of the prosthetic leg.

Multiple amputation. Refers to an amputation of two or more limbs.

Muscle contracture. Shortened muscles due to lack of use.

Myoelectric technology. A field in which electronic sensors are used to pick up the feedback of muscle fiber contractions as the muscles move naturally. This automatically controls the action of the prosthetic limb.

Myoplasty. A procedure during amputation surgery in which the muscles and muscle coverings are sewn together over the end of the bone or to the bone.

Neuroma. A small ball of nerve fibers that forms on the cut end of a nerve.

Occupational therapist (OT). A specialist with training in working with the musculoskeletal system, especially the upper extremities. An occupational therapist can also help teach adaptive skills to master tasks and activities of daily living.

Opposition post. A device that restores function of the opposable thumb and fingers, so items can be grasped more easily.

Orthopedist. A medical doctor who has additional training in treating disorders of the bones and joints.

Orthosis. Devices used to provide support to (or limit the motion of) weakened joints or limbs.

Orthotist. A professional who fits and builds braces or orthopedic supports.

Patella. The kneecap.

Phantom limb pain. Pain that feels as if it comes from the missing limb. The intensity and type of pain may vary from sharp tingly "pins and needles" to crushing, agonizing pain.

Phantom limb sensation. Feelings or sensations that seem to come from the missing limb; the range of sensation varies from simply feeling that the leg is still present, to a tingling or unpleasant itching. Any sensation that could normally be felt in the limb can be a part of phantom limb sensation.

Phocomelia. A congenital condition in which the hand or foot is attached near, or directly to, the trunk of the body because of absence of the limb.

Physiatrist. A physician who specializes in physical medicine and rehabilitation. The physiatrist deals with the diagnosis, evaluation, and treatment of persons with impairments or disabilities that involve the musculo-skeletal, neurologic, cardiovascular, or other body systems.

Physical therapist (PT). One who specializes in the rehabilitation of the major muscles of the trunk and extremities.

Ply. The thickness of the material used in the special stocking sometimes worn on the residual limb.

Posterior. The back side.

Prosthetic sock. A sock, generally worn with a below-knee prosthesis, that provides additional padding for bony surfaces.

Prosthesis. An artificial replacement for a body part; an artificial limb.

Prosthetist. A professional who builds and maintains artificial limbs.

Proximal. Anatomically, a position close to the center of the body; opposite of "distal."

Psychiatrist. A medical doctor with additional training in emotional and mental disorders; the only type of psychotherapist that can prescribe drug treatment.

Psychologist. A mental health professional who has a doctorate degree in psychology. Aside from practicing psychotherapy, psychologists are also able to administer psychological tests.

Pylon. A metal shaft that provides support from inside the prosthesis.

Quadrilateral amputation. The removal of all four extremities.

Radius. The shorter and thicker of the two forearm bones, the radius lies on the thumb-side of the arm.

Registered nurse (RN). A professional with nursing training who works under the supervision of a physician. He or she may have additional training in specialty areas.

Rehabilitation. The process of restoring a more independent, "normal" life for a person who has become ill or who has a disability.

Residual limb. The part of the limb that remains after the amputation; a more sensitive term than "stump."

Revision. The alteration of the residual limb through surgery to make it more functional or attractive.

Shinbone. *See* Tibia.

Shoulder disarticulation. An amputation in which the entire arm is removed, but the shoulder is left intact.

Skin breakdown. Damage that occurs to normal skin including irritation, blisters, and rashes.

Social worker. A professional with a degree in social work, who is trained to counsel and access community resources.

Stump. *See* Residual limb.

Syme's amputation. An amputation in which the foot is removed, the shin bones are flattened, and the heel pad is sewn back in place.

Terminal device. The "hand" of an upper-limb prosthesis. This device can be as simple as a mechanical hook, or as complex as a myoelectrically controlled hand.

Tibia. The inner and larger of the two bones of the lower leg; also called the "shinbone."

Transfemoral amputation. Any amputation that occurs between the knee and hip.

Translumbar amputation. Usually performed on those who have undergone severe trauma from an accident, or for those with cancer in related parts of the body, a translumbar amputation is made through the lumbar vertebra (lower back); formerly known as a hemicorpectomy.

Transpelvic amputation. Removal of part of the pelvis and, consequently, every connected structure of the lower extremity. Formerly referred to as a hemipelvectomy.

Transtibial amputation. Any amputation that occurs between the knee and ankle.

Trauma. A wound, especially one that is the result of a sudden physical injury.

Trilateral amputation. The removal of three extremities.

Tumor. An abnormal new growth of tissue.

Ulna. One of the two bones extending from the elbow to the wrist, the ulna lies on the little-finger side of the forearm.

Unilateral amputation. The removal of one upper or one lower extremity.

Vascular. Pertaining to blood vessels.

Volume change. Refers to a change in the size of the residual limb due to either shrinking or swelling.

BIBLIOGRAPHY

Adapted Physical Activity: An Interdisciplinary Approach, eds G. Doll-Tepper, C. Dahms, and H. von Selzman. Berlin, Germany: Springer-Verlag, 1990.

Aitken, G.T. *The Child with an Acquired Amputation.* Washington, D.C.: National Academy of Sciences, 1972.

The American Amputee Foundation National Resource Directory. Little Rock, AR: American Amputee Foundation, 1987.

The Americans with Disabilities Act: An Easy Checklist. Pamphlet E-69. Chicago, IL: National Easter Seal Society, 1992.

Atchison, W. M. "Psychological Impact of Amputation." Dissertation submitted to the Union Graduate School, Cincinnati, OH, 1988.

Awareness is the First Step Towards Change: The Air Carrier Access Act. Pamphlet PR-47. Chicago, IL: National Easter Seal Society.

Awareness is the First Step Towards Change: The Americans with Disabilities Act. Pamphlet PR-44. Chicago, IL: National Easter Seal Society.

Awareness is the First Step Towards Change: Tips for Disability Awareness. Pamphlet PR-42. Chicago, IL: National Easter Seal Society.

Awareness is the First Step Towards Change: Tips for Portraying People with Disabilities in the Media. Pamphlet PR-43. Chicago, IL: National Easter Seal Society.

Bader, N. "Meeting the Challenge of the Americans with Disabilities Act."*Business News,* Summer 1993, pp. 26–28.

Bandler, R., and John Grinder. *The Structure of Magic.* Palo Alto, CA: Science and Behavior Books, Inc., 1975.

Baraja, R.H., R.A. Sherman, J. Ernst, B. Dodd, S. Turner, R. Brown. *What to Expect When You Lose a Limb."* Fort Gordon, GA: Department of the Army, 1985.

Basmajian, J.V. *Therapeutic Exercise*, 4th Edition. Baltimore, MD: Williams and Wilkins, 1984.

Baugh, B. "Caveat Emptor?" *Journal of Orthotics and Prosthetics*, Vol. 4 No. 4, July 1992, pp. 180–181.

Bender, L.F. *Prostheses and Rehabilitation After Arm Amputation*. Springfield, IL: Charles C. Thomas, Publisher, 1974.

Benfield, L. and D.W. Head. "Discrimination and Disabled Women." *Journal of Humanistic Education and Development*, 23(2), 1984, pp. 60–68.

Benson, Herbert. *The Relaxation Response*. New York: William Morrow & Co, 1975.

Birk, Randi. "Learning to Cope With External and Internal Stressors." *Learning to Live Well With Diabetes*, eds Marion J. Franz, Donnell D. Etzwiler, Judy Ostrom Joynes, Priscilla M. Hollander. Minneapolis, MN: DCI Publishing (Division of ChroniMed Inc.), 1991.

Bourne, E.J. *The Anxiety and Phobia Workbook*. Oakland, CA: New Harbinger Publications, Inc., 1990.

Bradshaw, J. *Healing the Shame that Binds You*. Deerfield Beach, FL: Health Communications, Inc., 1988.

Bradway, J.K., J.M. Malone, J. Racy, J.M. Leal, and J. Poole. "Psychological Adaptation to Amputation: An Overview." *Orthotics and Prosthetics*, 38(3), Autumn 1984, pp. 46–50.

Brandon, N. *How to Raise Your Self-Esteem*. New York: Bantam Books, 1987.

Chapman, Beverly. "Wrong Word Can Be Crippling to People With Disability," *San Diego Union Tribune*, February 16, 1992.

Children With Hand Differences: A Guide for Families. Grand Rapids, MI: Mary Free Bed and Rehabilitation Center, 1989.

Client Information Booklet. Sacramento, CA: California Department of Rehabilitation.

Colgrove, M., H. Bloomfield, and P. McWilliams. *How to Survive the Loss of a Love*. New York: Bantam Books, 1976.

Congenital Limb Deficiencies: An Early Intervention Guide for Professionals. Park Ridge, IL: The Association of Children's Prosthetic-Orthotic Clinics.

Crowther, H. "New Perspectives on Nursing Lower Limb Amputees." *Journal of Advances in Nursing*, 7(5), 1982, pp. 453–460.

Darty, T.E., and S.J. Potter. "Sexual Work with Challenged Women: Sexism,

Sexuality, and the Female Cancer Experience." *Journal of Social Work and Human Sexuality*, 2(1), 1983, pp. 83–100.

Deits, B. *Life After Loss: A Personal Guide Dealing with Death, Divorce, Job Change, and Relocation.* Tucson, AZ: Fisher Books, 1988.

Diagnostic and Statistical Manual of Mental Disorders, 3rd Edition, revised. Washington, D.C.: American Psychiatric Association, 1987.

Dise-Lewis, J. E. "Psychological Adaptation to Limb Loss." *Comprehensive Management of the Upper-Limb Amputee*, eds D.J. Atkins, and R.H. Meier, III.) New York: Springer-Verlag, 1989, pp. 165–172.

Earle, E.M. "The Psychological Effects of Mutilating Surgery in Children and Adolescents." *Psychoanalytic Study of Children*, 34, 1979, pp. 527–546.

Finston, P. *Parenting Plus: Raising Children with Special Health Needs.* New York: Penguin Books, 1990.

Frankel, Victor. *Man's Search for Meaning.* Boston: Beacon Press, 1962.

Freedman, Rita J. *Bodylove: Learning to Like Our Looks—and Ourselves.* New York: Harper and Row Publishers, 1988.

Friedmann, L.W. *The Psychological Rehabilitation of the Amputee.* Springfield, IL: Charles C. Thomas Publishers, 1978.

Friedmann, L.W. *The Surgical Rehabilitation of the Amputee.* Springfield, IL: Charles C. Thomas Publishers, 1978.

Frierson, R.L., and S.B. Lippmann. "Psychiatric Consultation for Acute Amputees: Report on a Ten-Year Experience." *Psychosomatics*, 28(4), 1987, pp. 183–189.

Frye, V. and M. Peters. *Therapeutic Recreation: Its Theory, Philosophy, and Practice.* Harrisburg, PA: Stackpole Books, 1972.

Furst, R.L., and M. Humphrey. "Coping With the Loss of a Leg." *Prosthetics and Orthotics International*, 7(3), 1983, pp. 152–156.

Gailey, R.S. "Recreational Pursuits for Elders with Amputation." *Topics in Geriatric Rehabilitation*, 8(1), 1992, pp. 39–58.

Gailey, R.S. et al. "A Survey of Recreational Activities Participated in by Lower Extremity Amputees," University of Miami, School of Medicine, Department of Orthopaedics and Rehabilitation, Division of Physical Therapy, Coral Gables, FL, 1992.

Garee, B., ed. "Single-Handed: Devices and Aids for One Handers and Sources of These Devices." Bloomington, IL: Accent Special Publications, Cheever Publishing, Inc., 1990.

Garrett, J.F., and E.S. Levine. *Psychological Practices with the Physically Disabled*. New York: Columbia University Press, 1962.

Garrett, J.F., and E.S. Levine. *Rehabilitation Practices with the Physically Disabled*. New York: Columbia University Press, 1973.

Gerhards, F., I. Florin, and T. Knapp. "The Impact of Medical, Re-educational, and Psychological Variables on Rehabilitation Outcome in Amputees." *International Journal of Rehabilitation Research*, 7(3), 1984, pp. 283–292.

Goldberg, R.T. "New Trends in the Rehabilitation of Lower Limb Amputees." *Rehabilitation Literature*, 45, 1984, pp. 1–11.

Handley, R., with P. Neff. *Beyond Fear*. New York: Rawson Associates, 1987.

Hewett, S., J. Newson, and E. Newson. *The Family and the Handicapped Child*. London, England: George Allen and Unwin Ltd., 1970.

Hopkins, M.T. "Patterns of Self-Destruction Among the Orthopedically Disabled." *Rehabilitation Research and Practice Review*, 3(1), 1971.

Huston, T. "Feeling Good: Helping Patients Rediscover the Spirit of Life." *Orthotics and Prosthetics Almanac*, January 1994, pp. 32–43.

International Classification of Impairments, Disabilities, and Handicaps. Geneva, Switzerland: World Health Organization, 1980.

James, J.W. *The Grief Recovery Handbook: A Step-By-Step Program for Moving Beyond Loss*. New York: Harper and Row Publishers, 1988.

Jampolsky, G.G. and C. Huff. *Teach Only Love: The Seven Principles of Attitudinal Healing*. New York: Bantam Books, 1983.

Jeffers, S. *Feel the Fear and Do It Anyway*. San Diego, CA: Harcourt Brace Jovanovich, Publishers, 1987.

John-Roger, and P. McWilliams. *You Can't Afford the Luxury of a Negative Thought*. Los Angeles, CA: Prelude Press, Inc., 1991.

Jensen, T.S., B. Krebs, J. Neilson, P. Rasmussen. "Phantom Limb, Phantom Pain and Stump Pain in Amputees During the First Six Months Following Limb Amputation." *Pain*, 17(3), 1983, pp. 243–256.

Jevne, R.F. and A. Levitan. *No Time for Nonsense: Self-Help for the Seriously Ill*. San Diego, CA: Luramedia, 1989.

Kashani, J.H. "Depression Among Amputees." *Journal of Clinical Psychiatry*, 44(7), 1983, pp. 256–258.

Kegel, B., J.C. Webster, and E.M. Burgess. "Recreational Activities of Lower

Extremity Amputees: A Survey." *Archives of Physical Medicine and Rehabilitation,* 61, 1980, pp. 258–264.

Krohn, K. "Recreational Therapy." (A taped discussion), San Diego, CA., 1993.

Kübler-Ross, E. *On Death and Dying.* New York: MacMillan, 1970.

Lerner, H.G. *The Dance of Anger.* New York: Harper and Row Publishers, Inc., 1985.

Levy, W.S. *Skin Problems of the Amputee.* St. Louis, MO: Warren H. Green, Inc., 1983.

Living and Learning After Your Leg Amputation. Harmarville Rehabilitation Center, Pittsburgh, PA., 1983.

Malone, J. "Rehabilitation for Lower Extremity Amputation." *Archives of Surgery,* 116, 1981, pp. 93–98.

Marinelli, R.P., and A.E. Dell Orto. *The Psychological and Social Impact of Physical Disability.* New York: Springer Publishing Company, 1984.

Maurer, J.R., and P.D. Strasberg. *Building a New Dream: A Family Guide to Coping with Chronic Illness and Disability.* Reading, MA: Addison-Wesley Publishing Co., 1989.

McKay, M., and P. Fanning. *Self-Esteem: The ultimate program for self-help.* Oakland, CA: New Harbinger Publications, 1987.

Melzack, R. "Phantom limbs." *Scientific American,* 266:4, 1992, pp. 120–126.

Michael, J.W. "The Progress of Science," *Journal of Orthotics and Prosthetics,* Vol. 4 No. 4, July 1992, p. 177/17.

Mills, J.W. *Coping with Stress.* New York: John Wiley and Sons, Inc., 1982.

Mital, M.A., and D.S. Pierce. *Amputees and Their Prostheses.* Boston: Little, Brown and Company, 1971.

Murphy, R.F. *The Body Silent.* New York: W.W. Norton, 1990.

Parkes, C.M. "Psycho-Social Transitions: Comparison Between Reactions to Loss of a Limb and Loss of a Spouse." *British Journal of Psychiatry,* 1975, pp. 204–210.

Racy, John C. "Psychological Adaptation to Amputation." *Atlas of Limb Prosthetics: Surgical, Prosthetic, and Rehabilitation Principles,* 2nd Edition, eds. J.H. Bowker, and J.W. Michael. American Academy of Orthopedic Surgeons. St. Louis, MO: Mosby Yearbook, Inc., 1992.

Ratto, L.L. *Coping With Being Physically Challenged.* New York: The Rosen Publishing Group, Inc., 127, 1991.

Register, C., *Living With Chronic Illness: Days of Passion and Patience.* New York: Bantam Books, 1987, p. 261.

Reinstein, L. "Rehabilitation of the Lower Extremity Cancer Amputee." *Maryland State Medical Journal,* 29, 1980, pp. 85–87.

Reinstein, L., J. Ashley, and K. Miller. "Sexual Adjustment After Lower Extremity Amputation." *Archives of Physical Medicine and Rehabilitation,* 59, 1978, pp. 501–504.

Ringe, L.B. "Body Attitudes, Self-Esteem, and Physical Disability." *Dissertation Abstracts International,* Illinois Institute of Technology, 26(4), 1981, pp. 177–185.

Ritchie, J.A. "Children's Adjustive and Affective Responses in the Process of Reformulating a Body Image Following Limb Amputation." *Maternal–Child Nursing Journal,* 6(1), 1977, pp. 25–35.

Rogers, J., A. MacBride, B. Whylie, and S.J.Freeman. "The Use of Groups in the Rehabilitation of the Amputee." *International Journal of Psychiatry in Medicine,* 8, 3, 1977–1978.

Samelson, C.F., and W.G. Fischer. "Group Psychotherapy Sessions with Lower Extremity Amputees in a Physical Medicine Rehabilitation Setting." *Proceedings of the Annual Convention of the American Psychological Association,* 7(part 2), 1972, pp. 703–704.

Sanders, G.T. *Lower Limb Amputations: A Guide to Rehabilitation.* Philadelphia, PA: F.A. Davis Co., 1968.

Setoguchi, Y., and R. Rosenfelder. *The Limb Deficient Child.* Springfield, IL: Charles C. Thomas Publisher, 1982.

Sherman, R.A., A. Richard, N. Gall, G. Norman, and J. Gormly. "Treatment of Phantom Limb Pain with Muscular Relaxation Training to Disrupt the Pain-Anxiety-Tension Cycle." *Pain,* 6(1), 1979, pp. 47–55.

Sherman, R.A., C.J. Sherman, L. Parker. "Chronic Phantom and Stump Pain Among American Veterans: Results of a Survey." *Pain,* 18(1), 1984, pp. 83–95.

Simpson, E.B. "Individual Variations in Psychological Reaction to Amputation." University of California, San Francisco/Berkeley, CA: Biomechanics Laboratory, 1959.

Stein, S.B. *About Handicaps.* New York: Walker and Company, 1974.

Stromer, D.C., S.A. Grand, A. Sheldon, and M.J. Purcell. "Attitude Towards Persons with a Disability: An Examination of Demographic Factors, Social Context, and Specific Disability." *Rehabilitation Psychology,* 29(3), 1984, pp. 131–145.

Talbot, D., *The Child with a Limb Deficiency: A Guide for Parents*. Child Amputee Prosthetics Project, UCLA; Shriners Hospital, Los Angeles, CA., 1979.

Thompson, C.E. *Raising a Handicapped Child*. New York: Ballantine Books, 1986.

Thompson, D.M., and D. Haran. "Living with an Amputation: What it Means for Patients and Their Helpers." *International Journal of Rehabilitation Research*, 7(3), 1984, pp. 283–292.

Troup, I.M., and M.A. Wood. *Total Care of the Lower Limb Amputee*. Dundee, Scotland: Pitman Publishers, 1982.

Valliant, P.M., I. Bezzubk, L. Daley, A. Lorne, and E. Marjatta. "Psychological Impact of Sport on Disabled Athletes." *Psychological Reports*, 56(3), 1985, pp. 923–929.

Washam, V. *The One-Hander's Book: A Basic Guide to Activities of Daily Living*. New York: The John Day Company, Inc., 1973.

Weiss, S.A., S. Fishman, and F. Krause. "Severity of Disability as Related to Personality and Prosthetic Adjustment of Amputees." *Psychological Aspects of Disability*, 18(2), 1971, pp. 67–75.

Wilson, J.L. "Anticipatory Grief in Response to Threatened Amputation." *Maternal–Child Nursing Journal*, 6,(3), 1977, pp. 177–186.

Wolf, S., C.M. Wolf, and G. Spielberg. *The Wolf Counseling Skills Evaluation Handbook*. Omaha, NE: National Publication, 1988, pp. 7–13.

Wright, B.A. *Physical Disability—a Psychological Approach*. New York: Harper and Row Publishers, 1960.

Yapko, M.D. *Free Yourself From Depression*. Emmaus, PA: Rodale Press, 1992.

Youngs, B.B. *How to Develop Self-Esteem in Your Child: 6 Vital Ingredients*. New York: Ballantine Books, 1991.

GROUPS AND ORGANIZATIONS

Amputee Coalition of America (ACA)
(800) 355–8772
The ACA is a national network of individuals, support groups, and health-care professionals that strives to improve the lives of those with amputation through education, consumer empowerment, and outreach.

American Amputee Foundation (AAF)
PO Box 250218
Hillcrest Station
Little Rock, AR 72225
(501) 666–2523
The AAF is a national information and referral source for those with amputation. It provides the names of relevant organizations, publications, prosthetic and orthotic providers, and sports associations. Supportive services also include peer counseling and some financial aid.

National Association for Advancement of Orthotics and Prosthetics (NAAOP)
1275 Pennsylvania Avenue NW
Washington, DC 20004–2404
(202) 624–0064
(202) 737–2517 FAX
Composed of prosthetists, orthotists, and consumers, the NAAOP is dedicated to improving life for those with amputation and other disabilities through technological advancement, lobbying and legislation, education, and advocacy.

National Amputee Fund (NAF)
6147 University Avenue
San Diego, CA 92115–5796
(619) 582–0196
(800) 770–5090
A nonprofit organization that provides funding for prostheses and prosthetic-management care for persons in need. NAF accepts donations of checks and charitable trusts from individuals and corporations.

The War Amputations of Canada
2827 Riverside Drive
Ottawa, Ontario
K1V 0C4 Canada
(613) 731–3821

*The War Amputations of Canada
offers social, educational, and
financial assistance to persons
with amputations.*

National Center for Medical Rehabilitation Research (NCMRR)

Building 61E – Room 2A0E
9000 Rockville Pike
Bethesda, MD 20891
(301) 402–2242
(301) 402–0832 FAX
*A division of the National Institutes
of Health, NCMRR has the most
up-to-date information on govern-
ment-funded prosthetic research.*

American Academy of Orthotists and Prosthetists (AAOP)

c/o National Office for Orthotics
  and Prosthetics
1650 King Street – Suite 500
Alexandria, VA 22314
(703) 836–7118
*Composed of professionals in the
fields of orthotics and prosthetics, the
AAOP provides advanced continuing
education and improved quality of
prosthetics and orthotic care.*

American Orthotic and Prosthetic Association (AOPA)

c/o National Office for Orthotics
  and Prosthetics
1650 King Street – Suite 500
Alexandria, VA 22314
(703) 836–7118
*The AOPA is a trade association that
represents the majority of orthotic
and prosthetic businesses.*

American Board for Certification (ABC)

c/o National Office for
  Orthotics and Prosthetics
1650 King Street – Suite 500
Alexandria, VA 22314
(703) 836–7118
*The ABC is an independent body
that issues credentials for orthotists
and prosthetists.*

National Handicapped Sports (NHS)

451 Hungerford Drive – Suite 100
Rockville, MD 20850
(301) 217–0960
(301) 217–0963 (TDD)
*The nation's largest organization that
provides sports and recreation programs
and information to people with physical
disabilities. The NHS is a member of the
U.S. Olympic Committee.*

National Amputee Golf Association (NAGA)

PO Box 1228
Amherst, NH 03031–1228
(800) 633–NAGA (U.S. and Canada)
(603) 672–7140 (FAX)
*"We are a national amputation
support group with the golf course as
our meeting place." The purpose of
NAGA is to provide recreational
rehabilitation to those with
amputation through golf.*

National Sports Center for the Disabled (NSCD)

Winter Park Resort
PO Box 36
Winter Park, CO 80482
(303) 726–4101
*The emphasis of the NSCD is rehabili-
tation through recreation. Skiing is
the main wintertime activity, while
mountain biking, hiking, and white-*

water rafting are a sampling of the Center's summertime sports.*The program directors of NCSD travel to ski areas throughout the country and world to help develop skiing programs for those with disabilities.*

Wheelchair Sports, U.S.A.
3595 East Fountain Boulevard —
  Suite L-1
Colorado Springs, CO 80910
(719) 574–1150
The purpose of Wheelchair Sports, U.S.A. is to provide opportunities for those individuals with impaired mobility as a result of permanent lower-extremity immobility to compete in team and individual sports at local, regional, national, and international levels.

A Touch of Love
(800) 493–5462
A support group for families with limb-deficient children, A Touch of Love offers emotional support, an information network, and a limb bank for children whose families are unable to absorb the cost of their prosthetic devices. This group, largely sponsored by Inner Wheel, is not affiliated with any one clinic. Parents and children associated with A Touch of Love meet four times a year to socialize and exchange information.

National Rehabilitation Information Center (NARIC)
8455 Colesville Road – Suite 935
Silver Spring, MD 20910–3319
(301) 588–9284
(800) 346–2742
NARIC provides information and referral services on all aspects of disability and rehabilitation. For a nominal fee, NARIC information specialists provide customized database searches of their bibliographic database, REHABDATA, quick reference and referral services, and document delivery. NARIC also publishes a free newsletter, "NARIC Quarterly," and several resource guides.

FURTHER INFORMATION

PROSTHETICS AND GENERAL INFORMATION

The American Amputation Foundation National Resource Directory. Little Rock, AR: The American Amputee Foundation, 1991.

Bowker, John, and John Michael, eds. *Atlas of Limb Prosthetics: Surgical, Prosthetic, and Rehabilitation Principles,* 2nd Edition. American Academy of Orthopedic Surgeons. St. Louis, MO: Mosby Yearbook, Inc., 1992.

Garee, Betty, ed. *Single-Handed: Devices and Aids for One Handers and Sources of These Devices.* Bloomington, IL: Accent Special Publications, Cheever Publishing, Inc., 1990.

Novotny, Mary, and John W. Michael. *You Have a Choice: Improving Orthotic and Prosthetic Outcomes.* The American Academy of Orthotists and Prosthetists, Alexandria, VA, 1992.

Washam, Veronica. *The One-Hander's Book: A Basic Guide to Activities of Daily Living.* New York: The John Day Company, 1973.

PSYCHOLOGICAL ASPECTS

Benson, Herbert. *The Relaxation Response.* New York: Avon Books, 1975.

Bloomfield, Harold H. *Surviving Loss: Overcoming Hurt and Heartbreak.* Chicago, IL: Nightingale-Conant Corporation, 1985.

Bourne, Edmund James. *The Anxiety and Phobia Workbook.* Oakland, CA: New Harbinger Publications, Inc., 1990.

Brandon, Nathaniel. *How to Raise Your Self-Esteem,* New York: Bantam Books, 1987.

Burns, David D. *The Feeling Good Handbook.* New York: Penguin Books, 1989.

Deits, Bob. *Life After Loss: A Personal Guide to Dealing With Death, Divorce, Job Change, and Relocation.* Tucson, AZ: Fisher Books, 1988.

Gawain, Shakti. *Creative Visualization.* New York: Bantam Books, 1978.

Handley, Robert, with Pauline Neff. *Beyond Fear.* New York: Rawson Associates, 1987.

James, John W., and Frank Cherry. *The Grief Recovery Workbook.* New York: Harper and Row Publishers, 1988.

Jampolsky, Gerald G., and Cherie Huff. *Teach Only Love: The Seven Principles of Attitudinal Healing.* New York: Bantam Books, 1983.

Jeffers, Susan. *Feel the Fear and Do it Anyway.* San Diego, CA: Harcourt Brace & Company, 1987.

Jevne, Rona Fay, and Alexander Levitan. *No Time for Nonsense: Self-Help for the Seriously Ill.* San Diego, CA: Luramedia, 1989.

John-Roger, and Peter McWilliams. *You Can't Afford the Luxury of a Negative Thought.* Los Angeles, CA: Prelude Press, Inc., 1991.

Lerner, Harriet Goldhor. *The Dance of Anger.* New York: Harper and Row Publishers, 1985.

McKay, Matthew, and Patrick Fanning. *Self-Esteem: The ultimate program for self-help.* Oakland, CA: New Harbinger Publications, 1987.

Mills, James Willard. *Coping with Stress: A Guide to Living.* New York: John Wiley and Sons, Inc., 1982.

Register, Cherie. *Living With Chronic Illness: Days of Passion and Patience.* New York: Bantam Books, 1987.

Yapko, Michael. *Free Yourself from Depression.* Emmaus, PA: Rodale Press, 1992.

RELATING WITH OTHERS

Kegel, Bernice. *Sports for the Leg Amputee.* Redmond, WA: Medic Publishing Co.

Maurer, Janet, and Strasberg, Patricia. *Building a New Dream: A Family Guide to Coping with Chronic Illness and Disability,* Reading, MA: Addison-Wesley Publishing Company, Inc., 1990.

Paciorek, M.J., and J.A. Jones. *Sports Recreation for the Disabled.* Indianapolis, IN: Masters Press, 1994.

Palaestra: The Forum of Sport, Physical Education and Recreation for Those With Disabilities. To subscribe to this quarterly magazine, write: Palaestra, PO Box 508, Macomb, IL, 61455.

The following pamphlets are available through the National Easter Seal Society, 70 East Lake Street, Chicago, IL, 60601:

—*The Americans with Disabilities Act: An Easy Checklist.* Pamphlet E-69.

—*Awareness is the First Step Towards Change: The Air Carrier Access Act.* Pamphlet PR-47.

—*Awareness is the First Step Towards Change: The Americans with Disabilities Act.* Pamphet PR-44.

—*Awareness is the First Step Towards Change: Tips for Disability Awareness.* Pamphlet PR-42.

—*Awareness is the First Step Towards Change: Tips for Portraying People with Disabilities in the Media.* Pamphlet PR-43.

An excellent series of books and pamphlets written by Reverend Harold Wilke, who was born without arms, is available through Healing Community, 521 Harrison Avenue, Claremont, CA, 91711.

CHILDREN WITH LIMB DIFFERENCES

Finston, Peggy. *Parenting Plus: Raising Children with Special Health Needs.* New York: Penguin Books, 1990.

Gordon, Thomas. *P.E.T.: Parent Effectiveness Training.* New York: Plume Books, 1970.

Novotny, Mary, and C.M. Perryman. *Upper-Limb Prosthetic Options for Kids: Below-Elbow,* (videotape). Rehabilitation Institute of Chicago, and The Area Child Amputee Center, Mary Free Bed Hospital & Rehabilitation Center, Grand Rapids, MI, 1992.

Ratto, Linda Lee. *Coping with Being Physically Challenged.* New York: The Rosen Publishing Group, 1991.

Satir, Virginia. *The New Peoplemaking.* Mountain View, CA: Science and Behavior Books, Inc., 1988.

Stein, Sara Bonnett. *About Handicaps.* New York: Walker and Company, 1974.

Superkids: A Newsletter for Families and Friends of Children with Limb Differences. To subscribe, write to "Superkids" 60 Clyde Street, Newton, MA, 02160.

Talbot, Darlene. *The Child with a Limb Deficiency: A Guide for Parents.* Child Amputee Prosthetics Project, UCLA, Shriners Hospital, Los Angeles, CA, 1979.

Thompson, Charlotte E. *Raising a Handicapped Child.* New York: Ballantine Books, 1986.

Youngs, Bettie B. *How to Develop Self-Esteem in Your Child: 6 Vital Ingredients.* New York: Ballantine Books, 1991.

The following booklets are available through the Area Child Amputee Center, Mary Free Bed Hospital & Rehabilitation Center, 235 Wealthy SE, Grand Rapids, MI 49503; Phone (616) 454–7988:

—*Children with Limb Loss: A Handbook for Families—Ages Birth to Five Years,* 1990.

—*Children with Limb Loss: A Handbook for Families—Ages Six to Twelve Years,* 1990.

—*Children with Limb Loss: A Handbook for Adolescents and Their Families,* 1990.

—*Children with Hand Differences: A Guide for Families,* 1989.

—*Children with Limb Loss: A Handbook for Teachers,* 1989.

INDEX

2